CHILD ABUSE AND NEGLECT

A DIAGNOSTIC GUIDE

For physicians, surgeons, pathologists, dentists, nurses and social workers

Vincent J. Palusci, MD, MS

Howard Fischer, MD

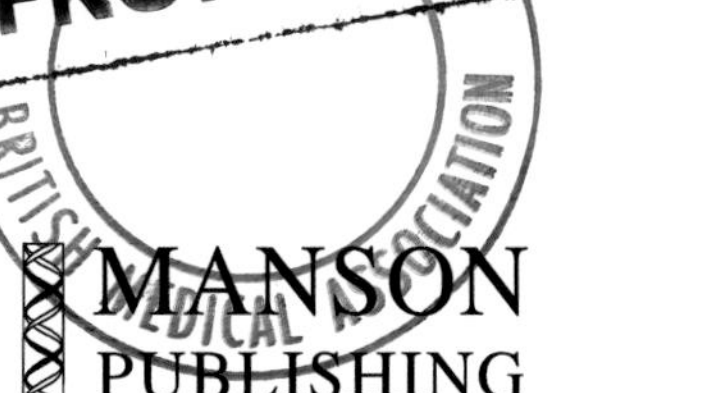

MANSON PUBLISHING

Dedication

For Roz, John, and Katie
For Barbara, Marcelle, and Suzanne
With our love, respect, and admiration.

ISBN: 978-1-84076-123-8

A CIP catalogue record for this book is available from the British Library.

For full details of all Manson Publishing titles please write to:
Manson Publishing Ltd, 73 Corringham Road, London NW11 7DL, UK.
Tel: +44(0)20 8905 5150
Fax: +44(0)20 8201 9233
Website: www.mansonpublishing.com

Commissioning editor: Jill Northcott
Project manager: Julie Bennett
Copy editor: Susie Bond
Proof reader: Carrie Walker
Layout: DiacriTech, India
Colour reproduction: Tenon & Polert Colour Scanning Ltd, Hong Kong
Printed by: Butler Tanner & Dennis, Frome, England

CONTENTS

LIST OF CONTRIBUTORS

Russell A. Faust, PhD, MD is an otolaryngologist at Nationwide Children's Hospital and a member of the Departments of Otolaryngology – Head and Neck Surgery and Oral Biology at the Ohio State University College of Dentistry in Columbus, Ohio. His clinical expertise is in endoscopic skull base and sinus surgery, and he has research interests in the role of microbial biofilm in chronic diseases of otolaryngology. He is a member in the International Society for Prevention of Child Abuse and Neglect, the American College of Legal Medicine, the American Society of Law, Medicine, and Ethics and has lectured before the American Bar Association.

Howard Fischer, MD is Professor of Pediatrics at Wayne State University School of Medicine in the Carman and Ann Adams Department of Pediatrics and Division Co-Chief of Ambulatory Pediatrics and Adolescent Medicine at Children's Hospital of Michigan. He was the medical director of the Children's Hospital of Michigan Child Protection Team for 14 years and is a member of the Ray Helfer Society.

Colleen M. Fitzpatrick, MD was a pediatric surgery fellow at the Children's Hospital of Michigan.

Pamela Wallace Hammel, DDS, DABFO is a Forensic Dental Consultant for the Children's Hospital of Michigan, Detroit, the Macomb County Medical Examiners Office, Mt. Clemens and the Oakland County Medical Examiners Office, Pontiac, Michigan. She is a Fellow of the American Academy of Forensic Sciences, and a Fellow of the American College of Dentists, the International College of Dentists and the Pierre Fauchard Academy.

Earl R. Hartwig, MD is Associate Professor of Pediatrics and Emergency Medicine at Wayne State University School of Medicine and a Child Protection Team Physician at Children's Hospital of Michigan.

Aparna Joshi, MD is a staff radiologist at Children's Hospital of Michigan and an Assistant Professor of Radiology at Wayne State University School of Medicine in Detroit, Michigan. She has co-authored an introductory textbook of pediatric radiology for pediatric health care providers.

Scott Langenburg, MD, FACS, FAAP is Assistant Professor of Surgery at Wayne State University and Pediatric Surgeon and Trauma Director for the Children's Hospital of Michigan.

Lisa Markman, MD is Assistant Clinical Professor of Pediatrics at the University of Michigan Medical School and Co-Medical Director of the Child Protection Team at the University of Michigan Medical Center in Ann Arbor, Michigan. She is a fellow of the American Academy of Pediatrics and a scholar member of the Ray E. Helfer Society.

Dena Nazer, MD is medical director of the Child Protection Center at Children's Hospital of Michigan and Assistant Professor of Pediatrics at Wayne State University School of Medicine. She is a Fellow of the American Academy of Pediatrics, a member of the Academic Pediatric Association, and a scholar member of the Ray E. Helfer Society. Her current research interests include epidemiology of child abuse using the National Child Abuse and Neglect Data System (NCANDS). She attended the 2007 Summer Research Institute at Cornell University and received the Sarniak Endowment Fund Award from the Children's Research Center of Michigan to study seasonal variations in the incidence of child maltreatment using NCANDS.

Vincent J. Palusci, MD, MS is Professor of Pediatrics at the New York University School of Medicine and Director of Research at the Frances L. Loeb Child Protection and Development Center at Bellevue Hospital in New York City. He is a Fellow of the American Academy of Pediatrics, a founding member of the Ray E. Helfer Society, and a member of the board of directors of the American Professional Society on the Abuse of Children. With Stephen Lazoritz, MD, he edited *The Shaken Baby Syndrome: A Multidisciplinary Approach*, published by the Haworth Press in 2002. In 2004, he received the Ray E. Helfer Award from the National Alliance of Children's Trust Funds and the American Academy of Pediatrics for his work in child abuse prevention.

John D. Roarty, MD, MPH is an Assistant Professor of Ophthalmology at the Kresge Eye Institute of Wayne State University and Chief of Ophthalmology at Children's Hospital of Michigan.

Carl J. Schmidt, MD, MPH grew up in Latin America where he graduated from medical school at the Universidad Anahuac. After 2 years of general surgery training and 2 years of graduate school in neurobiology, he trained in pathology at the Medical College of Ohio in Toledo, OH, now the University of Toledo Medical Center. He did his fellowship in forensic pathology at the Wayne County Medical Examiner's Office in Detroit, where he became the chief medical examiner in 2003. His main interests are pediatric trauma, forensic toxicology, and the neurobiology of addiction. He is Clinical Assistant Professor in the Department of Pathology at the Wayne State University School of Medicine. He has participated in a program sponsored by the US Department of Justice since 1998 that provides assistance for forensic issues in Latin America.

Philip V. Scribano, DO, MSCE is an Associate Professor of Clinical Pediatrics and Chief of the Division of Child and Family Advocacy at the Ohio State University College of Medicine. He is the Medical Director of the Center for Child and Family Advocacy at Nationwide Children's Hospital in Columbus, Ohio.

Thomas L. Slovis, MD is Professor of Radiology and Pediatrics at Wayne State University School of Medicine and former chief of the Department of Pediatric Imaging at Children's Hospital of Michigan. He has served as President and Chairman of the Board of the Society of Pediatric Radiology and is the American editor of *Pediatric Radiology* and editor of *Caffey's Pediatric Diagnostic Imaging*, 10th and 11th editions. He trained as a pediatric resident under the tutelage of Drs Henry Kempe, Henry Silver, and Ray Helfer.

Lynn C. Smitherman, MD, FAAP, is Assistant Professor of Pediatrics at Wayne State University School of Medicine in the Carman and Ann Adams Department of Pediatrics and is Clinical Chief of the Division of Ambulatory Pediatrics at Children's Hospital of Michigan.

Mary E. Smyth, MD is Medical Director of the Child Advocacy and Protection Team at William Beaumont Hospital in Royal Oak, Michigan and Clinical Assistant Professor in the Department of Pediatrics at Wayne State University School of Medicine. Dr Smyth is a fellow of the American Academy of Pediatrics, a member of the State of Michigan Department of Human Services Medical Advisory Team and the Michigan Chapter of the American Professional Society on the Abuse of Children (MiPSAC) Board of Directors.

ACKNOWLEDGMENTS

We are very grateful to Children's Hospital of Michigan, Bellevue Hospital Center, William Beaumont Hospital, and a number of colleagues for providing illustrative material. These include our chapter authors, as well as Kirk Barber MD, Waldo Nelson Henriquez Barraza MD, Jaenlee F. Carver MD, Martin Finkel DO, Deepak Kamat MD, PhD, Abu Khan MD, Alexander C. Leung MD, Laura Mankley MD, Margaret McHugh MD, MPH, Stephen Messner MD, Hisham Nazer MD, Sushma Nuthakki MD, Daniele Pacaud MD, Tor A. Shwayder MD, and the CHM Medical Photography Unit. Figures are reproduced with permission of the author and/or publisher

List of Image Contributors

Abu Khan 237. Alexander C. Leung 217-218. Aperna Joshi 251-258, 260-293, 296-315, 317-324.404-413, 508-567. Carl Schmidt 404-413, 508-567. Children's Hospital of Michigan 22-23, 37, 80-85, 107-108, 110-116, 119-127, 134-157, 164, 166-188. Daniele Pacaud 219. Deepak Kamat 225. Dena Nazur 190, 192, 248. Earl Hartwig 1-14, 18-21, 25-34, 38-49, 51-65, 67-79, 86-104, 189, 193, 196, 200-202, 206, 209, 212-215, 222, 226, 240-241. Hisham Nazer 245-247. Howard Fischer 15-16, 35, 117-118, 128-133, 160-163, 197-198, 568, 577. Jaenlee F. Carver 249. John Roarty 325-362. Kirk Barber 236, 238-239. Laura Mankley 210-211. Lynn Smitherman 569-576. Margaret McHugh 415-416, 432-433, 451-454, 456-458, 465, 479. Mary Smyth 17, 36, 66, 109, 165, 191, 203-205, 207, 216, 242-243, 250, 440, 459-461, 475-476, 502-503. Pamela Hammel 373-403. Philip Scribano 363-372. Stephen Messner 194-195. Sushma Nuthakki 244. Thomas Slovis 259, 294-295, 316. Tor A Shwayder 199, 208, 220, 223-224, 227-232, 234-235. Vincent Palusci 24, 50, 105-106, 158-159, 221, 414, 417-431, 434-439, 441-450, 455, 462-464, 466-474, 477-478, 480-501, 504-507. Waldo Nelson Henriquez Barraza 233.

PREFACE

The doctor who treats children, whether a generalist, pediatrician or one of a large number of specialists, has a moral and legal obligation to both dignose supected child maltreatment and to report it to the proper authorities. These obligations may bring the doctor into contact with the child protection system as well as with the courts. Any doctor or dentist who has testified in court will agree that the legal system operates under different rules, assumptions and standards of proof than does the medical system. The practitioner needs to be prepared for court testimony, and a foundation of knowledge about child maltreatment is essential.

This atlas is the product of cooperation among general pediatricians, child abuse pediatricians, social workers, psychologists, ophthalmologists, surgeons, emergency physicians, otorhinolaryngologists, and forensic dentists. It reflects our current, and increasing, knowledge base in this field. The reader will doubtless note that the contributors stress the importance of including a broad range of possibilities in their differential diagnoses. A color atlas is an ideal format for presenting high-quality representative photographs of diagnostic possibilities. A broad differential diagnosis is important, so that one does not call a non inflicted condition child abuse, nor mistake an inflicted injury for a more innocent condition. We would like to thank our contributors for the many images they have shared which have often been taken under difficult circumstances and over several years. We hope that this endeavor will prove useful to those who care for our most precious resource – our children.

Howard Fischer and Vincent Palusci

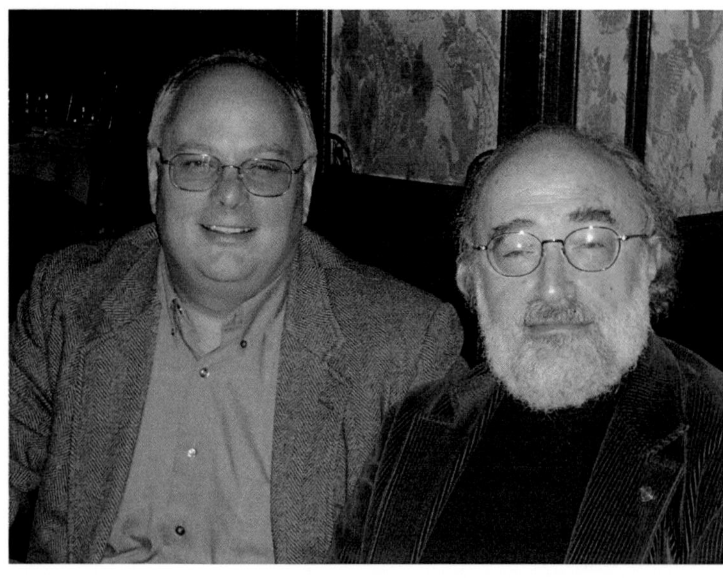

Chapter 1

INTRODUCTION

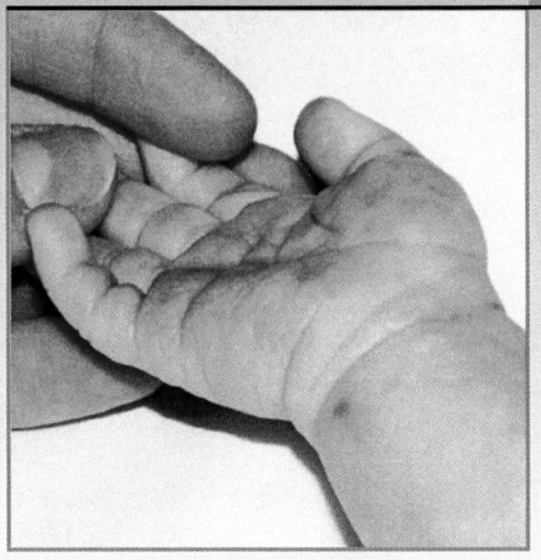

Vincent J. Palusci
MD, MS

In the 48 years since the publication of Dr C. Henry Kempe's landmark article, 'The battered child syndrome', the subject of child maltreatment has become a universal topic, not restricted to one professional community or to one type of professional for its identification[1]. As the field has grown, child welfare professionals have had to broaden their intellectual and personal perspectives not only to identify and report maltreatment, but also to provide interventions to prevent further abuse. Mandated reporters play a pivotal role in the identification and treatment of the health consequences of such victimization and should understand how to identify and report medical concerns in suspected maltreatment. Medical practitioners need information about what is known about its epidemiology and the process of its medical diagnosis, including key elements of the history, physical examination, and laboratory testing. This section will serve as an overview of the manifestations and reporting requirements to assist mandated reporters in accurately identifying and reporting suspected child abuse and neglect.

The epidemiology of child maltreatment and the role of the physician

The victimization of children through abuse and neglect remains an all too common occurrence[2]. In 2002, 12.3 per 1,000 children in the United States were victimized, and young children and infants had the highest rates[3]. While there are trends suggesting decreasing incidence, the United States child abuse and neglect reporting system continues to document over 900,000 substantiated victims of child maltreatment annually, with over 1,400 deaths[4–6]. Overall, injuries place a heavy burden on children, and inflicted injuries affect far too many[7,8]. Health care costs for inflicted injures are difficult to estimate, but estimates place the total costs associated with abuse at over $9 billion annually in the United States[6]. Maltreated children suffer from a variety of behavior problems and mental disorders, in addition to physical injuries[9–11]. The Adverse Childhood Experiences study has noted the powerful relationship between adverse childhood experiences and several conditions of adulthood, including risk of suicide, alcoholism, depression, illicit drug use, and other lifestyle changes[12]. While the exact pathways are still being explored, childhood abuse is thought to affect adult health by putting people at risk for depression and post-traumatic stress disorders, difficulties in relationships, and negative beliefs and attitudes towards others[13,14].

Studies in the United Kingdom have shown similar rates and risk factors for child maltreatment. In a population-based study in Wales over 2 years in the late 1990s, severe physical abuse, defined as death, traumatic brain injury, intracranial hemorrhage, Munchausen by proxy, internal injuries, fractures, burns, and bites, was seen in large numbers of infants (54 per 100,000 annually). When data from both child protection registers and a pediatrician surveillance system were combined, this rose to 114 per 100,000[15]. A random survey of 2,869 young adults throughout the United Kingdom noted that maltreatment during their childhood was experienced by 16% of the sample[16]. Of these, 7% had serious physical abuse, 6% had emotional abuse, 11% had sexual abuse with contact, 6% had absence of care, and 5% had absence of supervision. Using a cohort from the Avon Longitudinal Study of Parents and Children (ALSPAC), approximately 7% of the children had been placed on the child protection register before their 6th birthday, and several risk factors were noted to be associated with registration (parental unemployment, public housing, overcrowding, lack of car ownership, and a poor social network)[17]. In a later analysis, the strongest risks for registration were found to be socioeconomic deprivation and from other factors in the parents' own background[18].

Physicians have historically had an important role in the assessment and reporting of suspected child abuse and neglect, while treatment and prevention activities have relied on mental health professionals, and community and governmental services[19]. However, medical providers often viewed child abuse and neglect as a social rather than medical problem until the mid-twentieth century after the publication of several landmark articles in the medical literature and the development of the medical specialty of child abuse pediatrics[20]. In a recent survey, two-thirds of pediatricians reported treating injuries from child abuse, two-thirds had treated injuries from other community violence, and one-half treated injuries related to domestic violence. Those receiving recent education on abuse were more confident in their ability to identify and manage it[21]. Physicians assist the community response to child abuse and neglect by collaborating with community agencies (such as child advocacy centers and social services agencies) and governmental entities (such as police and child protective services) that have the resources, responsibility, and authority to protect children to improve their lives[22].

Identification of injuries

Several physical findings have been observed in child abuse and neglect. A comprehensive medical assessment includes a well-documented history as to how an injury occurred, physical characteristics of a witnessed traumatic event, the role of the caregiver, any symptoms present, and what medical care was sought[3]. Specific statements by the family and child should also be copied into the medical chart for potential use later in the legal system. The medical history should be reviewed to identify previous trauma, injury, chronic illness, and medications. A developmental history should document the child's best level of functioning and abilities, and social history should include those who routinely supervise the child, those who have been with the child during any recent events, and discipline practices or other stressors in the home. A physical examination should note the presence of and document any bruises, burns, or other skin lesions and requires complete undressing of the child and comprehensive assessment of multiple organ systems. Particular emphasis is placed on the anogenital examination if sexual abuse is suspected. It is important to know whether any findings are specific (strong causal link to abuse or neglect) or nonspecific (associated with a variety of causes, including maltreatment). For skin lesions, lesions may be documented using notes, hand-drawn diagrams, or photographs, although law enforcement and child protection workers often have resources to assure high-quality photodocumentation. Even if photographs are taken, the physician should also contemporaneously document any skin injuries identified[23]. Suspicion of internal injury requires medical imaging, with computerized tomography (CT) generally used for abdomen, chest, and acute head trauma. Magnetic resonance (MR) imaging is indicated for less acute or chronic head injury and soft tissue imaging. Plain radiographs continue to be important to identify fractures and can be ordered contemporaneously with CT or MR[24,25]. Protocols have been developed to direct the physician and radiologist as to the numbers, types, and repetition of dedicated radiographic images required for such assessments for suspected child abuse[24]. Abnormalities in serologic tests for liver function have been correlated with inflicted abdominal trauma, and experimental serologic markers are being identified for traumatic brain injury[26]. Tests for sexually transmitted infections vary by disease and can be obtained as blood tests for serology or swabs for culture or nonculture tests[27]. Tests for potential underlying medical conditions take a variety of forms and are used as indicated in the differential diagnosis for specific potentially abusive conditions.

Physical abuse

Physicians have noted specific injuries that stem from abuse and neglect, with early identification of maltreatment as a disease in the medical literature by John Caffey and others[28–30]. In the 1950s, Paul Woolley and William Evans in Detroit noted the presence of significant injuries that were inconsistent with parental explanations[31,32]. Discussions of diagnoses in the medical literature began to focus upon injuries from physical abuse, with Silverman's identification of fractures[33,34] and Henry Kempe's landmark article[1] naming the battered child syndrome prominent among them. Since that time, articles in the medical literature on maltreatment have escalated in number, having concentrated on physical abuse in the 1960s and 1970s, and later sexual abuse, domestic violence, neglect, and Munchausen by proxy[35–47]. A better understanding of these threats to child health and development led to clearer definitions of victimization, such as those adopted by the World Health Organization[48].

The leading cause of abusive mortality and morbidity is inflicted traumatic brain injury[49,50]. With mortality rates of 10–50% and more than 90% of survivors having significant handicap, physical abuse to the head has been noted to have patterns of injuries that are distinct from accidental or medical causes. At least 1,400 cases of fatal

Table 1 **Physical findings after child physical abuse**[a]

Skin	Pattern bruises or scars Symmetric immersion burns, especially with well-demarcated edges Pattern contact burns Any bruises or burns in a nonambulating infant Multiple injuries in differing stages of healing/battered child syndrome Nonpattern bruises of the abdomen, thorax, or soft tissues of the extremities
Head, eyes, ears, mouth, and neck	Bruises on the earlobes Perforated tympanic membranes without middle ear infection Retinal hemorrhages, especially multiple layers and not limited to the posterior pole Soft tissue swelling of the scalp Intra-oral bruising Torn labial frenulum Circumferential or ligature bruises or scars Subdural hemorrhage, especially interhemispheric
Thorax/abdomen/anogenital	Duodenal hematoma Liver laceration Kidney laceration Pancreatic injury
Anus/genitals	See *Table 2*

[a]In the absence of specific nonabusive history of trauma or specific underlying medical condition.

abusive head trauma occur annually in the United States, and there is growing sophistication in our ability to differentiate these fatalities from those from nonabusive causes[51]. The evaluation of abusive head trauma and other injuries has been greatly enhanced by the development of specialized imaging and diagnostic techniques, which has allowed better understanding of the wide range of injuries from child abuse and neglect[52,53]. New diagnostic technologies developed in the last century, from radiographs to sophisticated computer-assisted imaging techniques, such as CT or 'CAT' scans and MR, have proved invaluable in visualizing internal bleeding and injury[54]. In one study, infants and children under 3 years with interhemispheric subdural hemorrhage were found to have a greater than 99% probability of intentional trauma[55].

There are several physical injuries that are specific for abuse (*Table 1*). The most common physical injury from abuse affects the skin by bruising (see Chapter 2, Bruises) or burning (Chapter 3, Abusive burns). Any skin lesion beyond temporary reddening should be considered as potential physical abuse when (1) the injury is inflicted and nonaccidental, (2) the pattern of injury fits biomechanical models of abusive trauma, (3) the pattern corresponds to infliction with an instrument that would not occur through play or in the environment, (4) the history provided is not in keeping with the child's development, or (5) the history does not explain the injury[56]. The aging of bruises in children has received considerable attention and current guidelines are severely limited in their ability to precisely time when an injury occurred. Similar to the assessments of burns, electrical and radiation injuries have also been identified to aid in their assessment. Pattern, depth (degree), and healing of burns helps in determining their specificity for maltreatment. Developmental and other considerations need to be entertained as there are a host of potential confounders or 'mimics' which need to be reviewed when coming to a diagnosis (Chapter 4, Cutaneous conditions mimicking child abuse). Some children as young as 10 months of age, for example, have been shown to have the developmental capability to climb into the bath, suggesting that nonspecific burn patterns could be attributed to actions by the child rather than the parent in some cases[57]. Specific patterns of fracture (Chapter 5, Imaging child abuse) have been associated with physical abuse, with posterior rib fractures, rarely injured bones and long bone fractures in nonambulatory children being specific for abuse[24]. There is also a growing body of knowledge of abdominal and chest trauma available to identify these often 'silent' injuries with potentially devastating consequences and to differentiate abuse from accidental trauma (Chapter 9, Abusive abdominal trauma). Abdominal injuries are the second leading cause of death after maltreatment, but are difficult to assess given their occult nature, relative lack of bruising, and potential for significant delay in symptoms after injury. Recent studies suggest that abdominal CT imaging and/or liver function and pancreatic testing should be carried out in all abusive head trauma victims to identify occult abdominal trauma, given that 25% or more of even fatal abdominal trauma cases can have few or no visible external bruises[46]. Other specific injuries in other organ systems, such as eyes, ears, nose, throat, and dentition, are reviewed elsewhere in this text (Chapter 6, Ocular trauma; Chapter 7, Otolaryngologic manifestations of abuse and neglect; and Chapter 8, Recognition of child abuse by dentists, heath care professionals, and law enforcement). A unique form of maltreatment in which parents create or feign illness in their children to receive medical care is also discussed (Chapter 13, Munchausen syndrome by proxy).

Sexual abuse

Sexual abuse has been defined as sexual contact or exploitation of children by adults, to which children cannot give consent, and which violate social laws or taboos. 'Sexual assault' is a comprehensive term encompassing several types of forced sexual activity, while the term 'molestation' means noncoital sexual activity between a child and an adolescent or adult. 'Rape' is defined as forced sexual intercourse with vaginal, oral, or anal penetration by the offender. 'Acquaintance rape' or 'date rape' refers to when the assailant and victim are of similar age, know each other, but the victim has nonconsensual contact. 'Statutory rape' involves sexual contact by an adult with a minor, as defined in state law, regardless of assent.

A major injury of sexual abuse is emotional. While most young children with proven sexual abuse have few physical injuries, patterns of anogenital injury and sexually transmitted diseases have been identified[58,59]. Assessing sexual abuse requires detailed knowledge of anogenital anatomy and sexually transmitted infections (STIs) in children, both of which have important differences from adults (Chapter 10, Anogenital findings and child sexual abuse). Specialized skills and examination techniques have had to be developed for correct assessment[27,60–69].

Pediatricians caring for sexual abuse victims should be trained in the procedures required for documentation and collection of evidence and protecting the child from further victimization[23,70,71]. The examination begins with a comprehensive general examination followed by detailed visualization of the genital, anal, and oral cavities[72-75]. New procedures, such as colposcopy and videocolposcopy, offer ways to better document and record findings, allowing the child to be more relaxed and cooperative during examination, and begin the process of emotional healing[76]. Sexualized behaviors, which can suggest sexual knowledge inappropriate for the child based on age and development, are often nonspecific[77,78]. Recent research suggests that few physical findings, such as lacerations and transections of the hymen, and bruising and other injury to the anus and genitals, have high specificity[58]. Several physical findings that were once thought to indicate trauma are now considered nonspecific, accidentally acquired, or congenital variations[58,75].

While all STIs should raise the suspicion of sexual contact, infections with *Neisseria gonorrhoea* and *Treponema pallidum* are most specific for mucosal sexual contact and must generally be reported[27,66]. The presence of STIs needs to be evaluated on a case-by-case basis, and the possibility of nonsexual or vertical transmission considered. Other infections to be considered include *Chlamydia trachomatis*, *Trichomonas* species, human immunodeficiency virus, and hepatitis B virus[27]. The pediatrician should be knowledgeable about the potential sources of infection, body sites, types of contact and testing strategies and complete testing before treatment eradicates microbiologic evidence. Physicians need to carefully consider the types and timing of any prophylaxis for STI or pregnancy based on the age and development of the child, the type and timing of contact, and risk factors for disease in the alleged perpetrator[27,61].

Psychological maltreatment

Psychological maltreatment (PM) is commonly associated with other forms of abuse, but may also occur in isolation in a small number of cases. By definition, PM is a repeated pattern of interaction between a parent and child that harms the child's emotional well-being. Spurning, belittling, degrading, ridiculing, or shaming can psychologically harm children[11]. Terrorizing and otherwise exploiting the child increases the harm further. The denial of emotional closeness leads to physical and developmental delays in young children and failure to thrive in infants. Rejecting the child, isolating the child, and being inconsistent in parenting styles leads the child to feel insecure in his home relationships. An emerging form of PM includes the child's witnessing violence in the home, be it between the parent and spouse, within the community, or even on television or movies[11,79].

Increasingly, behavioral problems, depression, post-traumatic stress, and other psychological conditions are being identified after PM. The true prevalence is not known, but fewer than 10% of mandated child maltreatment reports in the United States specifically include PM. PM may first lead to post-traumatic stress disorder and later lead to juvenile delinquency, depression, or mental illness in adolescence or during adulthood[14]. Parental factors contributing to PM include poor parenting skills, inappropriate expectations, substance abuse, mental illness, psychological problems, poor social skills, lack of empathy, social stress, domestic violence, and other family dysfunction. Children at increased risk are those in families with divorce or separation, unwanted pregnancy, behavior problems, or physical or emotional delays, or who are socially isolated or emotionally handicapped[11,79]. Psychological neglect has been significantly associated with behavior problems and poor cognitive development even after controlling for poverty[79–81].

The psychologic effects specific to maltreatment may be very difficult to recognize in the medical office. Sometimes the poor parent–child relationship is seen and the verbal stigmata of PM exposed, but often there are little or no physical findings demonstrating the emotional harm, other than weight loss, excessive weight gain, or family discord. The quiet, depressed child is not often identified as a victim of neglect as readily as is the hyperactive, aggressive child[82]. The pediatrician needs to evaluate the harm or potential harm to the child's mental health, while realizing that it many take several years for sufficient harm to become apparent. Documentation must be objective, with appropriate use of psychological tests and mental health referrals for the evaluation. In the young child, behavioral changes, such as sleep problems, eating problems, and school problems are early but nonspecific events, and any assessment should include multiple domains, including function at home, school, and at play. These effects are further modified by the intensity, frequency, and severity of the exposure, as well as the developmental stage and resilience of the child[11].

Neglect

Child neglect is the most common form of child maltreatment, affecting 60% or more of children reported annually to Child Protective Services[6]. Dr Ray Helfer rightly reminded pediatricians about the significant harms caused by the 'litany of smoldering neglect' and the de-emphasis of neglect which has caused mandated reporters to have second thoughts about reporting neglect because little, if anything, would supposedly be done by overwhelmed, understaffed child protective services agencies[82]. Neglect is the omission or lack of a minimal level of care by the parents or caregivers that results in actual or potential harm to the child[6]. Neglect is often associated with poverty, but poor families are not necessarily neglectful[83]. Many subtypes of neglect often occur concurrently, but our understanding of its outcome is often aided by identifying subtypes that can direct potential interventions. Physical neglect is the lack of food, clothing, or shelter, while emotional neglect is a form of psychological maltreatment, and educational neglect refers to the lack of proper educational resources. Medical providers are most likely to encounter and treat medical care neglect and failure to thrive[84].

In a small number of cases, neglect can be fatal (Chapter 11, Child maltreatment fatalities). Although poorly identified on death certificates, child death review teams consistently identify supervisional and medical neglect as causing as many as or even more deaths than does physical abuse[85]. Physical conditions caused by neglect include 'accidental' injuries, ingestions, inadequately treated illnesses, dental problems, malnutrition, and neurological and developmental deficits. Manifestations in neglectful families include noncompliance or nonadherence to medical recommendations, delay or failure in seeking appropriate health care, hunger, failure to thrive and unmanaged morbid obesity, poor hygiene, and physical and medical conditions contributing to poor cognitive and educational achievement[86]. Poor supervision is less well defined, but has been broken down into broad categories of not watching the child closely enough, inadequate substitute child care, failure to protect from third parties, knowingly allowing the child to participate in harmful activities, and driving (with a child passenger) recklessly or while intoxicated[86–90]. A comprehensive response requires that the physician address the actual or potential harms that have occurred to the child and make appropriate referrals to community services to address what is usually a variety of social and economic issues. Important screening questions which can elicit further avenues of intervention include inquiring as to the family's access to food, their access to appropriate medical and dental services and medicines, substance abuse during and after pregnancy, homelessness, housing, environmental safety, depression, domestic violence, and degree of supervision[86].

Failure to thrive, otherwise known as the lack of normal physiological development associated with malnutrition in infancy, is a nonspecific sign of maltreatment (Chapter 12, Failure to thrive). It has historically been grouped into organic, nonorganic, and mixed varieties[90]. Nonorganic failure to thrive (NOFTT) is more realistically called malnutrition due to neglect. To the extent that many cases fall into the mixed category, such divisions are less important. A comprehensive history and physical examination should guide management and initial laboratory testing. In the face of normal basic metabolic measurements, a careful observation of parental feeding practices and the child's intake and output is often illuminating. Height and weight need to be precisely measured over multiple visits and compared to currently accepted norms, some of which are modified by race, prematurity, or other medical conditions. With acceptable weight gain under direct supervision and a lack of significant medical cause for malnutrition, a presumptive diagnosis of nonorganic failure to thrive can be made.

Medical diagnosis

The physician should be able to recognize and report potential child maltreatment, using standard methods of obtaining history, physical examination, and selected laboratory and imaging tests. He or she must also be cognizant that multiple forms of maltreatment may co-exist, understand the importance of certain risk factors, assist in choosing the appropriate location and timing of evaluation, and appropriately refer children and families to specialized medical and social services. In health care, a clinical assessment of child victimization begins with a medical encounter that usually follows a predictable pattern of information gathering, physical assessment, testing, and clinical diagnosis followed by treatment and/or referral[27,91–93].

Medical history, a cornerstone of medical diagnosis in general, still plays the most important part in the diagnosis of child abuse and neglect. It is that history, taken with physical examination findings and other studies in the context of the family, which offers a sound basis for diagnosis and treatment recommendations[27,94]. First, the main reason for the medical encounter or 'chief complaint' is recorded from the child or family, followed by delineation of appropriate elements of the medical history. Inquiring and recording the specific complaints and disclosures of maltreatment by the child and parent, if any, in their own words is vitally important to the ultimate protection of the child. An accurate and detailed history is very important in assessing the potentially abused child, and it is important to take a history from the child directly. Explain to the parents or caregiver the importance of this direct questioning and try to appropriately prevent them from attempting to fill in details. Only after you feel you have gleaned all the information from the child that you reasonably can should you then address the caregiver for clarification or additional details. History obtained directly from the child, particularly when obtained in the course of taking a medical history to provide a diagnosis and treatment plan, may be admissible. Remember to begin with open-ended questions and progress to more focused, but nonleading questions. Use age and developmentally appropriate terminology and avoid expressions of shock and disbelief. With accidental injuries, there is often a very detailed history as opposed to abusive injuries where the history is often vague and changes when retold. Most parents can provide a reasonable history for significant bruises on their child and the absence of history with significant bruising should raise concern. Behavioral and emotional issues are important in this assessment. Certain nonspecific behaviors, developmental delays, and history of abuse should be recorded as part of the medical history, aiding in assessing harm and planning for appropriate treatment[77]. However, a simple set of screening questions for sexual abuse, for example, for the general pediatric encounter has yet to be widely implemented[95].

After examination (as noted above), the physician then arrives at an assessment or diagnosis using standard diagnostic categories, such as the International Classification of Disease[96] or a specialized diagnostic scheme for certain types of abuse[58]. Medical diagnosis of child abuse and neglect follows commonly accepted practices for other medical diagnoses. While the use of such coding does not guarantee reimbursement, it highlights the standard approach to maltreatment as a concern of the health care provider and allows collection of population data[91]. Unique to child maltreatment diagnosis is a determination of certainty, with only a low level of certainty required to meet general standards of a 'reasonable cause to suspect' that maltreatment has occurred for mandated reporting (*Table 2*). When maltreatment is suspected, the practitioner can request additional diagnostic tests for the child, such as radiographs, blood work, or microbiologic identification. Furthermore, the practitioner can begin treatment of acute injuries, ensure protection of the child from further harm, and arrange referrals to appropriate physical or mental health specialists for further evaluation and treatment[52,97].

Significant differences exist between standards for medical diagnosis and those for legal adjudication. Medical diagnosis is defined as 'the act of distinguishing one disease from another' or 'the determination of the nature of a case of disease'[98]. The constellation of the patient's history, physical examination, and laboratory findings may result in

Table 2 **Relationship among medical findings, diagnostic certainty, and need for reporting**[a]

History of maltreatment	None or any	Disclosure by child or report by third party	Inconsistent or nonspecific	None	Plausible consistent alternative
Specificity of examination or laboratory findings	Specific	Normal or nonspecific	Normal or nonspecific	Normal or nonspecific	Normal or nonspecific
Diagnostic certainty	Definitive	Likely or probably	Possible	No basis for concern	No basis for concern
Reporting	Yes	Yes	Yes	No	No

[a]This is for guidance only. All cases require assessment of the need for reporting and are affected by other factors, such as delay in seeking care, inconsistency over time, or development, seriousness of injury, prior injury, or other child maltreatment.

multiple potential diagnoses, often leading the practitioner to a treatment plan without 100% or even probable certainty of the diagnosis. These criteria differ significantly from legal standards, by which a level of certainty must be carefully crafted to include 'credible' evidence, a 'preponderance' of the evidence, 'clear and convincing' evidence, or evidence 'beyond a reasonable doubt.' These standards of evidence in the legal system are defined by a state's case law and/or statute and are distinct from those in medical practice. As one might imagine, differences in interpretation of certainty can lead to difficulties in communication between legal and medical practitioners.

Documentation

The evaluation of a child suspected to have been abused includes the physician's documentation. This written record may be used to provide information to child protection workers, the police, and the court. A complete and accurate record will help these professionals with their evaluations. The doctor's note may provide the necessary material to refresh his or her memory when called to court months or years after having seen the child. The record should be legible. Important statements, either by the child or the parents, should be placed verbatim with quotation marks in the record. Abbreviations and medical jargon that will not be understood by nonphysicians should be avoided, or, if deemed important, followed by an explanation in parentheses. Opinions based on documented findings are appropriately included in the medical record; unsubstantiated snap judgments or 'gut feelings' are not.

Specific details that should be sought during the medical history and physical examination should be included in the physician's documentation. Height, weight, and head circumference should be measured and graphed as poor growth gain may be an indicator of neglect. An evaluation of the child's behavior and development may provide clues as to the child's motor abilities and whether he could have performed the action (e.g. rolling off a bed) that is said to have led to his injuries. Interactions between the parent and the child should be observed and noted. Instances of parental concern, indifference, or hostility deserve documentation. The physician's documentation should conclude with a diagnosis and an assessment of certainty, as needed, taking into account historical, psychosocial, physical examination, and ancillary investigation (laboratory, imaging) data available, as well as treatment plans, reports to authorities, and disposition.

Reporting

Medical diagnosis is not the same as reporting, and differing diagnostic certainties may lead to differing reporting outcomes (*Table 2*). The practice of health care professionals is regulated by a series of laws in the states' statutes and through licensing requirements specific to individual disciplines. Mandated reporters have legal responsibilities under child protection laws to report their concerns of child abuse and neglect to appropriate state agencies in all 50 states in the United States[6,99]. Although the forms of the legislation vary from state to state, these child protection laws stipulate that certain professionals must report their concerns of child abuse and neglect to appropriate governmental agencies when there is reasonable suspicion. The reporting requirements of these laws supersede the confidentiality of medical records and the patient–provider relationship. Mandated reporters generally include physicians, nurses, and other professionals working in hospitals, in addition to a variety of other licensed professionals who include dentists, teachers, counselors, law enforcement officers, and mental health professionals. Specific protections are usually given for reports made in good faith, and certain penalties are listed for the failure to report when child maltreatment would reasonably have been suspected.

Requirements vary from state to state, and no national or even international criteria exist for determining whether to report suspected abuse or neglect based on medical indications[6,100,101]. There are often differing interpretations as to whether a specific practice or injury must be reported[25]. General guidelines have been suggested which include the patient meeting the legal definition of being a child, the act or omission having been committed by the parent or caregiver, the history being inconsistent with the injury, or that other features of a reported episode fulfill other criteria for abuse or neglect. Multiple missed medical appointments, unreasonable delay in seeking medical treatment, abandonment, illnesses that could be prevented by routine medical care, and inadequate care have been identified as potential minimal criteria for a neglect report[102,103]. Statements made by the child or parent disclosing potential maltreatment, physical injuries, or death inconsistent with accident or medical disease, or sexually transmitted infections or pregnancy are generally accepted as a basis for suspected maltreatment reports[27].

It is important to note that child abuse reporting is one of the few instances in which health care professionals are required to contact a governmental agency in the routine course of their practice. While disease reporting has traditionally existed within the public health community (particularly when a contagious infection may pose a hazard to community health), reporting actions that are deemed to be 'crimes' has historically been less accepted by the medical community. Less clear statutory requirements have been enacted in the United States for reporting victimization of the elderly and vulnerable adults, and for domestic violence. Recent US federal legislation specifically allows state-mandated child abuse reporting and exempts such state reporting laws from federal privacy requirements under the Health Insurance Portability and Accountability Act of 1996. Penalties for not reporting range from fines in some states to criminal charges in others, but also include civil penalties so that the child and/or the child's guardian may litigate to redress financial losses sustained caused by the failure to report.

Teaching points

- Physicians, nurses, and other health professionals have improved their identification of the physical injuries associated with victimization and have developed increasingly sophisticated techniques for diagnosing and documenting physical abuse, sexual abuse, psychological maltreatment, and neglect.
- Physicians and other mandated reporters play a vital role in the identification, reporting, and treatment of child victims of abuse and neglect.
- There are specific patterns of injury associated with different forms of maltreatment, and mandated reporters need to learn about the specificity of historical information and physical findings to be able to accurately diagnose, document, and report suspected maltreatment.
- Using this atlas, physicians and others can fulfill their roles both as mandated reporters and as important members of the crew of the 'lifeboat' needed to save children in the sometimes turbulent 'ocean of life'[104].

Chapter 2

BRUISES

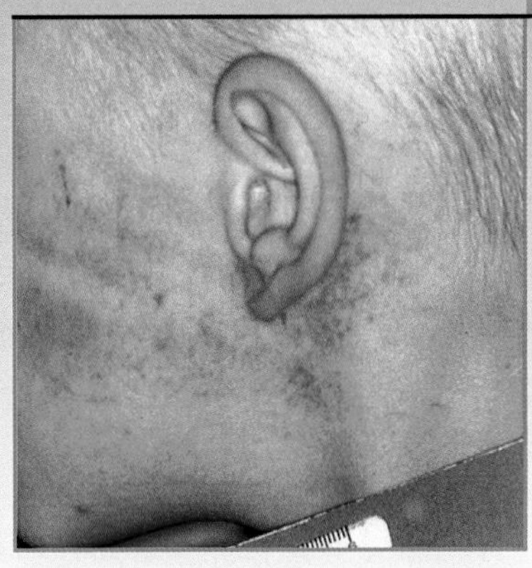

Earl Hartwig MD and
Howard Fischer MD

Bruises are seen with great regularity in children. They can represent injuries from accidental or noninflicted events, can be the sole manifestation of child abuse, or can be but one component of a pattern of abusive or neglectful injuries[1,2]. The physician must have at his or her disposal a method of distinguishing accidental bruises from those that are inflicted. The overarching question, when one is faced with any injury, is whether the history of how the injury occurred is compatible with the observed injury. To make such an assessment one should consider (1) the developmental stage of the child, (2) the site of the injury, and (3) the fashion in which the injury is said to have happened[1].

Introduction

The nonambulatory child does not have much opportunity for accidental bruising, although he may scratch himself accidentally with his fingernails. Until a child starts walking, his opportunities to bump into objects or to fall with sufficient force to produce bruising are virtually nonexistent – 'Those who don't cruise rarely bruise[3]' (**1–8**). Additionally, accidental bruising tends to occur in skin closely overlying bone, that is, the knees, shins, elbows, spinous processes, and forehead (**9–14**). Bruises that occur on fleshy parts of the body – the upper arm, the thigh, the genitals, or the soft tissues of the mouth – should raise suspicion of abuse (**15–21**). Traditionally, bruises at certain sites were considered pathognomonic for abuse based on the frequency with which they were seen in children suspected of abuse[4,5]. To wit, bruises on the buttocks are from spanking or paddling[6] (**22, 23**); genital and inner-thigh bruises inflicted for toileting accidents (**8, 24**); penile injuries from ligatures (a string or rubber band) placed to prevent wetting (**25–30**); slap marks to the cheeks (**23, 31–36**); and bruises to the upper lip and frenulum are from forcefully thrusting a bottle or pacifier (dummy) in the infant's mouth (**37**). Similarly, bruises on the neck, hands, and feet are usually not accidental and should therefore be considered attentively (**4, 5**). One must realize, however, that some of these bruises can, at times, be produced by other mechanisms of injury, including accidental. For example, a bruised frenulum may be sustained through a punch to the mouth or via an accidental fall to the floor, pavement, or ground[7]. Therefore, it is most important to elicit a careful history and determine if the injuries seen are compatible with the mechanism described by the caregiver.

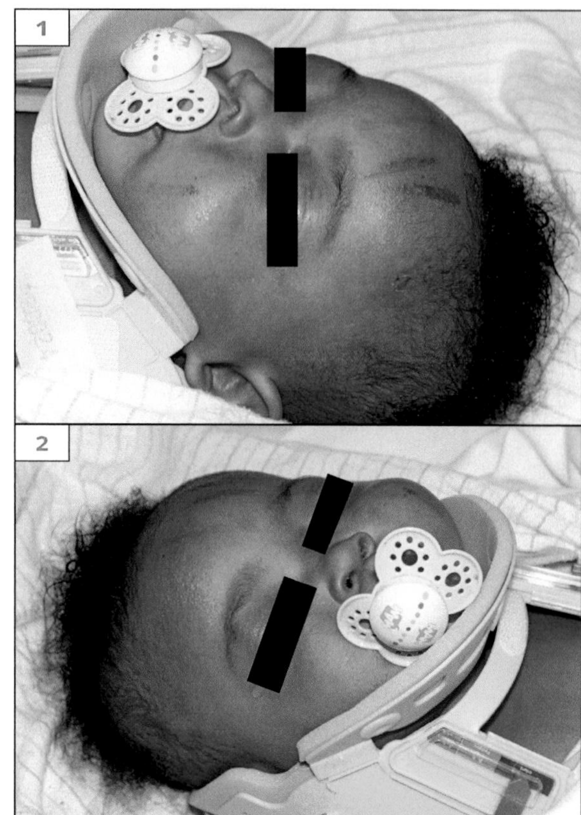

1, 2 Four-month-old female who was left with an 8-year-old uncle with 'behavioral problems' while she was sleeping. The 8-year-old has admitted to hitting the infant. Examination shows peri-orbital bruising and swelling bilaterally and linear abrasions of the forehead. Although infants may occasionally scratch themselves, such wide and deep abrasions are not seen in infants with self-inflicted injury. These were likely fingernail scratches from an older person. The diagnosis was nonaccidental injuries.

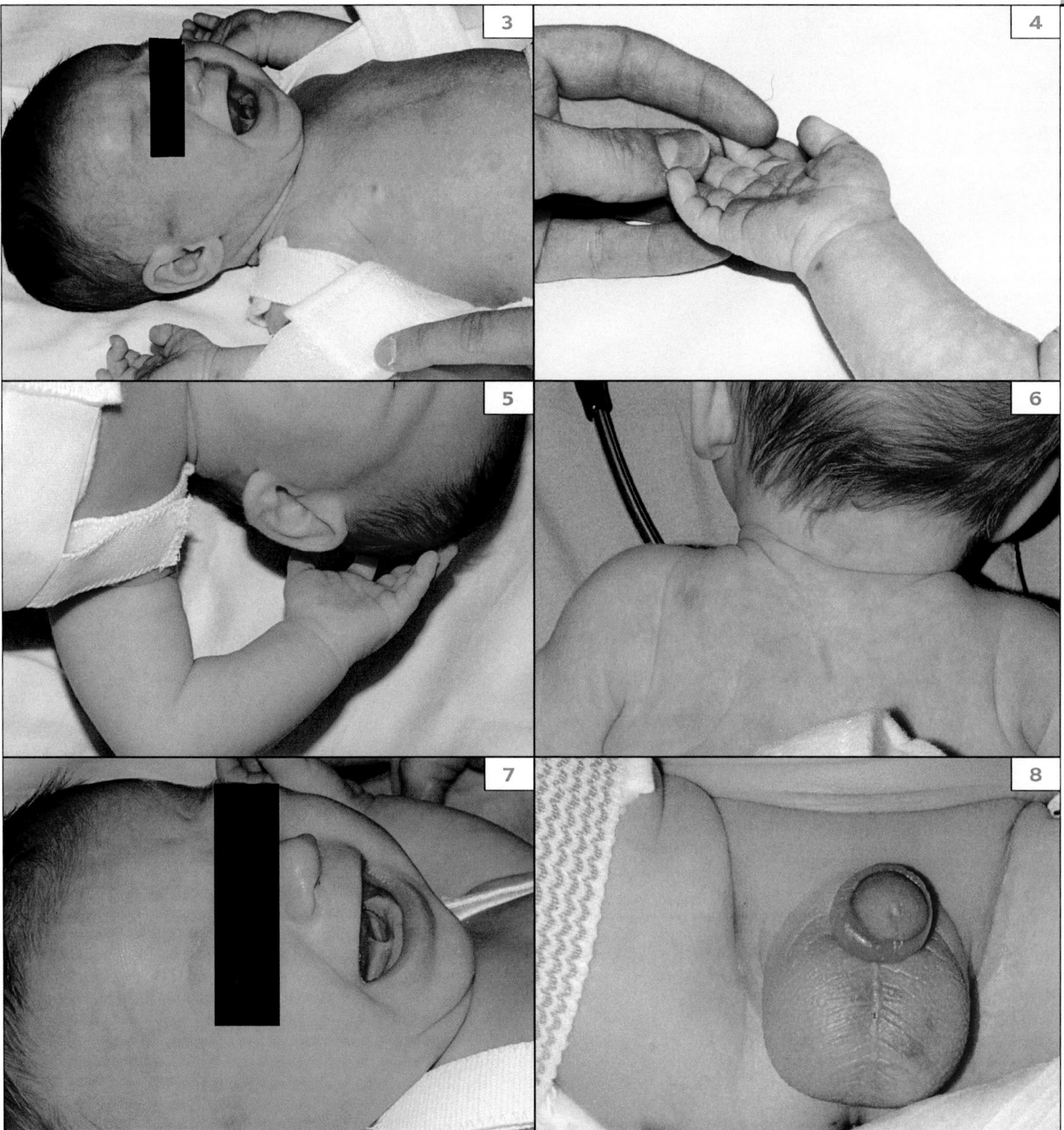

3–8 Seven-week-old male who presented with right thigh swelling noted that morning while the mother was changing the infant. The initial history reveals no possible trauma. After injuries were discovered, the father stated that he had the infant on his lap at 5 a.m. while playing a video game. He further stated that he dropped the infant's bottle and leaned forward to pick it up and may have injured the infant at that time. Retrospectively, the mother indicated the infant had been crying more over the past few days. Examination shows a linear bruise across right cheek consistent with a slap mark, abrasion over the bridge of the nose, foreskin edema and ecchymosis, left scrotal bruise, bruises on the palms of the hands, right wrist and forearm, right heel and ankle, left foot and right flank, upper left chest, upper back, left posterior shoulder, left and right sides of the neck. There is obvious swelling and pain of the right thigh. Skeletal survey shows healing left clavicular fracture and transverse right femur fracture. Laboratories reveal elevated liver transaminases (aspartate transaminase (AST) 263; alanine transaminase (ALT) 454). The diagnosis was that the findings were clearly not consistent with history provided and represent abuse.

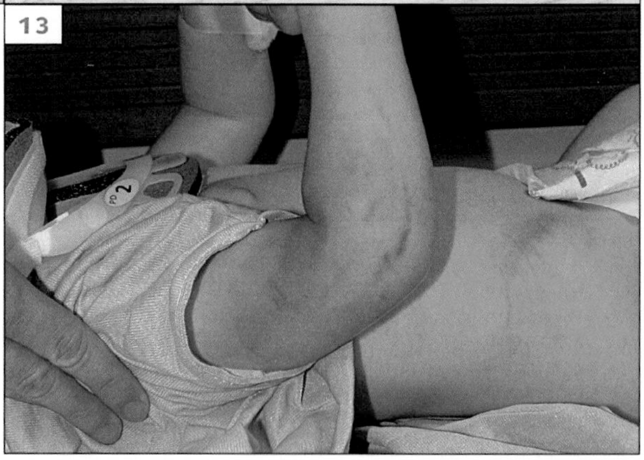

9–13 Eighteen-month-old female who was playing in the driveway and run over by the family car twice. A relative 'backed over the child' and believed she 'ran over something' then pulled forward and 'ran over her again' before realizing what had happened. Examination shows bruises of the lower extremities (likely old and accidental) and recent bruises of the abdomen and right arm. Work-up revealed elevated liver transaminases and a hypodense area in the liver on computed tomography, which may have represented a liver laceration. Radiographs also revealed a right pelvic (ala of the ileum) fracture.

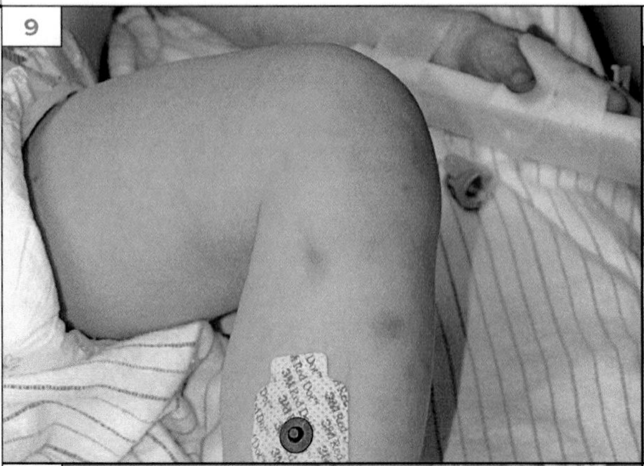

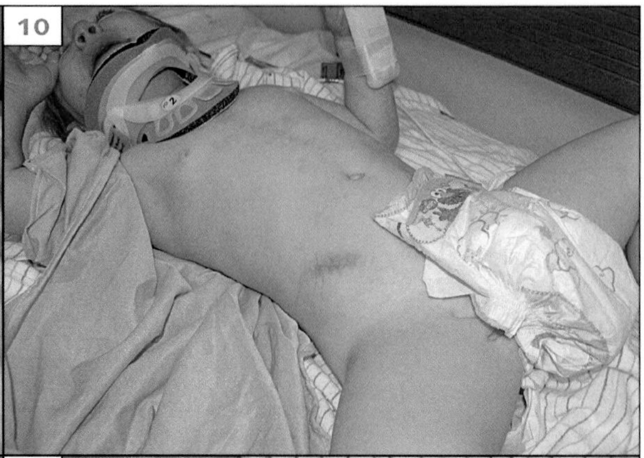

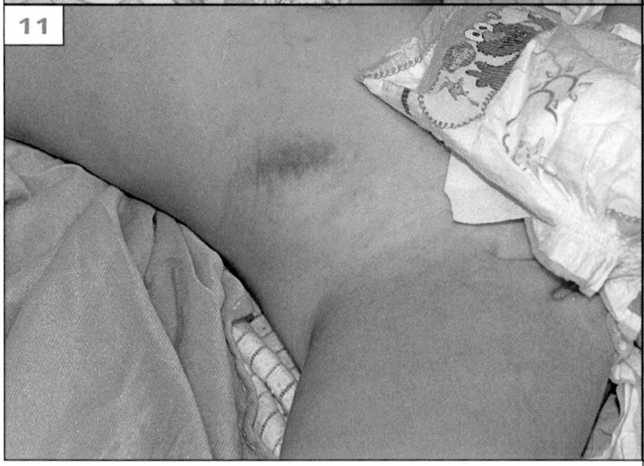

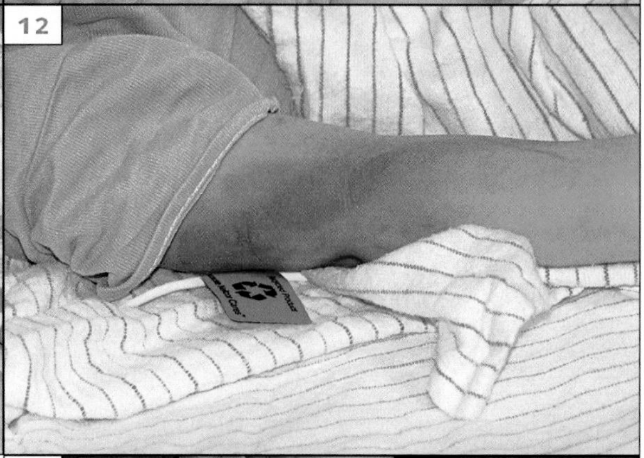

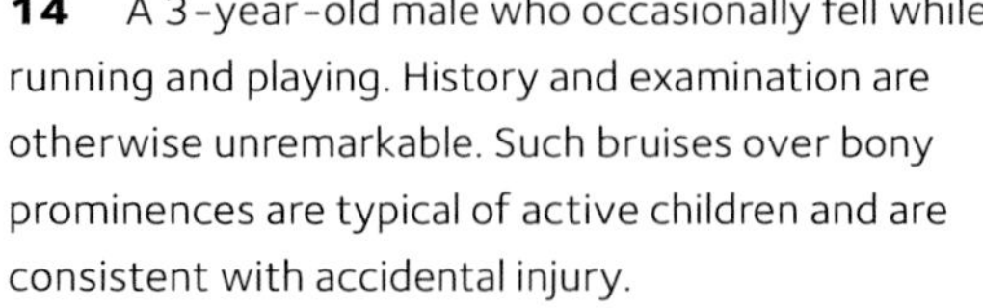

14 A 3-year-old male who occasionally fell while running and playing. History and examination are otherwise unremarkable. Such bruises over bony prominences are typical of active children and are consistent with accidental injury.

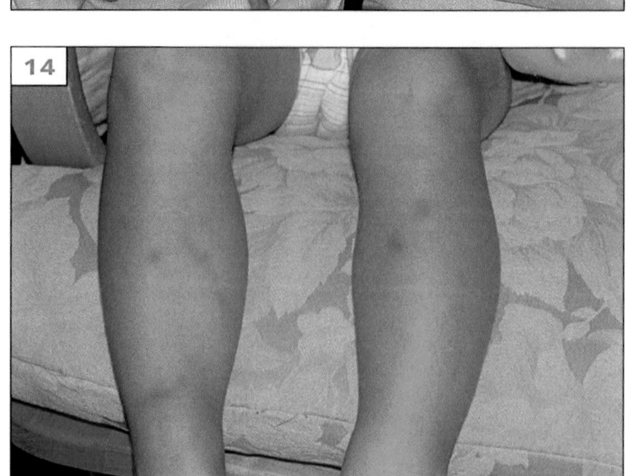

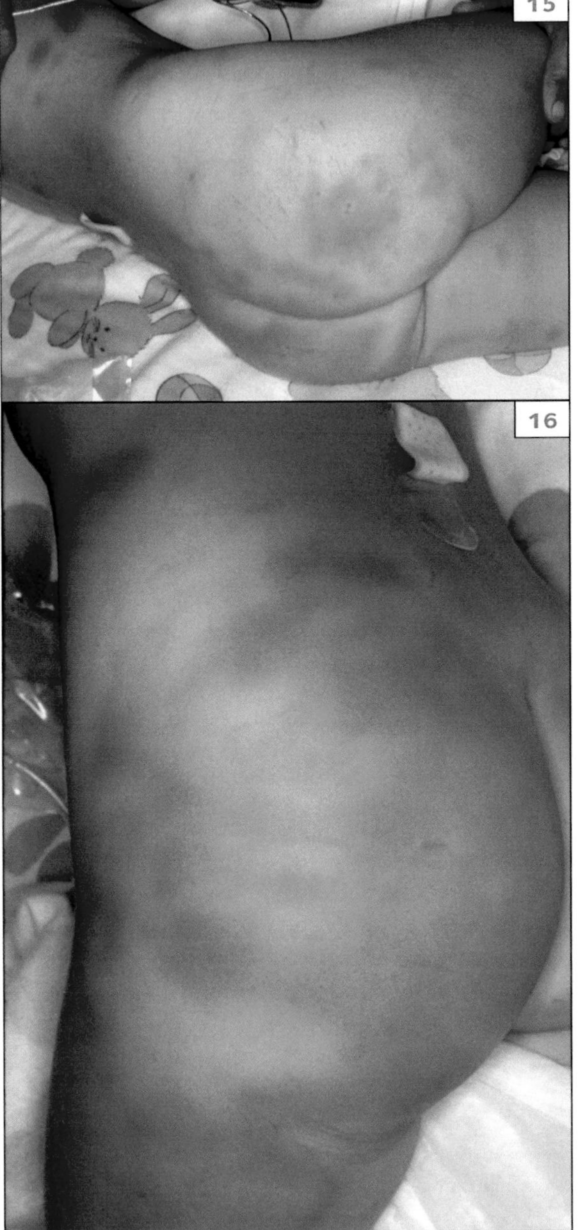

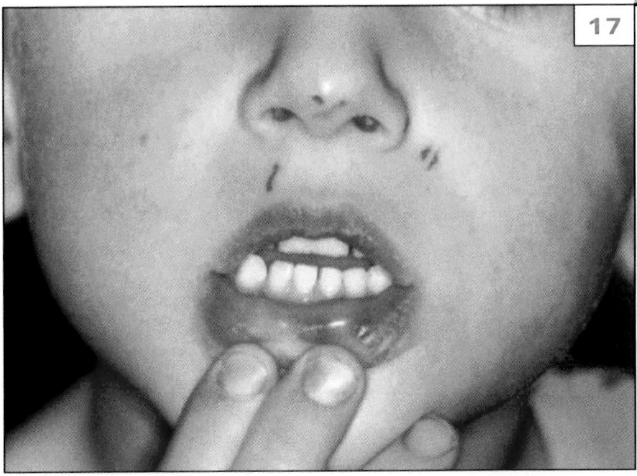

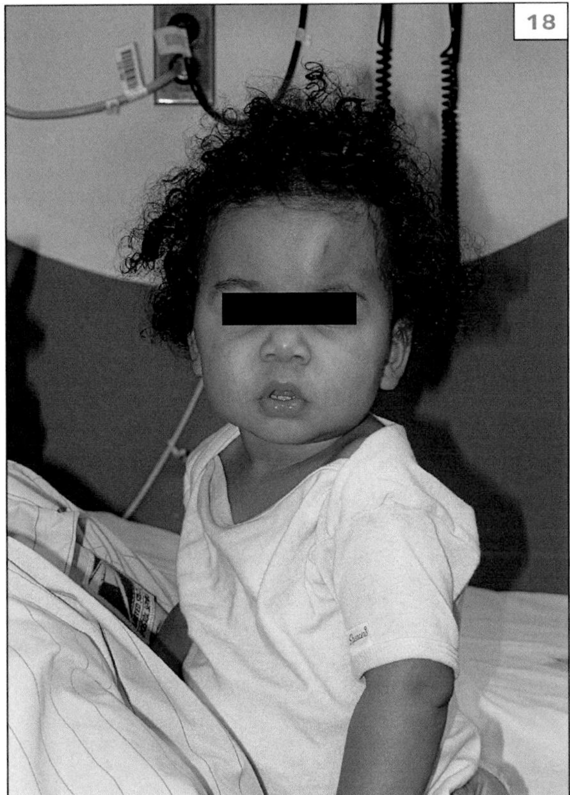

15, 16 Bruising of well-padded soft tissue area of the thigh with multiple amorphous bruises, some with differing colors. Coagulation studies were normal and the child was reported for suspected physical abuse, likely mechanism beating with a hand or object.

17 Injury of the soft tissues of the mouth with tooth imprints likely resulting from a blow to the mouth.

18 A 16-month-old mixed race male who presented after hitting a chair. A contusion was noted on the left forehead with linear ecchymosis. The remaining history and full examination were unremarkable for suspicious lesions. This vertical linear pattern is typical of a child who strikes (runs into) a corner of a wall, or in this instance, the edge of a chair. The diagnosis was closed head injury consistent with accidental injury.

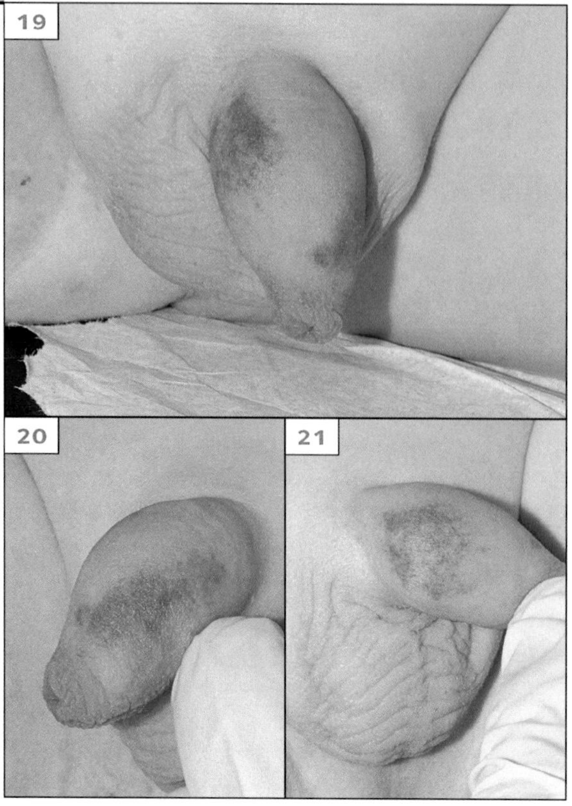

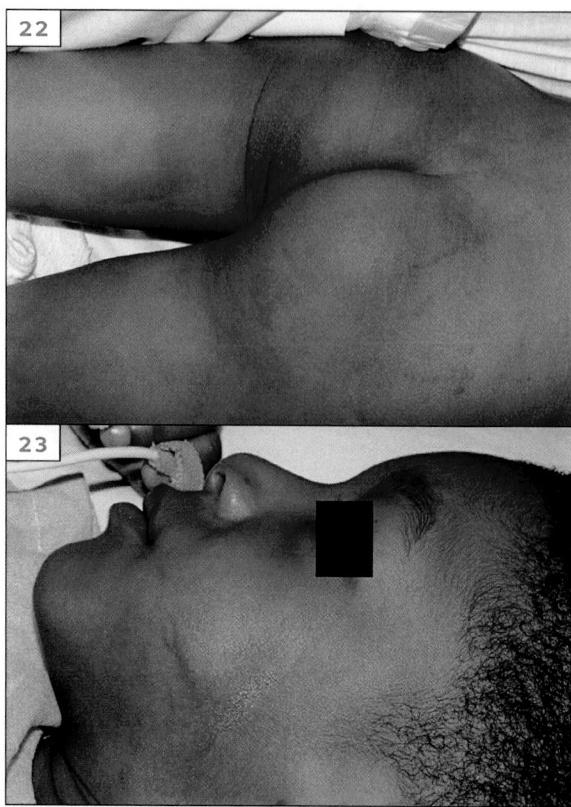

19–21 An 18-month-old male with swelling and redness of his penis noted 1 hour earlier with a diaper/nappy change. The child was with his grandparents for a short period just before his mother discovered the swelling. Examination revealed a subtle petechial rash on the upper face and penile bruise. Past history shows that the patient ingested sertraline hydrochloride at 9 months of age. The diagnosis was penile ecchymosis, suspicious for abuse.

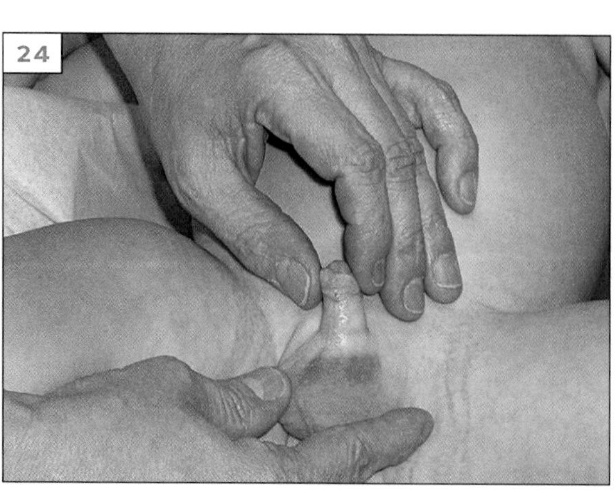

22, 23 A 6-year-old male was reportedly hit in the chest and abdomen by his father using his fist. According to the mother, the child was also whipped by the father 3 days previously with a belt. Six months before, the child was brought in by his father and treated for bilateral wrist fractures reportedly sustained by falling off the couch while playing football with the father. The mother and father are separated. Examination reveals a small bruise with swelling on the right eyebrow, a linear bruise on the right cheek consistent with slap mechanism, diffuse bruising and hyperpigmentation on the posterior thighs and buttocks, with swelling and induration of the right buttock. Further bruises were noted on the left forearm, left upper arm, right wrist, and hand. His stool was Hemoccult positive. The child had tenderness of the abdomen with elevated liver transaminases. The diagnosis was liver contusion with findings consistent with recent and old nonaccidental trauma.

24 This figure demonstrates genital injury. This is a well-protected area, especially in a child wearing a diaper/nappy. This child had normal coagulation tests and was reported for suspected physical abuse, likely mechanism pinching.

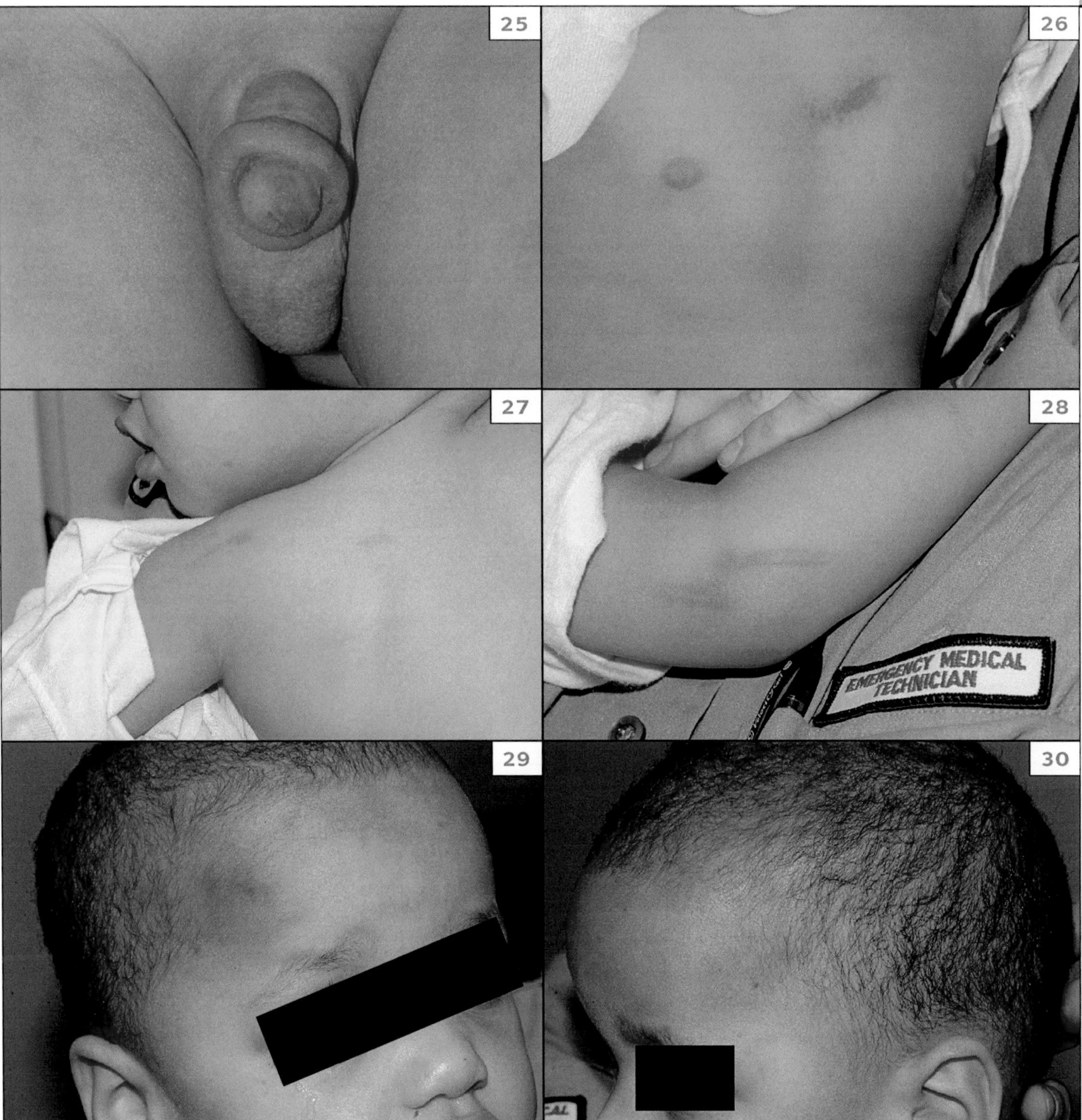

25–30 A 23-month-old male who presented with swelling of the penis. His mother indicated to the doctor that the patient's 7-year-old sister pulled on the penis the day before. Reportedly, the child was in the process of toilet training and the mother stated that the child walks around frequently without a diaper/nappy. The nursing notes from triage indicate, however, that the mother had stated that a 'man in the house' did this to her son. The child had been seen 14 days previously with a forehead and peri-orbital bruise reportedly from 'hitting his head on a vanity unit multiple times having a tantrum while he was sitting on a potty chair'. Two weeks earlier, an anonymous call was made to the child protective services regarding his bruises. Examination shows foreskin edema and swelling with possible ecchymosis of the glans penis, bruises noted on the forehead and scalp, as well as left posterior shoulder, left hip, left leg, and chest. Bruises were seen on the right forearm and left elbow that showed linear parallel marks consistent with a strike from a belt, cord, or other linear object. The diagnosis was nonaccidental trauma, penile injury consistent with ligature.

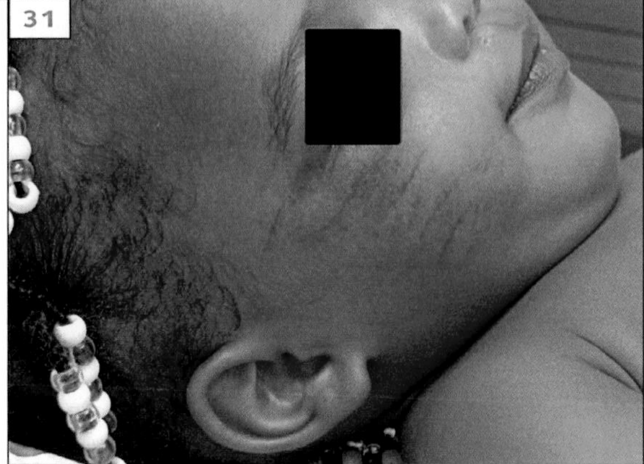

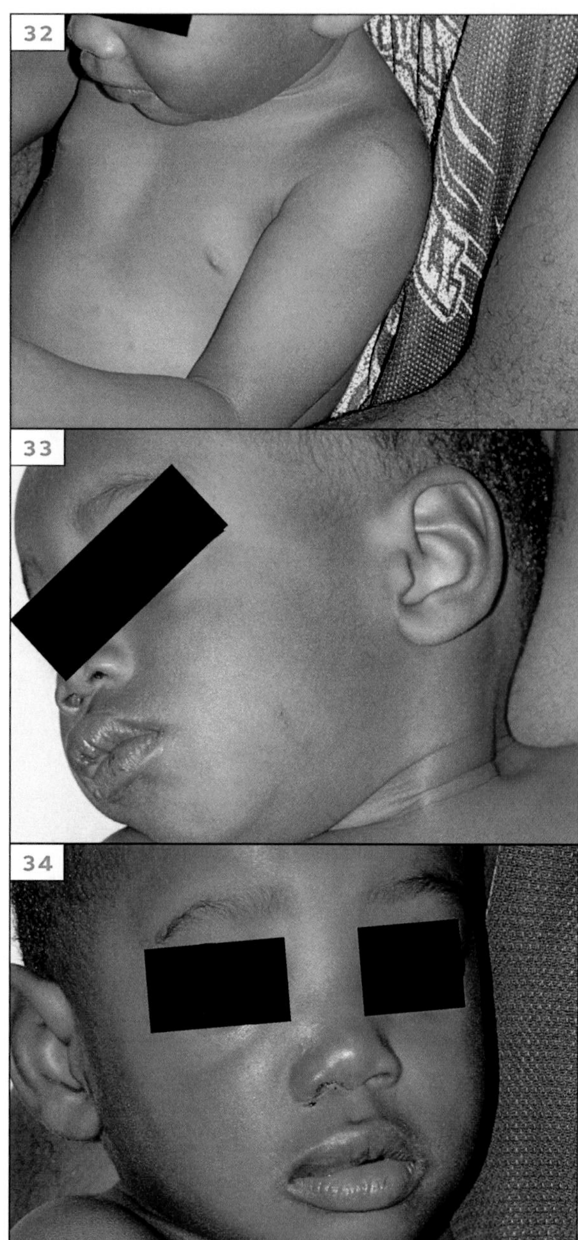

31 An 18-month-old female was picked up by the biological mother from the foster mother from a weekend visit 36 hours previously. A swollen red rash was noted on the right cheek at that time which had subsided somewhat. The biological mother questions potential abuse. Examination reveals a linear pattern to the bruise consistent with the 'negative imprint' of repeated hand slaps. The bruises continue to be swollen and tender and do not show any obvious aging or hemoglobin breakdown; this would be consistent with recent injury, including within the past 36 hours. The diagnosis was hand marks to the face consistent with child abuse.

32–34 An 18-month-old male was reportedly hit in the face with a belt and hanger by his 5- and 7-year-old brothers. Examination shows epistaxis with bruising and swelling of the right cheek and infraorbital area. There is also a linear bruise on the left cheek which may reflect a strike from a linear object (such as a hanger) or the 'reverse imprint' of a hand slap. There is also a circular pattern bruise noted on the left shoulder. The diagnosis was contusions consistent with child abuse.

35 This figure demonstrates a slap mark, as well as linear burns or scars on the face and neck.

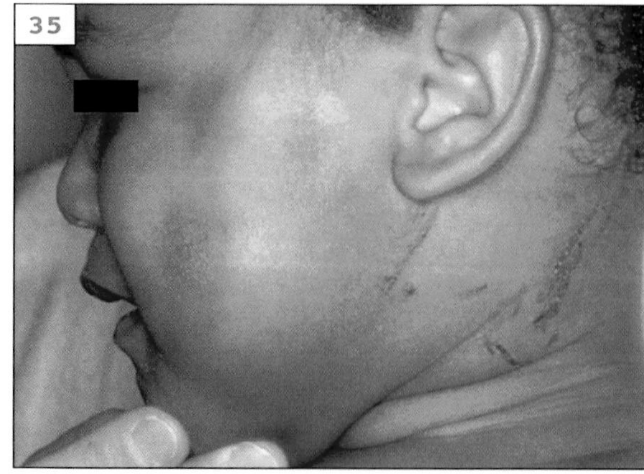

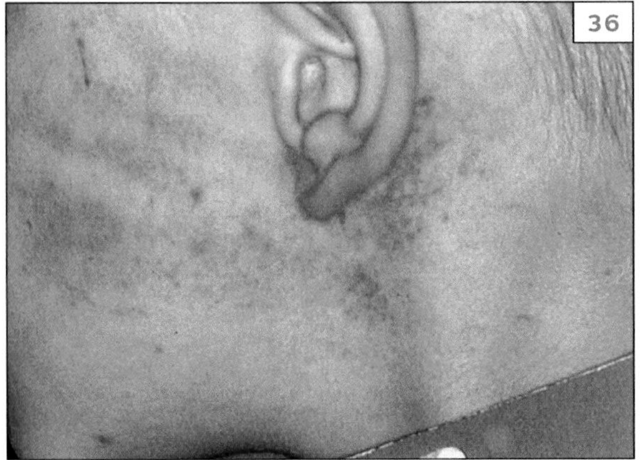

36 This figure demonstrates a slap mark on the face and neck with bruising of the ear and retroauricular area. One needs to look for retinal hemorrhage, hemotympanum and consider an intracranial injury with such an injury.

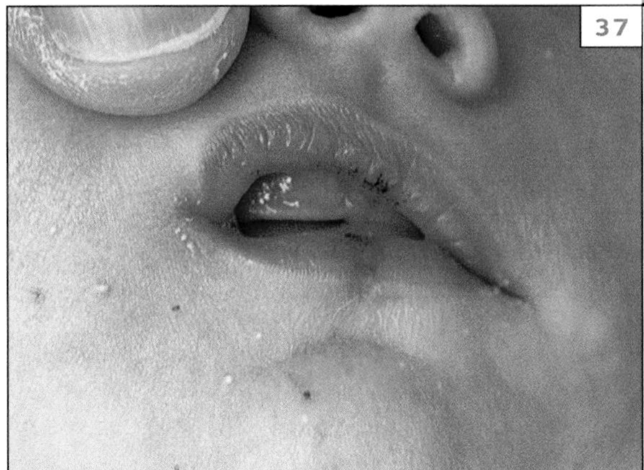

37 Injury to the upper lip and frenulum.

Pathophysiology

A bruise is an escape of blood into the skin, subcutaneous tissue, or both, following the rupture of blood vessels (usually capillaries) secondary to pressure and/or shearing forces associated with blunt trauma. This is in comparison to a petechia which is a pinpoint nonraised purplish red spot caused by intradermal or submucosal hemorrhage, and an ecchymosis which is a small hemorrhagic spot, larger than a petechia but also nonraised, in the skin or mucous membranes. Purpura is described as a small hemorrhage in the skin, mucous membranes, or serosal surfaces, which may be caused by a variety of factors including blood and blood vessel disorders, as well as trauma. Depending on the shearing forces involved, there may be associated abrasion or laceration as well (**38, 39**) with subsequent scarring (**40–42**). Given the frequency with which accidental bumps and falls occur in children, it is interesting to note that the majority of these injuries occur without any obvious bruising or swelling. At times, sustained pressure or minor injury may produce erythema and/or tenderness to the skin that resolves over several minutes to hours (**43–45**). With impact trauma, there may be a localized collection of blood with associated swelling, in which case the injury may be referred to as a hematoma. It is not uncommon, however, to see significant injury, such as underlying long bone fracture or marked hematoma involving the deeper subcutaneous fatty layer, with no visible bruising initially (**46, 47**). Hemorrhage into the deeper tissues may take several days to visualize with gradual extravasation and tracking to more superficial layers and may never show superficial discoloration. The area of discoloration can also increase or shift considerably from the site of impact with tracking of blood to adjacent tissues. The common example of this is a bruise or contusion that originates at the forehead or glabella and the blood and associated fluid subsequently shifts to produce peri-orbital bruising or swelling (see Chapter 4, Cutaneous conditions mimicking child abuse).

Bruising can take on a variety of appearances based upon the magnitude and type of force applied. Diffuse force or force dispersed through clothing layers may show a soft edge to the bruise or perhaps a petechial appearance (**48–50**). More localized force will produce a more homogeneous bruise with more discrete edges, and significant impact with a discrete object will frequently produce a pattern to the bruise (**38, 39, 51–66**). If an object strikes the skin with significant energy, pressure forces blood through small vessels to the edges of the skin area not exposed to (or under) pressure. There, rupture and extravasation of blood occurs and the subsequent bruise is actually a negative imprint or outline of the object used to strike the skin. The classic example of this is a hand slap across the face which results in a bruise resembling a line or parallel lines corresponding with the interdigital spaces (**23, 31, 33, 35**).

When a bruise or hematoma is new, there is frequently pain, tenderness, and swelling of the affected area. Pain and tenderness lessen over subsequent days and their presence can be helpful in grossly dating when an injury occurred. The initial appearance of a bruise can be variable, but generally will show more reddish coloration with superficial intradermal bleeding and will take on more of a bluish coloration with deeper subcutaneous bleeding. The actual coloration perceived by the naked eye depends upon irregularity and thickness of the surface layer, degree of light scattering properties of the collagen fibers, and reflective properties of the underlying structures. With time, there is degradation of hemoglobin pigment and subsequent color changes to the bruise with gradual fading as resorption of blood occurs.

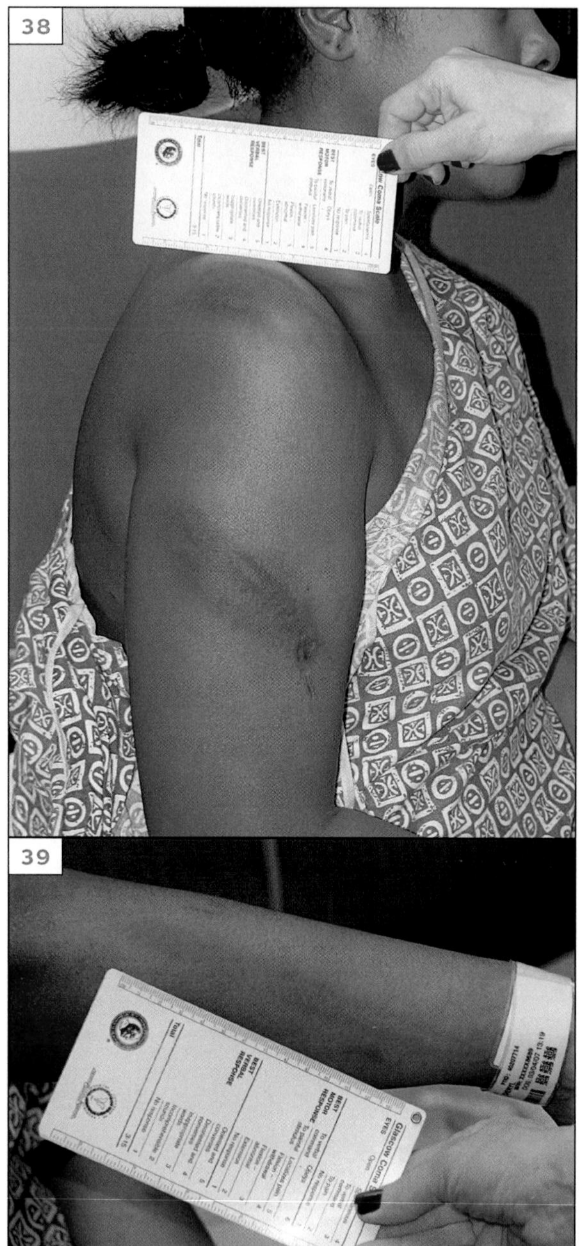

38, 39 A 14-year-old female who was hit repeatedly with a broomstick by her guardian. Examination shows reverse image bruises (outline of handle) on the right shoulder, upper and lower arm, and calf. A deep abrasion was noted on the right arm. Note that the 'reverse image' is less well demarcated over the more padded shoulder and upper arm than the lower arm. The diagnosis was child abuse.

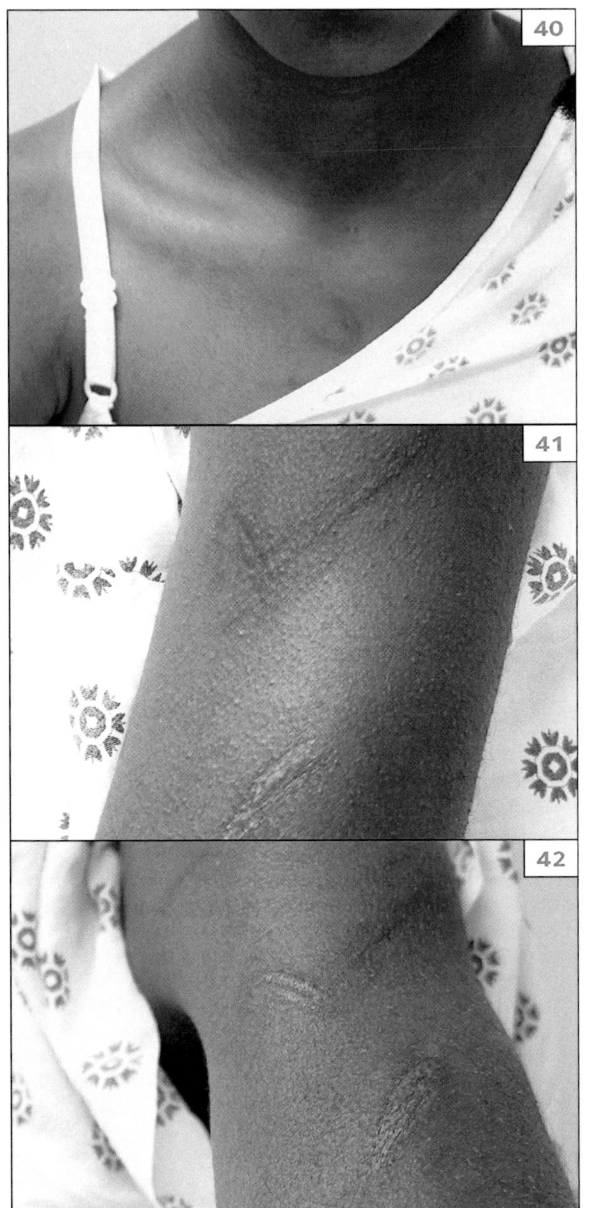

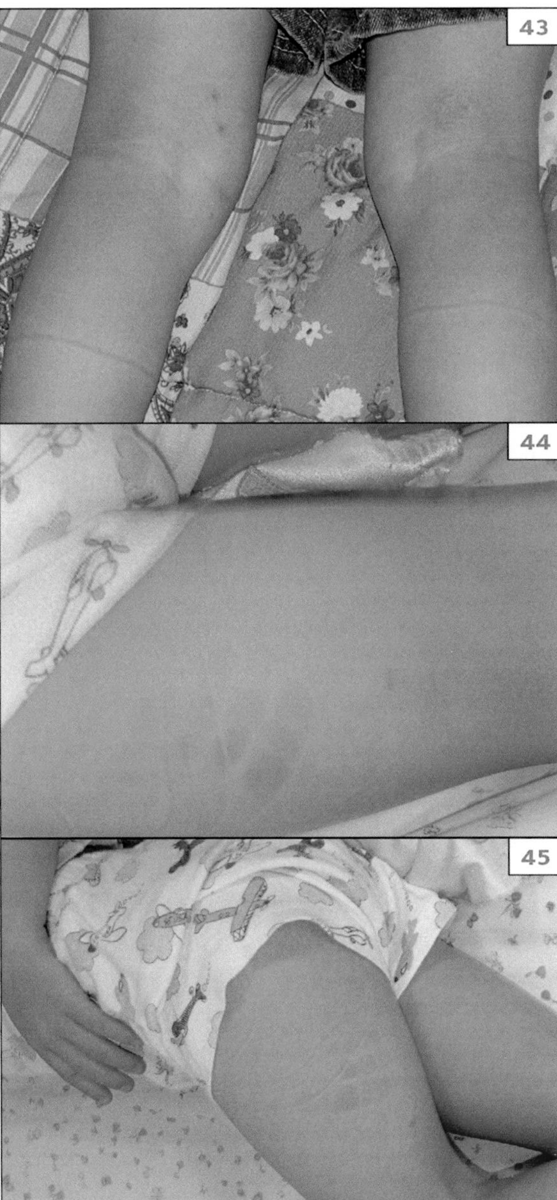

40–42 An 11-year-old female brought into hospital for suspicion of abuse. Examination reveals multiple recent linear and 'loop mark' bruises consistent with abuse. Well-healed, linear and 'loop marks' were also noted consistent with previous injury (belt or extension cord beating) with such force as to significantly abrade or lacerate the skin leading to the scarring seen. Such injury implies a great force used by the perpetrator. The diagnosis was recent and old injuries consistent with child abuse.

43–45 A 3-year-old male who was noted to have linear marks on the lower extremities after wearing socks with elastic overnight. This apparent bruising was no longer noticeable a few hours later. The lesions seen at the popliteal fossa represent atopic dermatitis and molluscum contagiosum. On a second occasion (44, 45), this hand imprint mark was noted after sleeping. The child's handprint mark disappeared after approximately 15 minutes. Note that there is a 'positive image' with sparing of the interphalangeal creases as opposed to the 'negative image' seen with forceful hand slap. The diagnosis was transient elastic band mark and handprint without ecchymosis.

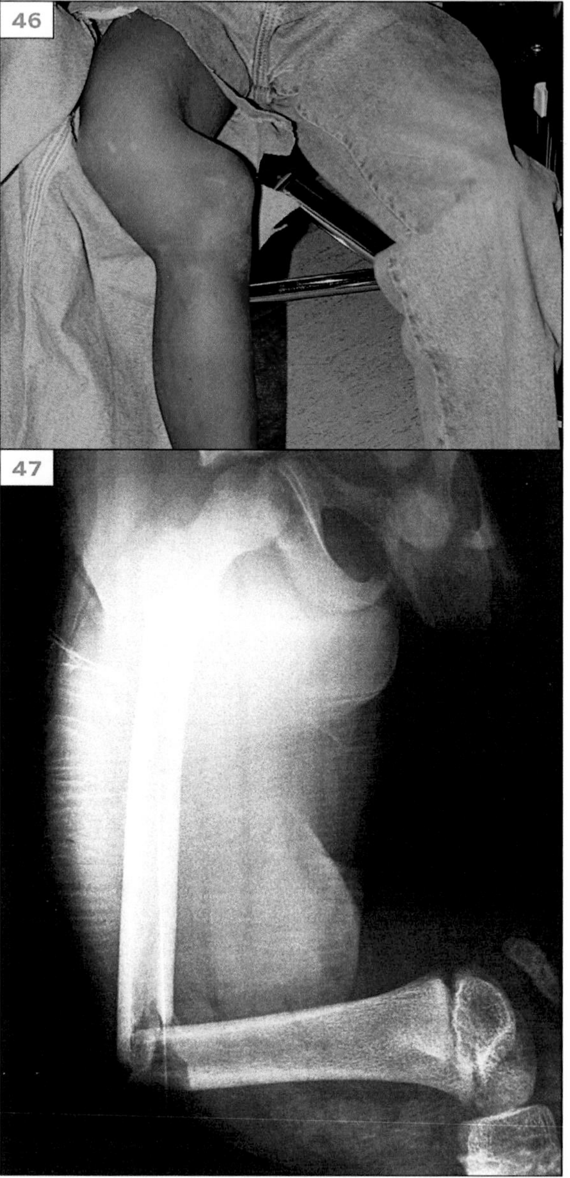

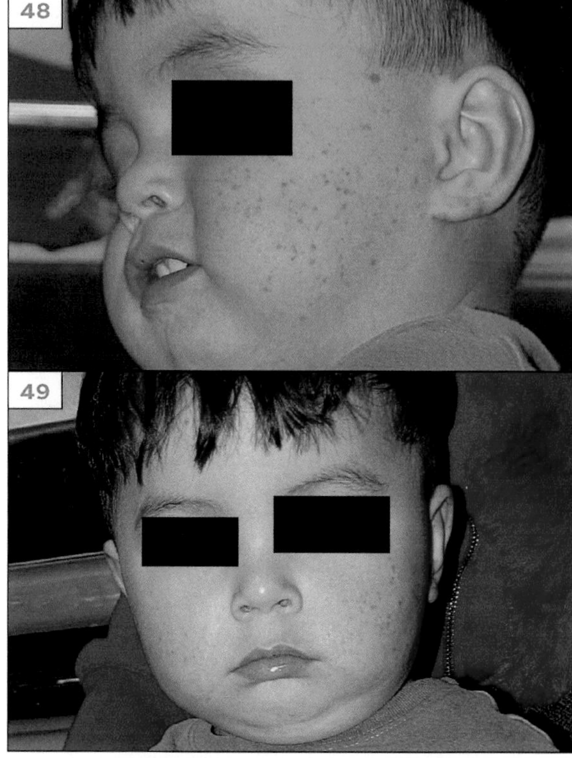

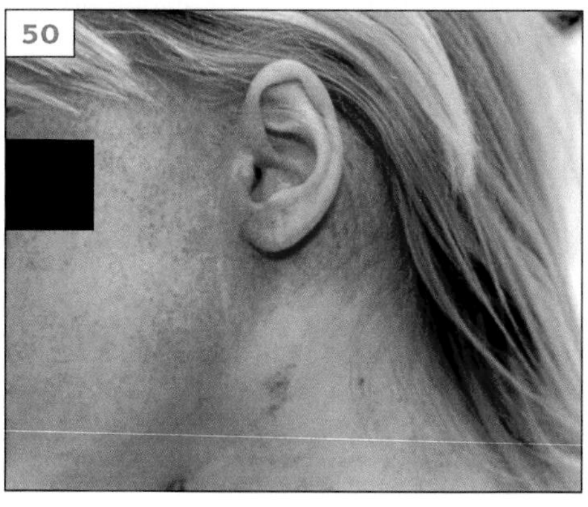

46, 47 A 6-year-old male who fell from a height sustaining fracture with deformity of the right leg. Although there was considerable underlying injury (see radiographs), there is no noticeable bruise on presentation. The diagnosis was accidental femur fracture.

48, 49 A 15-month-old male who fell 2 days previously on his cheek with no observed bruising. He gradually developed a small bruise with soft edges on the left cheek. He developed a hard cough and the parents noted a rash developing over the previous day. Examination showed a coarse petechial/purpuric rash on the left (previously injured) cheek and a subtle petechial rash on the right cheek. The diagnosis was petechial rash secondary to straining, more prominent on the left due to previous trauma.

50 Petechiae consistent with a diffuse force injury. This appearance is also seen in some cases of strangulation.

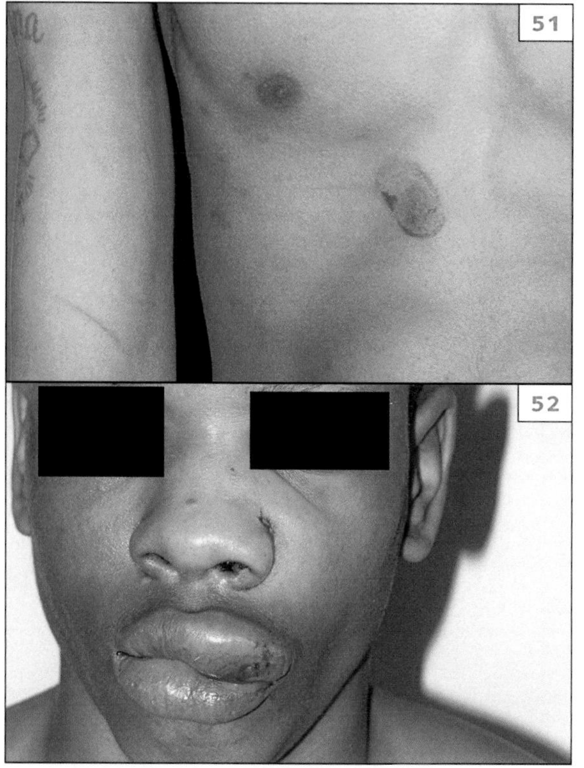

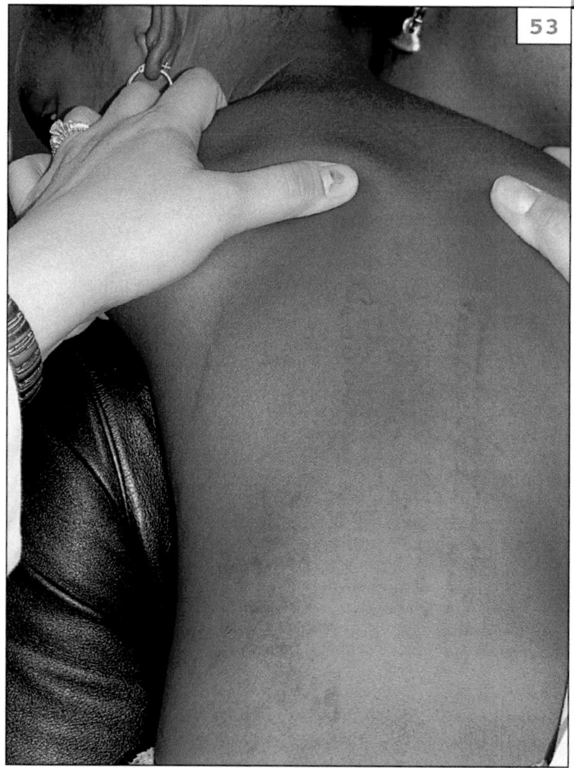

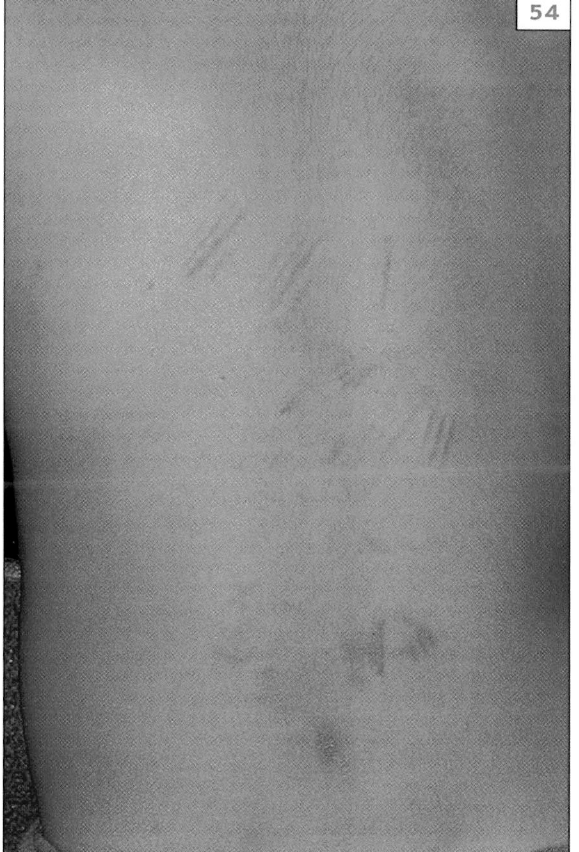

51, 52 A 17-year-old male was hit in the face and chest with a gun during an altercation. Swelling and bruises were noted on the face and lips. A well-demarcated bruise consistent with the handle of the pistol was noted on the chest. The diagnosis was physical assault.

53 A 2.5-year-old female who had recently returned to her mother after a 24-hour visit with her father was noted to have red marks on her back. The father admitted to 'spanking the child on the butt'. Examination showed a pattern bruise with linear distribution and repeated circles on the lower half of the back perhaps from a belt or strap with metal eyelets. The diagnosis was pattern bruising consistent with child abuse.

54 A 4-year-old male brought in for swelling of the frontal scalp and right parietal-occipital scalp area after 'being hit by a door'. These linear lesions found on the back were reportedly from 'falling on his toys'. The diagnosis was well-demarcated linear lesions on the back consistent with nonaccidental injury, possibly from a fork.

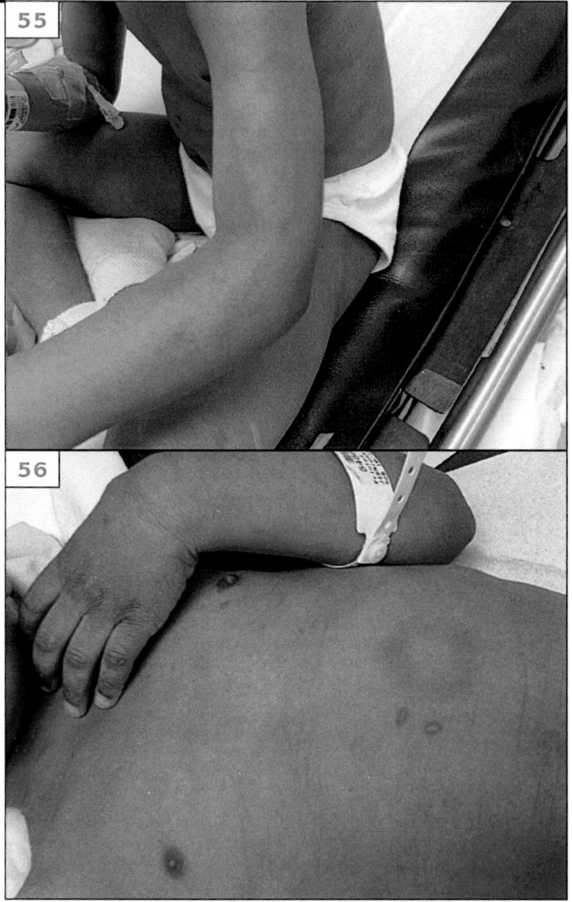

55, 56 Child's injuries consistent with loop marks from an extension cord and an old bite mark to the abdomen.

57 A 7-year-old male brought in by police for evaluation of marks to his body. Police were initially called for reported screams heard by neighbors. Subsequently, the father admitted to hitting the children with a belt. Physical examination reveals multiple bruises and old scars on the anterior chest, back, thighs, and arms. Linear bruises and loop marks are consistent with belt mechanism. Old scars and recent injuries were noted. The diagnosis was child abuse.

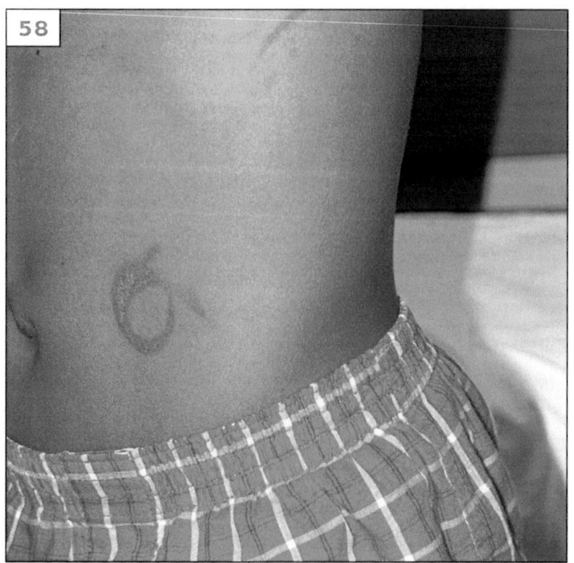

58 An 8-year-old male (sibling of the patient in 57) with linear bruises and scars on his back. He was also found to have scars on his chest and abdomen reportedly from the handlebar of a bicycle.

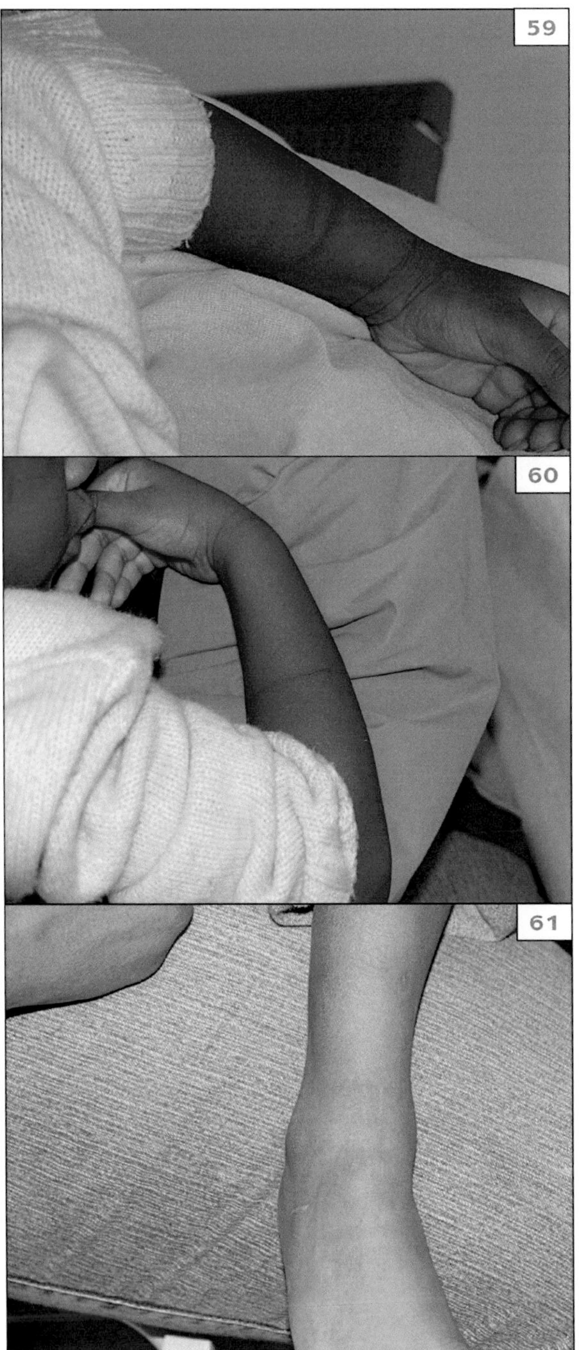

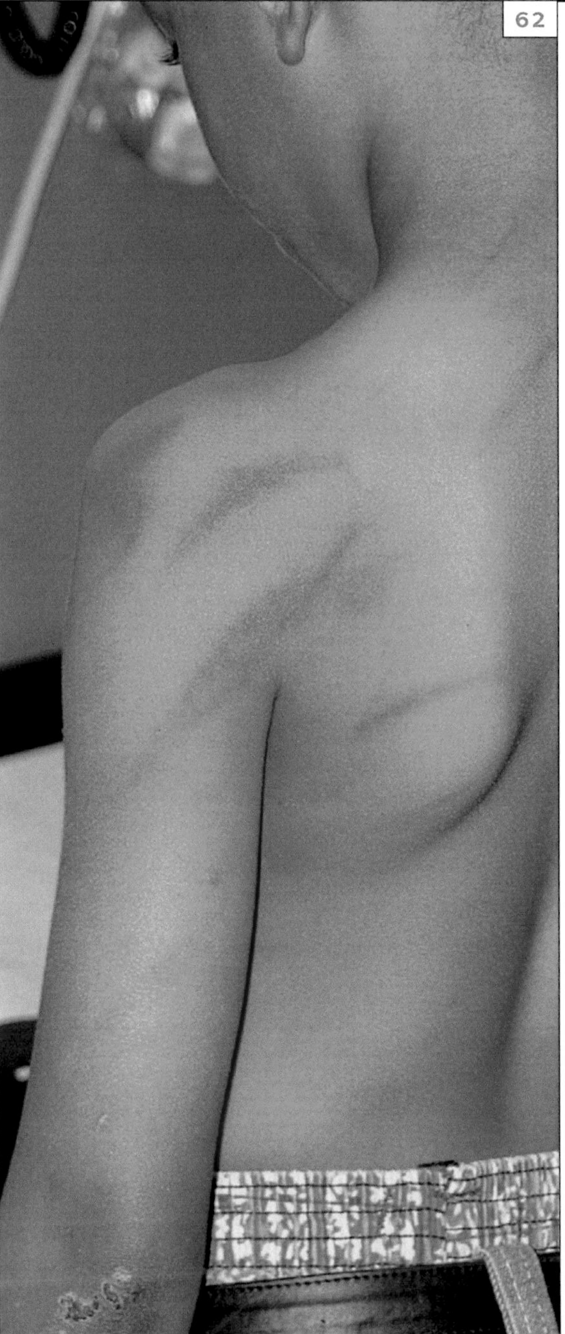

59–61 A 3-year-old female brought in with ear pain and found to have an incidental finding of circumferential bruising and abrasion on both wrists. Examination of the ankles revealed subtle hyperpigmentation in a similar circumferential pattern. There was no history provided by the mother for these lesions. The diagnosis was skin lesions suspicious for ligature marks or use of restraints.

62 A 7-year-old male who had been returned to his father's custody and alleged he was hit with a belt by his brother for letting the dog into the house. The injuries reportedly occurred 3 days previously. The child was noted to have bruising on the right face and left posterior shoulder, the latter being consistent with markings from a belt. The diagnosis was ecchymoses consistent with child abuse.

63

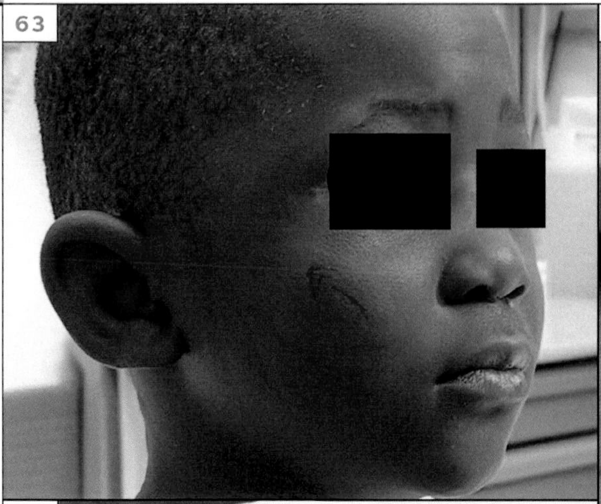

64

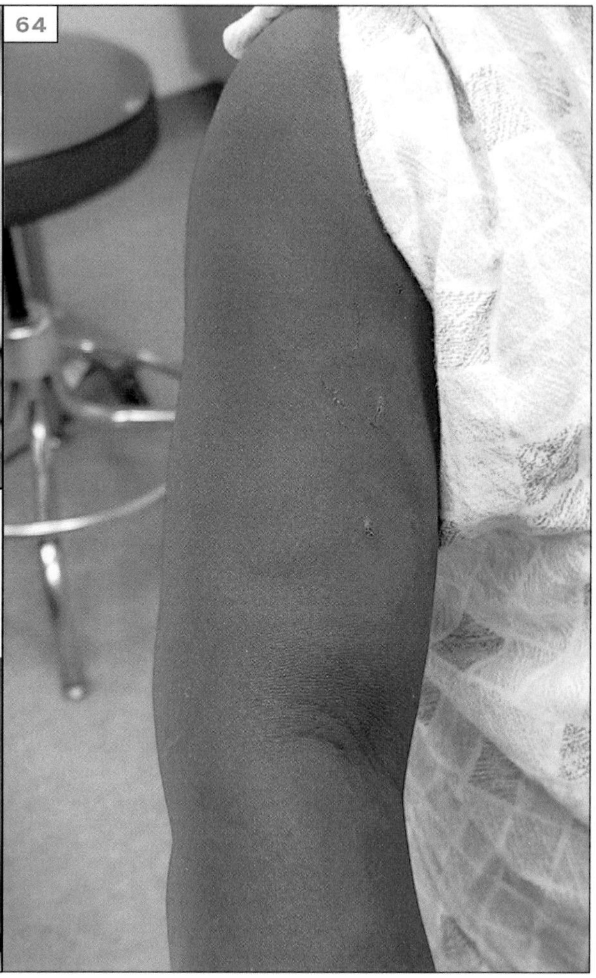

65

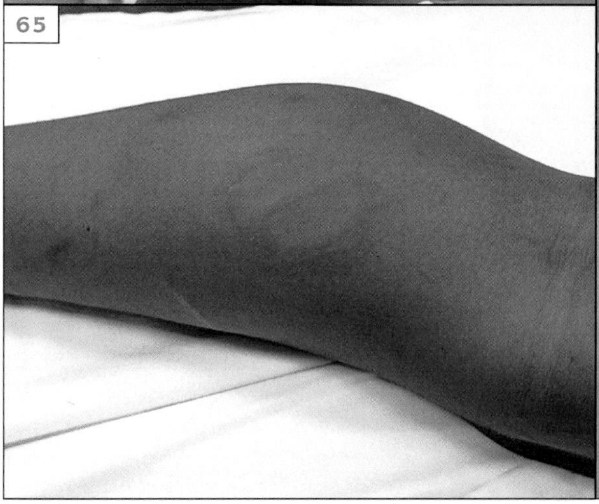

66

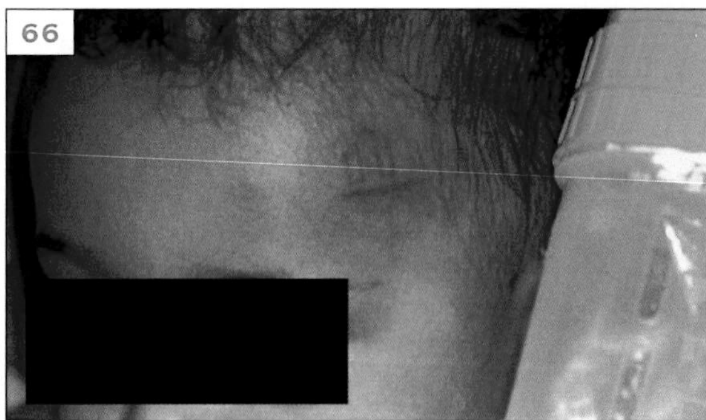

63–65 A 5-year-old male was referred by protective services for multiple bruises of the trunk and extremities. Mechanism of injury reported by the mother was a fall. Many linear lesions were noted and a well-demarcated lesion was noted on the calf. The diagnosis was bruising inconsistent with the history and inflicted trauma consistent with belt and belt buckle injury.

66 Imprint from baby bottle noted on the infant's forehead.

Dating bruises

Comparing the appearance of a bruise with the history described by the child's caregivers is important in many child abuse assessments. Physicians are often asked by child protection and law enforcement authorities, and by the courts, to offer opinions about the age of a child's bruise in order to assess the credibility of the history. Several factors affect the time of appearance and the color of a bruise. The rate of color change and time to resolution are also variable. A superficial bruise will appear immediately, while deep bruising may take days to appear. Areas where connective tissue is lax and blood vessels are poorly supported – the eyelids, for instance – will show bruises earlier than denser tissues (**67**). The color of a bruise depends upon the individual's skin color, the ambient lighting, and also the depth of the injury. In darker-skinned children, it may be helpful to compare the area in question with the surrounding skin or opposite side to appreciate the color change fully (**68–71**). The rate of color change as extravasated hemoglobin breaks down is a function of the depth of injury, the age of the patient (more rapid change in the young) and the environmental temperature. It is commonly believed that bruises resolve more quickly in children and superficial bruises resolve more rapidly than deeper ones[3].

The commonly used table of color changes in bruises over time attributed to Dr E. F. Wilson[8] did not, in fact, appear in Wilson's article, but was rather an interpretation of his work in adults and cadavers. It should be noted that he did also state that the dating of contusions is imprecise. At present, our knowledge base on color changes in bruises over time consists of only two prospective studies in living patients. Langlois and Gresham[9] took 369 photographs of the bruises of 89 people aged 10–100 years. All were white. Only bruises with known ages and origins were photographed. Photographs were taken of bruises from less than 6 hours to 21 days old. The conclusions of this study were:

- A bruise with any yellow in it must be older than 18 hours (**72, 73**).
- Red, purple, blue, and black could occur at any time.
- 'Even in the same subject, where two separate bruises have occurred on the same part of the anatomy and are identical in etiology and age, these need not display identical colours nor undergo changes of colour at the identical rate'.

This last statement challenges the long-held belief that bruises of different color in the same area must have been inflicted at different times. In 1966, Stephenson and Bialas in Nottingham[10] followed and photographed the appearance of accidental bruising in pediatric patients. Their subjects were 23 white children, ages 8 months to 13 years, with a total of 36 bruises. The bruises occurred in pedestrian or cyclist collisions with a motor vehicle or in falls of less than 2 m. They observed bruises of the arms, legs, face, and trunk from 1.5 hours to 14 days. The conclusions of this study were:

- Yellow was seen in bruises at least 24 hours old.
- Green was seen in bruises at least 48 hours old.
- Red was seen from the time of injury until day 7.
- Purple, blue, and brown were seen from the day of injury until day 14 (the duration of observation).

They also state 'Several different colours can be present at the same time within one bruise.' Two recent articles on the distribution and aging of bruises by Maguire *et al.*[11,12] stress that what was taught in the past about bruises had little basis in fact. They conclude that there is not adequate published evidence for offering an accurate opinion about the age of a bruise. This suggests that definitive opinions on this subject may be difficult to support in court.

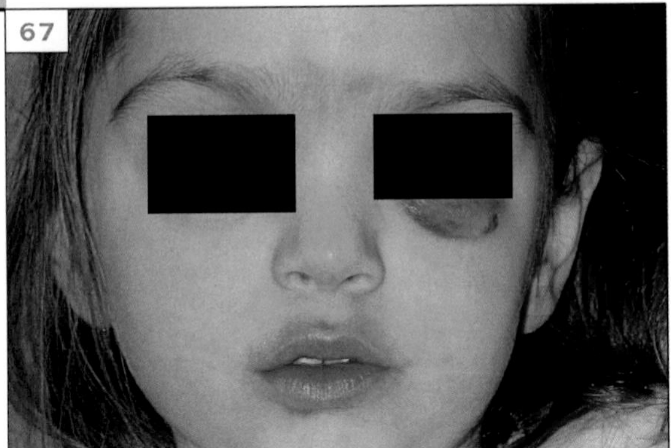

67 A 33-month-old female who reportedly fell and struck her eye on the edge of a table. Initially, there was bruising on the glabella and a small linear bruise noted on the left infraorbital area. At presentation, the parents noticed an increasing area of bruising and have fears about visual loss. A review of past history and a full examination reveal no further concerns. Note the ability of blood to descend and collect in the loose areolar tissue surrounding the eye, making the bruised area appear larger. The diagnosis was peri-orbital contusion without suspicion of abuse.

68–71 A 9-year-old male initially stated that he was hit on the arms by some 'kids' at school. Further questioning revealed that his mother's boyfriend had restrained his arms the previous day and struck him repeatedly over a 40–60-minute period. This was allegedly a punishment for being caught playing with matches. Examination shows a very uncomfortable child who has significant pain with movement of his arms. There is dependent tracking of blood with three-quarters circumferential bruising of the upper arms and extending down to the radial aspect of the forearms. The bruising of the upper arm appears deep within the muscle and some of the edges reflect the fascial planes of the muscle. There is some patterning which delineates the underlying blood vessels and outline of the radius and ulna. Coagulation profile and radiographs are unremarkable except for soft tissue swelling; the creatine phosphokinase (CPK) is noted to be elevated at 6600U/L. Hydration was emphasized with the family to prevent renal injury. The diagnosis was child abuse with bruising and underlying muscular injury.

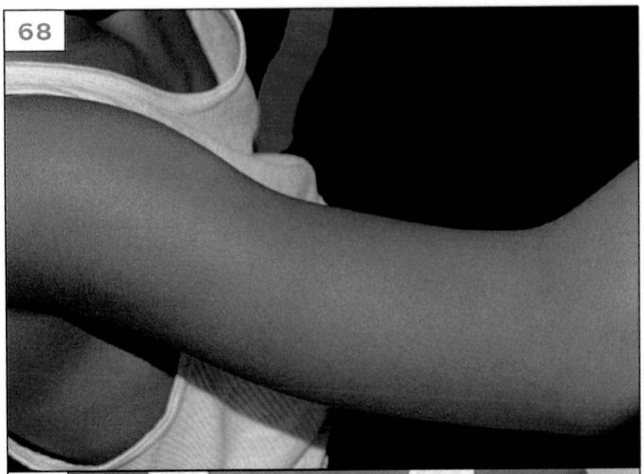

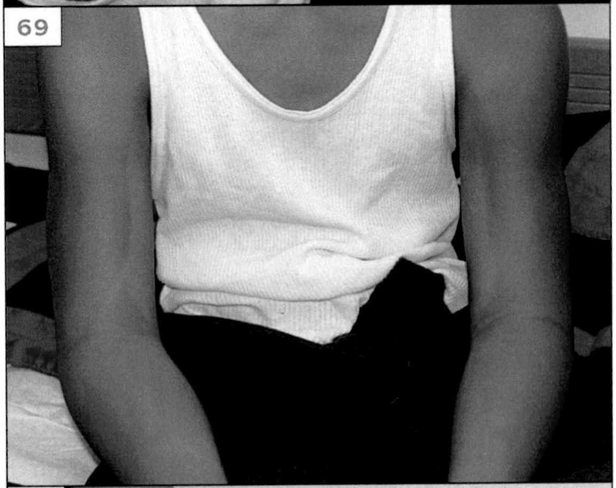

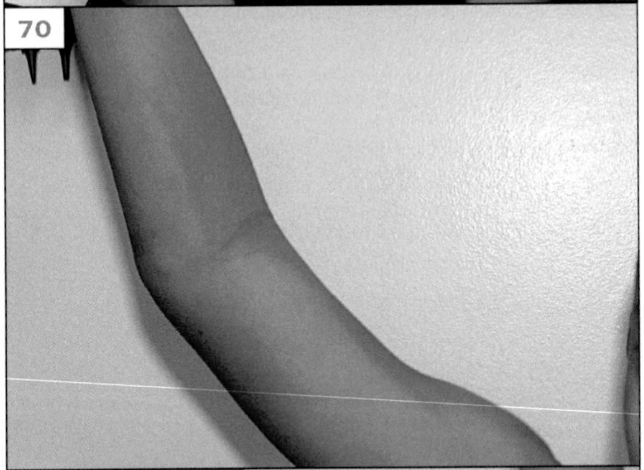

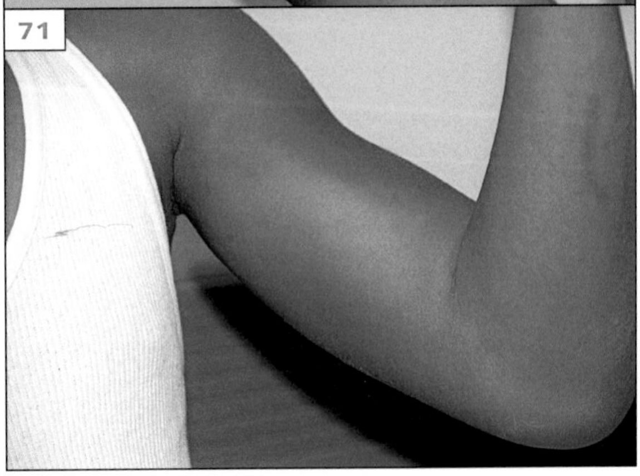

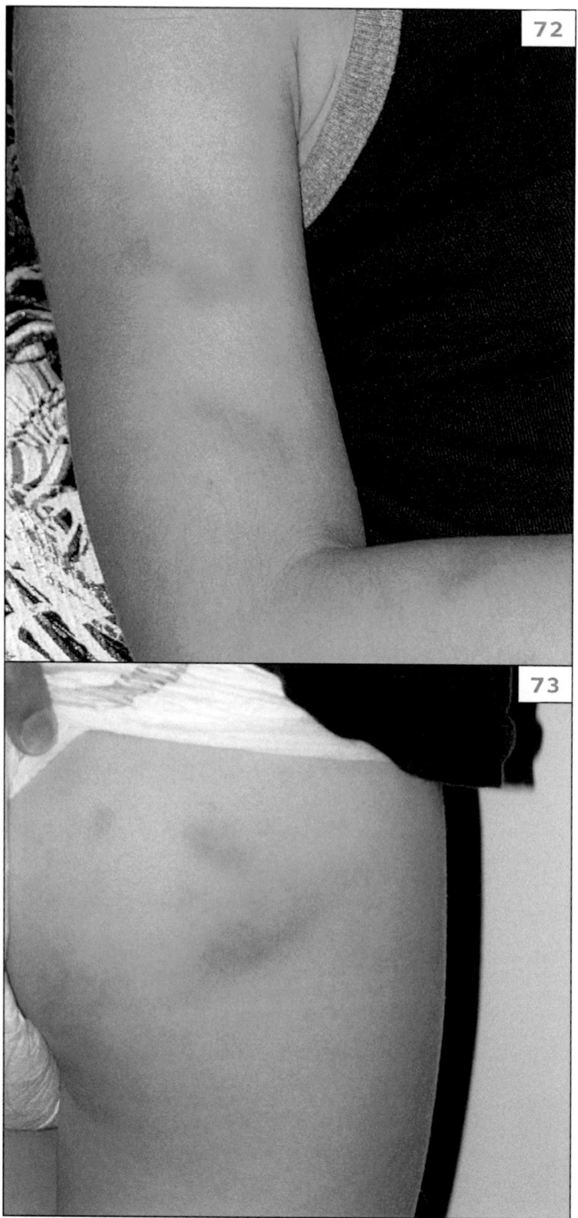

72, 73 A 3.5-year-old male who reportedly had a '200 pound industrial garage door' fall on him several days ago while on holiday in Yugoslavia. He was treated and released from a hospital there and now returns with persistent pain. Examination shows older bruising on the left infraorbital area and right arm and posterior thigh. Bruising shows yellow and green coloration consistent with hemoglobin breakdown. The diagnosis was bruising consistent with an old injury.

History and physical examination

The history should take into consideration the developmental stage of the child, and inconsistencies should elicit further questioning (68–71). Time delay in seeking care, particularly for more severe injuries, should also raise suspicion. The history of 'self-inflicted' injury, particularly in a young infant, and 'sibling-inflicted injury' are also concerning for abuse. When considering children with very severe or multiple bruises, especially when found in the usual or more expected areas, one should explore the possibility of acquired or inherited bleeding disorder (Chapter 4, Cutaneous conditions mimicking child abuse). History of excessive bleeding from the newborn screening heel stick, bleeding from the umbilical cord, circumcision, and delayed umbilical cord separation are early signs of possible bleeding disorder. Prior history of prolonged bleeding with accidental cuts, surgery, dental extractions, or previous excessive bruising or swelling with minor trauma, such as immunizations should be sought[13]. Petechial rash, recurrent epistaxis, mucosal bleeding, or gum bleeding with tooth brushing would also raise concern for a bleeding disorder. Similarly, family history of the above, consanguinity, or excessive menstrual bleeding in family members should be taken. Medication history should be sought (steroids, anticonvulsants that affect vitamin K, anti-platelet agents) with particular attention to over-the-counter (OTC) products (aspirin and nonsteroidal anti-inflammatory drugs (NSAIDs)) that may affect bleeding. Rodenticides frequently contain 'superwarfarin' substances and their presence in the home should be determined.

Although it may be very time consuming, an important consideration in the detection of abusive bruising is to be thorough in your physical examination. Clearly, subtle findings such as bruises to the back, digits, genitals, buttocks, or even the back of the ears cannot be seen unless the child is fully undressed and a thorough head to toe examination is performed. Such an examination is essential in all patients whose presentation may be associated with abuse (**74, 75**). This would include patients with sudden infant death syndrome, apparent life threatening events, failure to thrive, new onset seizures, and all patients presenting with trauma (fractures, burns, bruises, and lacerations). The importance of a careful skin examination is magnified when one realizes that even subtle findings on the skin can be markers for serious underlying injury (**3, 10, 11**). A careful head, eyes, ears, nose, and throat (HEENT) examination (Chapter 6, Ocular trauma and Chapter 7, Otolaryngologic manifestations of abuse and neglect) should look for the presence of scalp lesions, retinal hemorrhage, posterior ear injuries, hemotympanum, and epistaxis, all of which may help diagnose abusive head trauma (**76, 77**). Bruises to the upper chest and arms or paraspinal area of the back may be the only clue to an infant being shaken, and neck bruising may be the result of strangulation (**78–85**). Bruising to the thorax may be associated with rib fractures, pulmonary contusions, or hemothorax and those over the abdomen may lead to finding life-threatening underlying injuries to the liver, spleen, or viscera (**3, 6, 10, 11, 80, 81, 86, 87**). Subtle swelling and bruising over the head, trunk, or extremities may be a clue to an underlying bony injury. A well-lit room is essential for finding subtle bruises, particularly in dark-skinned children. Palpation of the scalp and parting of hair will help in finding bruises underlying hair. Attention should be paid to the scalp for bruises or lacerations, which are a sensitive indicator of abuse. The presence of lice and the general condition of the hair can be suggestive of malnutrition or neglect. During this process, any tenderness or masses that may indicate soft tissue injury, healing fractures, or hematomas should be noted; similarly, any asymmetries should be noted. Asymmetry may reflect skull fractures, hematomas, or soft tissue injury; alternatively, the differential diagnosis for head asymmetry includes plagiocephaly and craniosynostoses. Accidental injury to the head and scalp are rare in infants, very common in toddlers, tapering off with mastery of walking skills.[3,14] Evidence of epistaxis, intraoral or mucosal bleeding or bruising may be a clue to abuse or a bleeding disorder[14]. Neck, back, and chest bruising are very suspicious for nonaccidental injury.

Bruising in the categories below should raise your suspicion for abuse:

- Infants, especially under 9 months
- Multiple bruises and those associated with other injuries (fractures, burns)
- Ears and cheeks
- Handprint or other pattern bruises, including parallel lines and other geometric shapes
- Upper lip with frenulum injury
- Neck: choke marks
- Abdomen, chest and upper arms
- Small of the back
- Genital, buttock, and peri-anal areas
- Bruises to the feet and hands.

Bleeding in unusual patterns involving the above categories should still raise suspicion of nonaccidental injury, even in a child with known bleeding diathesis.

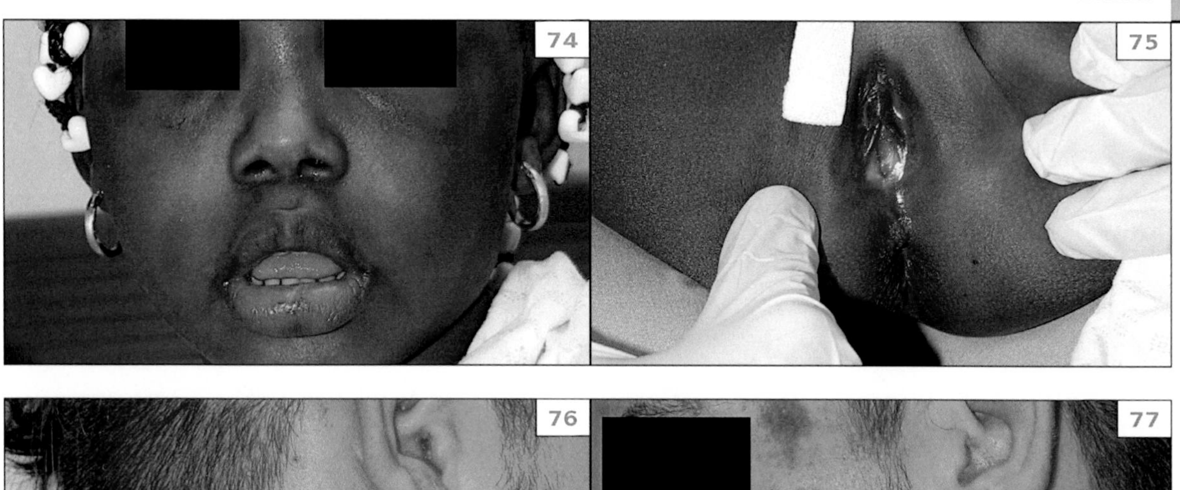

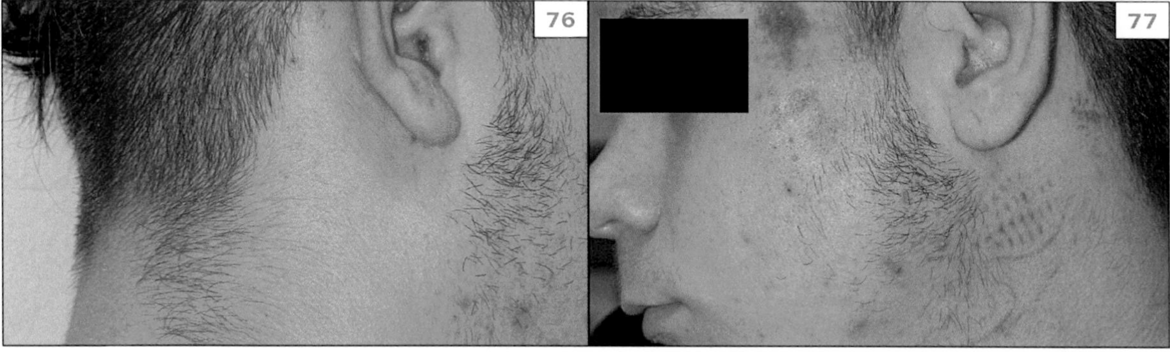

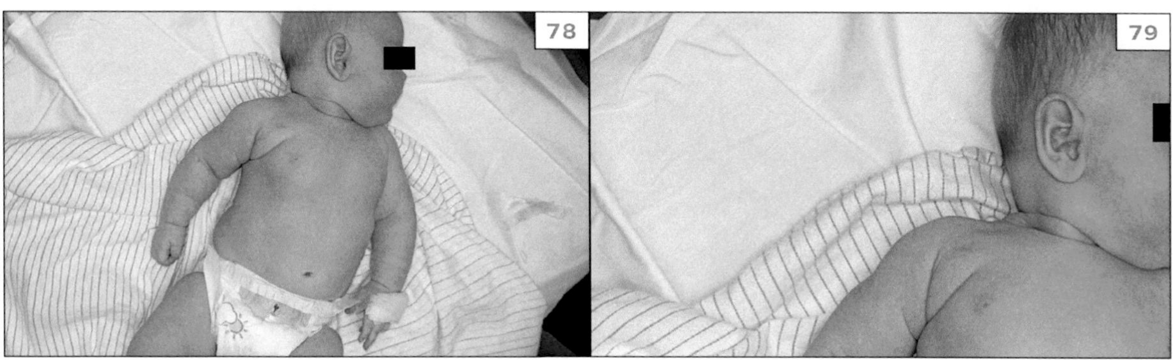

74, 75 A 3-year-old female who 3 hours previously was reportedly left with a 9-year-old foster brother for 20 minutes as the caregiver went into 'another room'. Blood was noted in the diaper/nappy area and the child had been unwilling to go to the bathroom. The foster brother admits to hand to genital contact only. Multiple bruises were found on the face, back, and left thigh. Anal fissures were noted at the 5, 6, and 12 o'clock positions. Genital examination revealed a posterior fourchette laceration and avascular scarring of the introitus with a thick whitish vaginal discharge. The diagnosis was physical and sexual abuse.

76, 77 A 16-year-old male had been assaulted, hit, and kicked with fists and feet. Examination showed bruising of the head and neck and the right infraorbital area (76), as well as the left face, ear, neck, and scalp (77). Bruising of the mastoid area or 'battle sign' may be associated with basilar skull fractures. The pattern mark on left neck is likely a shoe imprint. The diagnosis was physical assault with closed head injury.

78, 79 A 4-month-old female, previously well, found 'not breathing' at baby sitter's home. The sitter's husband shook the infant to 'make her breathe'. Infant was found to have left occipital subdural hematoma on computed tomography scan. A small bruise was noted on the right anterior shoulder. Work-up for coagulopathy was normal. The diagnosis was suspected shaken baby.

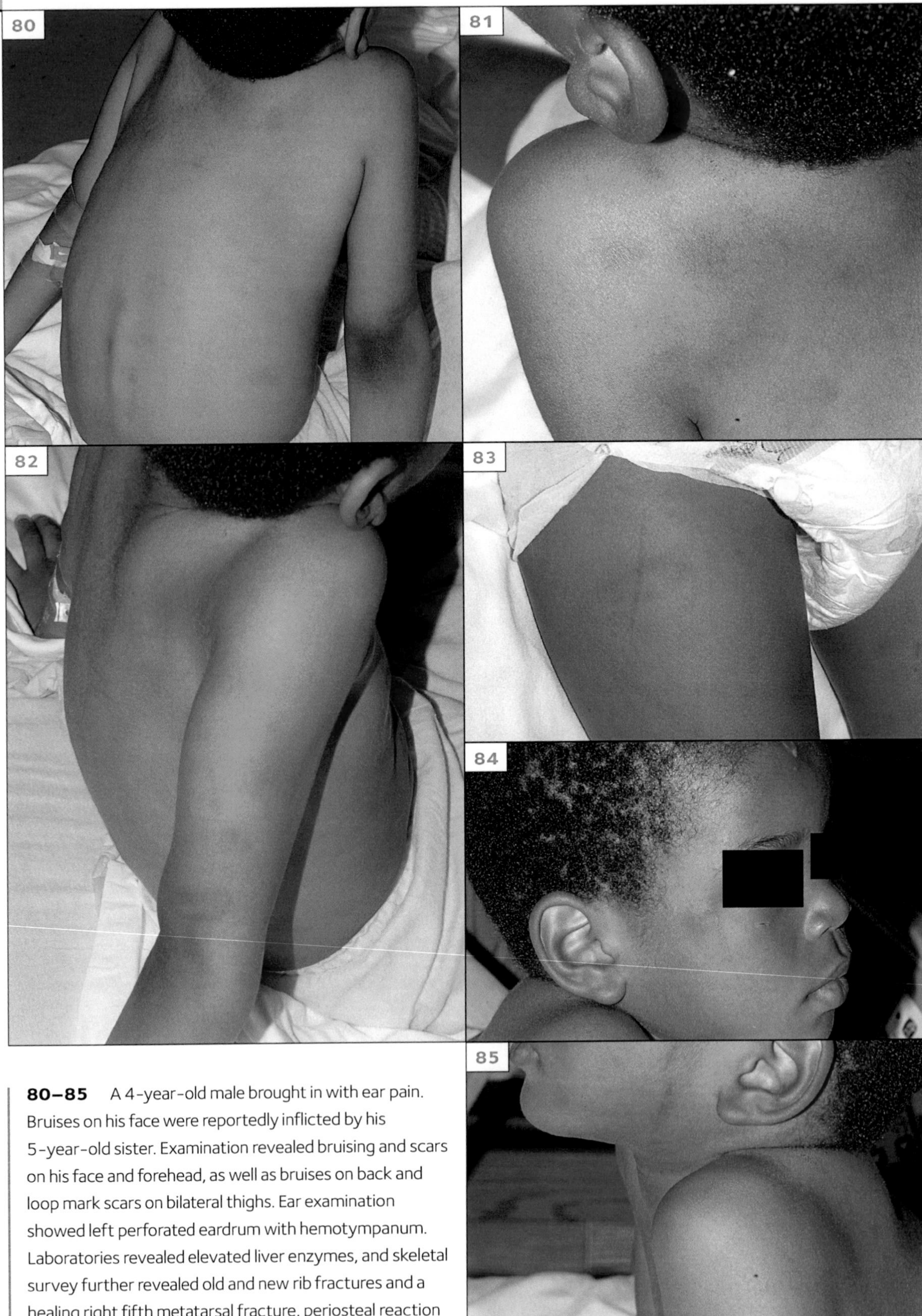

80–85 A 4-year-old male brought in with ear pain. Bruises on his face were reportedly inflicted by his 5-year-old sister. Examination revealed bruising and scars on his face and forehead, as well as bruises on back and loop mark scars on bilateral thighs. Ear examination showed left perforated eardrum with hemotympanum. Laboratories revealed elevated liver enzymes, and skeletal survey further revealed old and new rib fractures and a healing right fifth metatarsal fracture, periosteal reaction on the left radius, and right thumb's proximal phalanx.

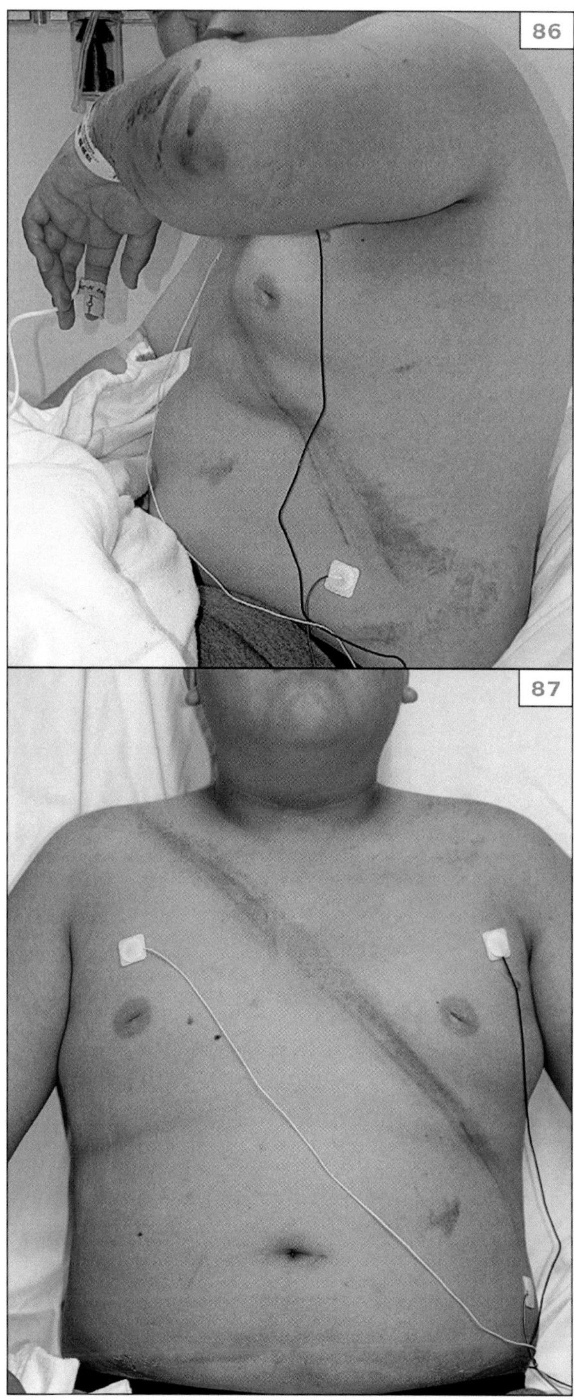

86, 87 A 12-year-old male who was a restrained passenger in a head-on motor vehicle collision presented for full evaluation. An abrasion and bruise were noted on the chest and abdomen consistent with lap and shoulder belt. Although the bruising requires little management, underlying chest and intra-abdominal injuries should be suspected and excluded.

Differential diagnosis

The physician must distinguish between inflicted bruises and accidental bruises.[1,14] He or she must also ascertain that he or she is, in fact, looking at a bruise and not one of many 'mimics'. A number of dermatologic conditions, coagulation disorders, collagen synthesis defects, as well as infections and folk medicine practices, may produce skin lesions that may easily be mistaken for bruises or increase the child's propensity for true bruising (Chapter 4, Cutaneous conditions mimicking child abuse).

Laboratory evaluation

A diagnosis of inflicted bruising may be apparent because of a typical body site involved, absence of appropriate history, a patently false history, or the pattern of bruising. In such cases, an evaluation for coagulation disorders is medically unnecessary. However, because abusive caregivers may allege that their child bruises easily or has a clotting disorder, it is now our practice to perform screening on nearly all children with suspicious bruises, particularly when pattern marks are not present. Such a screen should, as a minimum, consist of a complete blood count with platelets, peripheral smear, prothrombin time (PT) and a partial thromboplastin time (PTT). Should an abnormality be discovered as a result of screening, one must try to determine if that abnormality is sufficient to account for the bruising observed. Children with hemophilia, for instance, may also be victims of child abuse. In cases of uncertainty, even with a negative screen, we advise seeking a hematologist consultant. If extensive bruising is encountered, a creatine phosphokinase (CPK) should be obtained to assess for underlying muscle injury and potential for renal involvement (**68–71**). Work-up should also consider the underlying organs and appropriate laboratory tests (urinalysis (UA), liver enzymes, amylase, lipase) and imaging (chest x-ray, head or abdominal computed tomography (CT), skeletal survey) should be performed depending on the age of the child and the area involved (**88, 89**).

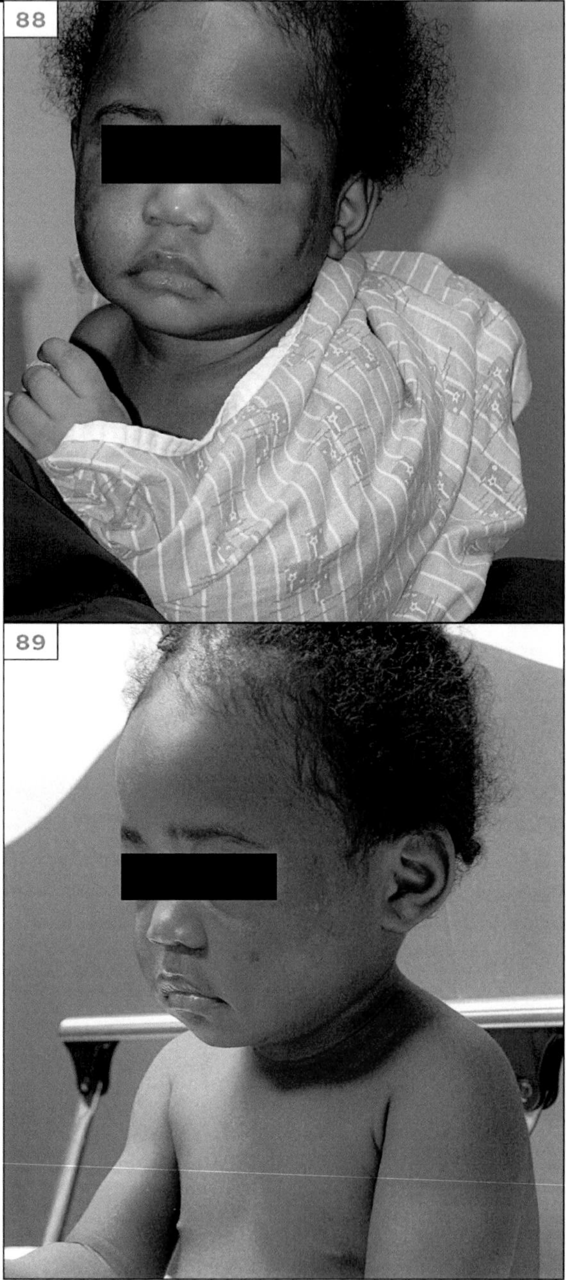

88, 89 A 16-month-old female whose twin was found dead on the morning of presentation with multiple unexplained injuries. The patient was brought in by police for a suspicious 'rash' on face. Examination shows considerable swelling and bruises of the forehead, cheeks, and peri-orbital areas. Bruising was also noted on the scalp. Considerable bruising, such as this, should lead to the suspicion of intracranial injury and further imaging should be carried out.

Management

Management of bruises is usually limited to comfort measures, such as cold compresses for pain and swelling and acetaminophen (paracetamol) or acetaminophen with codeine for pain or severe pain, respectively[15]. Avoid medications, such as aspirin and nonsteroidal anti-inflammatory agents, that may affect bleeding tendency. Management should be directed at diagnosing more serious underlying injuries that may have a greater impact on the child. Whenever abuse is considered in the differential diagnosis, it is helpful to review the child's past medical record. At many large institutions, an electronic medical record may be reviewed to determine if the child has had previous visits and if these encounters included physical findings or other concerns for abuse or neglect (**25–30**). A social service or protective services evaluation should then be considered if there still is concern for suspected abuse or neglect. Some jurisdictions may have a registry that contains prior reports of abuse or neglect for the same family (or child), even if the child has not been previously seen at your medical institution. Further concerns would then warrant assessment of the home environment or even removal of the child from the home until circumstances of the injury can be clarified.

Documentation

Most skin findings are transient and change or resolve over time, and preserving evidence for future review and medicolegal documentation is helpful. A diagram of the body, such as those used to document burn lesions and to estimate body surface area of burns, may be employed to aid in documentation of numerous lesions. The number, appearance and location of swelling, bruises, and other skin findings may also be difficult to describe in words even with lengthy documentation (**90–99**). Photodocumentation can accurately record the color, size, shape, and location of skin findings and can be very helpful in assisting the examiner in recalling such findings in the future for court testimony[16]. Photography may also be helpful in obtaining a second opinion without subjecting the child and family to repeated examinations. At times, photographs can help the practitioner identify lesions on review that may not have been easily identified on the initial examination. Physicians caring for abused children should have appropriate equipment at their disposal and familiarity with basic aspects of clinical photography or have such a service readily available to them for this purpose. This service can be provided by a medical photography department at your facility or through the use of photography through law enforcement personnel. With digital photography, we have the added benefit of being able to immediately review photos taken. This is especially useful for the less experienced photographer to ensure they are in good focus and accurately depict the lesion(s) in question. Recent articles have suggested that alternative light sources and more specialized photographic systems can even better document subtle findings[17,18].

As with the history and physical examination, taking photographs should keep the child's physical and emotional comfort in mind. This may be an extremely embarrassing experience for children of preschool age and older and should be explained carefully to both the child and caregiver. A child life specialist or experienced pediatric nurse can be of great value in facilitating this comfort through distraction techniques (**89**). This distraction can provide the child with a more comfortable experience and also limit child movement for better photographs without restraint. Efforts should be made to obtain consent from the caregiver and child, although this may not be necessary in cases of suspected abuse. You will need to consult with your local law enforcement for rules that may apply in your jurisdiction. Adequate lighting is essential for indoor photography especially when using cameras with autofocus. Your best angle to photograph a lesion is usually the same angle from which you can best visualize the lesion with the naked eye. When in doubt, photographing from different angles for comparison can be helpful particularly if immediate review is available. Photographs will also be less distorted if the camera and the child are at the same level. Make every attempt to document the lesions in question while minimizing the number of photographs taken and subsequent discomfort to the child.

When choosing a camera for clinical photography, there are several factors to be considered to improve your chances of success. Although a 35-mm camera in the right hands can produce excellent results, usually there is no means to review your pictures immediately for success. A digital camera avoids this concern, as well as the cost of film and processing. The ability to email digital photographs for review with child abuse experts can also be particularly helpful in difficult cases. The ideal camera would have good quality lenses, in particular a macrolens for close up times power and some (perhaps between three and eight times power) optical zoom to be able to take photographs from a distance as well. The ideal flash for medical photography is a ring flash that will allow for uniform lighting while minimizing shadows and glare. A top- or side-mount flash gives reasonable lighting, but produces considerable shadow and undesired glare which can be lessened only somewhat by shooting from a distance (5–10 feet (1.5–3 m) or more) (**100, 101**). Children are also more comfortable when the photographer is some distance away. At times, it may be beneficial to employ other external lighting, such as an overhead ceiling light, goose neck lighting, or colposcopy, particularly when photographing mucous membranes. Whether using standard film and processing or digital photography, one should make every effort to maintain an unbroken 'chain of evidence' with the film or electronic media in question. Although digital photography allows for considerable alteration of your photographs (cropping, lighten, darken, change color or saturation, etc.) to improve the image, there should be no attempt to alter any digital photographs that may be used in legal proceedings. The images may be identified as being altered and may limit the credibility of the findings.

When composing your photographs, include anatomic landmarks to clarify the exact location of the lesion. This can be followed by a close up of the lesion if necessary (**102–104**). When taking photographs of unknown marks or lesions, it is helpful to photograph a metric ruler adjacent to the lesion for measurement purposes. Photos should be labeled with the date and time, which can usually be achieved automatically with most cameras through use of a camera 'databack' or automatically through most digital photography software. Each photograph should also include the patient's name, medical record, name of the photographer, and the practitioner (if an outside photographer is used). There should always be careful and thorough written documentation of all the lesions in the event of lost or destroyed photographs.

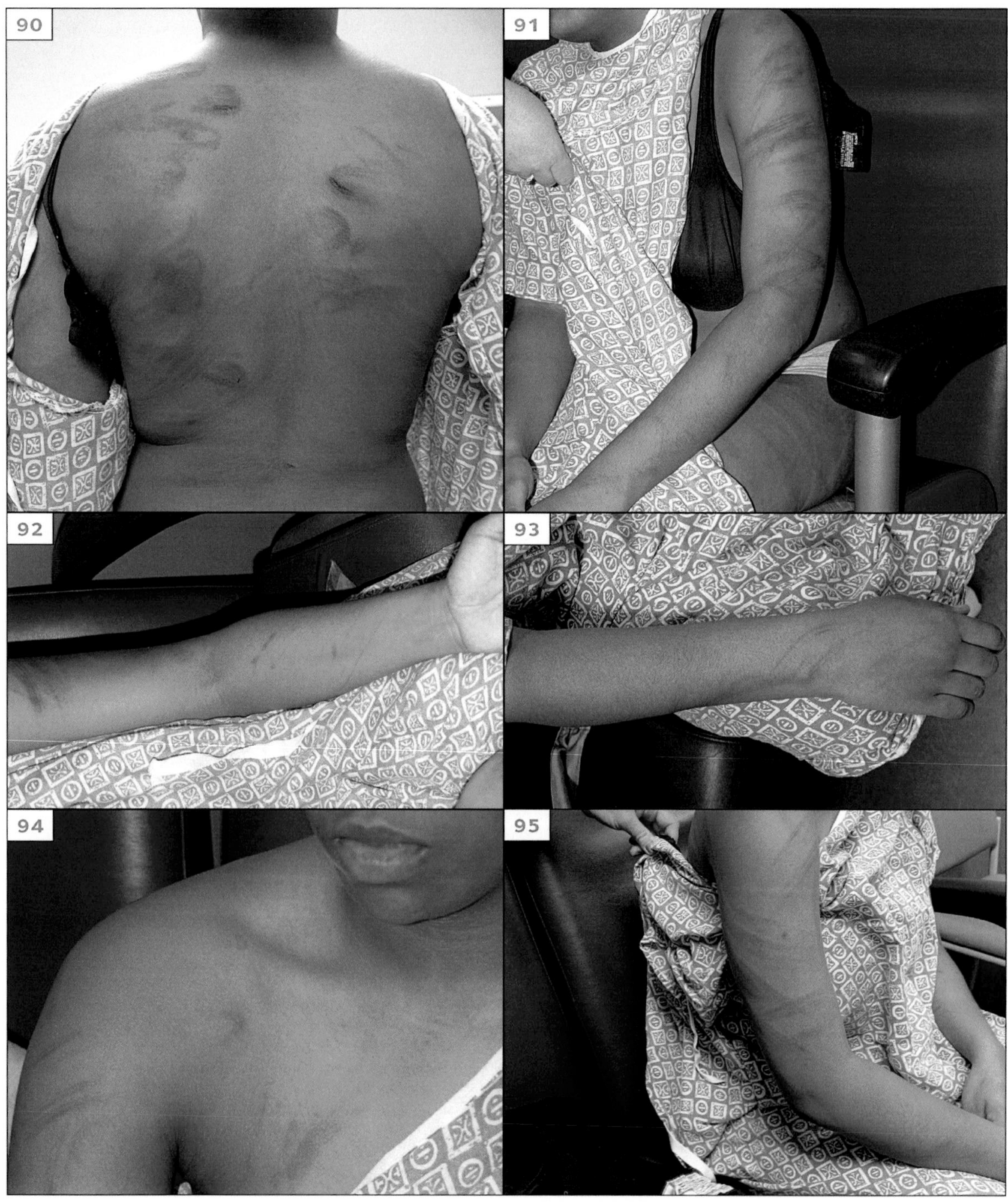

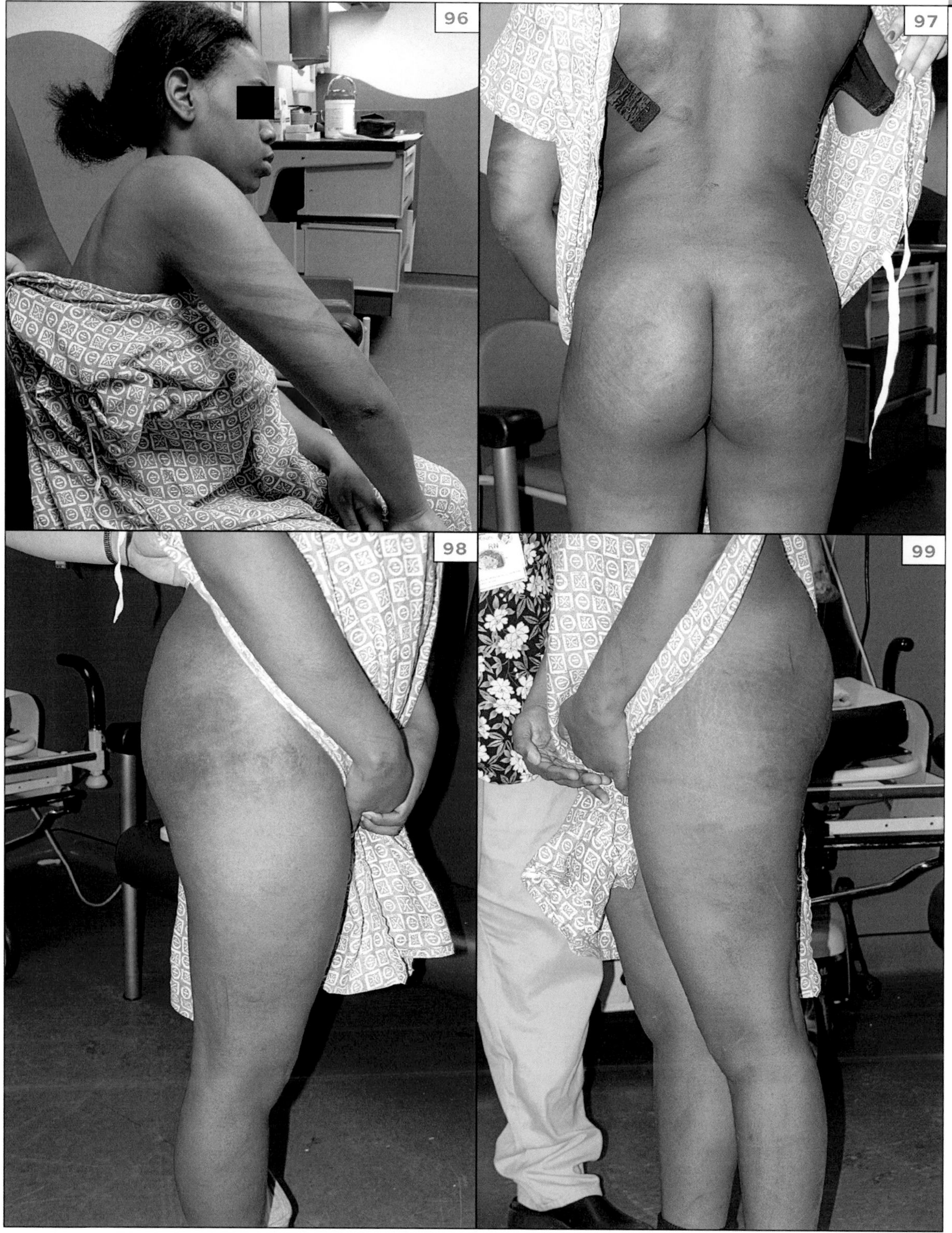

90–99 A 16-year-old female who reported being beaten by her uncle with an extension cord a few hours before presentation. She provided a history of previous extension cord and belt beatings. There were approximately 100 acute lesions in total and a few older scars noted as well. The diagnosis was multiple bruises consistent with abuse.

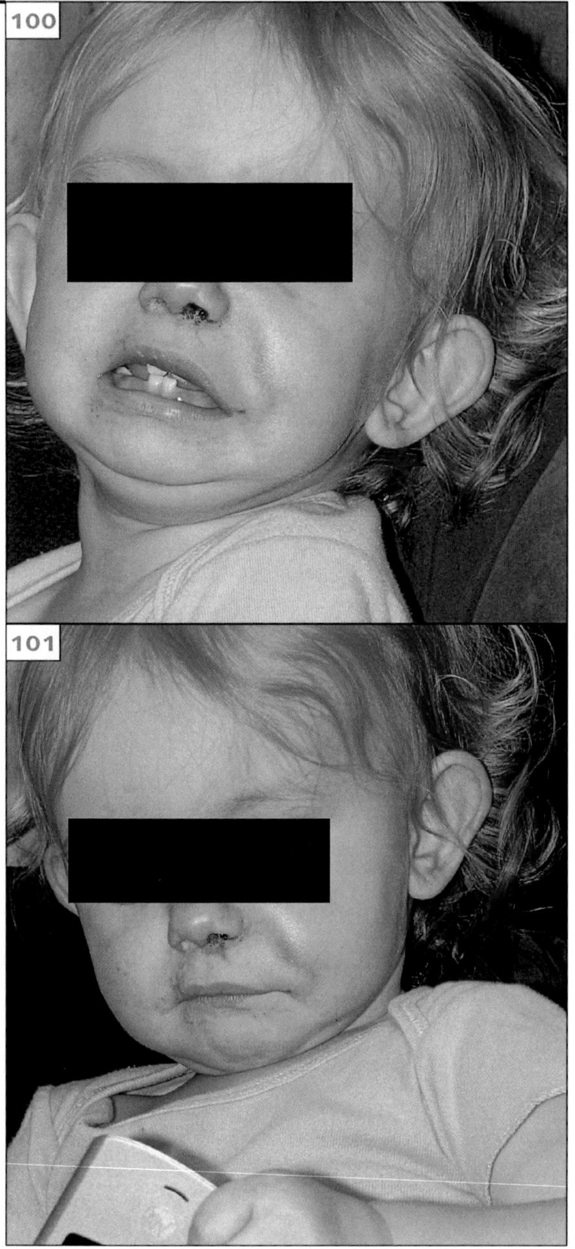

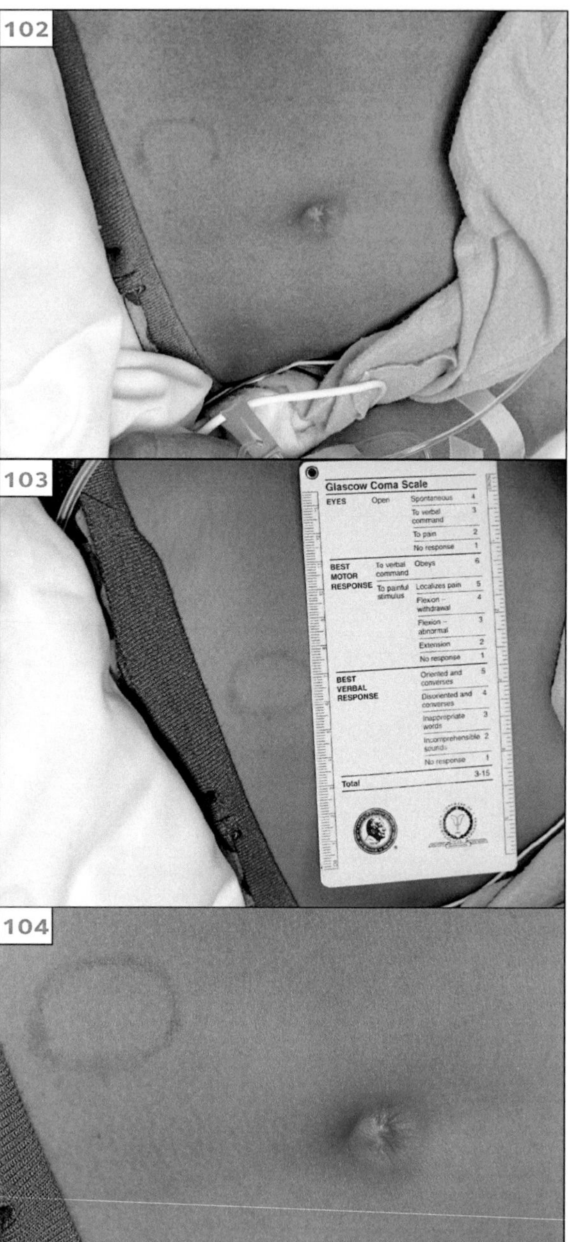

100, 101 A 16-month-old female who reportedly fell from a bed 20 hours before presentation. The child had epistaxis and swollen lip and otherwise appeared well. She was put to bed in the evening and upon awakening was noted to have dried blood in the nares and bruising of left cheek and infraorbital area. Examination further revealed a 3-cm laceration of the upper left gingiva with mucosal bruising. Work-up revealed no occult injuries. The diagnosis was gingival laceration with facial bruising. Considerable glare from a top-mount flash distorts the true color of the lesions.

102–104 An 8-year-old male who struck the handlebar on the right lower abdomen during a fall from his bicycle 12 hours previously. The patient presents with exquisite pain in the area. Work-up performed for intra-abdominal injury was negative. Lesion mimics a bite wound to the abdomen. The diagnosis was contusion with ecchymosis.

Teaching points

- The evaluation of any child presenting with history or physical evidence of trauma (swelling, bruises, burns, fractures), as well as other presentations that may represent child abuse (new onset seizures, failure to thrive, apparent life-threatening events, sudden infant death syndrome) is a time-consuming task for any physician in an office, urgent care, or emergency setting.
- As with many other medical conditions, however, the correct diagnosis and management plan requires a careful and complete history and very thorough head to toe physical examination.
- While there are several characteristics of bruises with varying degrees of specificity for abuse, the timing of those injuries based on the color of the bruise alone is problematic.
- Given the devastating potential of a missed case of child abuse, medical professionals must be willing to spend the time and effort needed for a comprehensive evaluation and documentation of potentially abusive injuries.

Chapter 3

ABUSIVE BURNS

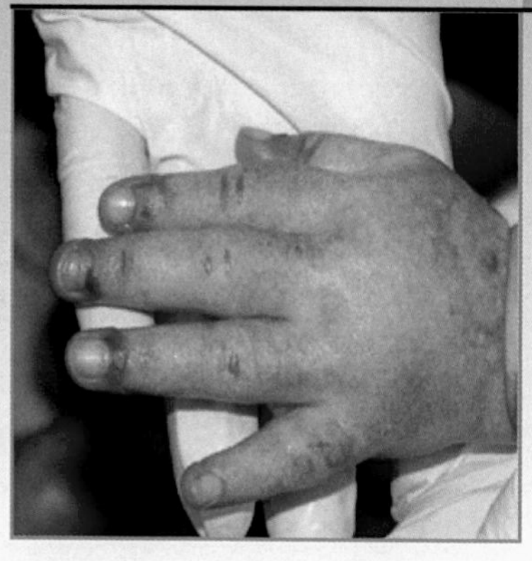

Lisa Markman MD

Execution by burning has a long history as a method of punishment for crimes such as treason, heresy, and witchcraft. For a number of reasons, this method of execution fell into disfavor among governments in the late 18th century. Today, it is considered a cruel and unusual punishment. Burning as a mechanism of child maltreatment, however, is still common, accounting for between 6 and 25% of all cases of abuse[1–4] and accounting for between 10 and 20% of all pediatric burn admissions[3–7]. Abusive burns cause severe injury, extreme pain, and enduring psychologic distress.

Introduction

Burns, unlike bruises, often lead to permanent physical scarring and disfigurement. 'The stigma of the burn does not end when the child is removed from the home of the abusing parent or discharged from the hospital; it may persist for years'[2] (**105, 106**).

The hospital admission rate for abusive burns is 55%; this is twice as high as the admission rates for all other forms of child abuse[3]. Although burn units have dramatically improved the survival of burn victims with an overall survival of 99%, abusive burns continue to have high morbidity and mortality when compared to accidental burns. Thombs reviewed over 15,000 burn admissions (909 suspected of being abusive) and found that compared to children with accidental burns, children with abusive burns had larger total body surface area burned (13 versus 9.7%), required longer intensive care unit stays, and were two to three times more likely to die[8]. These children are also more likely to require skin grafting (**107–111**)(*Table 3*)[9].

Abusive burn injuries, like other forms of child abuse, are seen in all socioeconomic classes and ethnic backgrounds. Studies have found, however, that there are certain characteristics common to burn victims and their abusers. Showers examined 132 cases of abusive burns and found the alleged perpetrator was female in 70% of cases. Women who are responsible for abusive burns are commonly single parents with several children. They are frequently impoverished, poorly educated, have a limited support system, and often have been the victims of abuse themselves (*Table 4*)[1,3,10–12].

Women are often the primary caregivers of children under 3 years of age and they are frequently the sole caregiver present during childhood behaviors that are thought to trigger burning, such as toilet training accidents and temper tantrums. Monteleone and Brodeur found that 70–90% of burns occur in the home at peak times of stress for the parents[2]. Educating caregivers on how to cope with stress, normal but difficult childhood behaviors, and what are reasonable expectations for young children may help caregivers cope during these stressful periods[3].

Childhood victims have common characteristics as well (*Table 5*). Children who are intentionally burned are usually between 1 and 4 years of age, with a peak incidence seen around 3 years of age[7,9,12]. Toddlers are frequently the victims of abuse because this is a difficult developmental stage, which includes a desire for independence, but a continued dependence on the caregiver. The family make-up of these children often reveals there are several children in the home, with the victim being the youngest[3]. Previous protective service involvement was found in 46–53% of children with intentional burns versus 4–11% of accidental burns[9,13]. Kumar[13] and Showers *et al.*[3] found a history of nonaccidental trauma in a sibling in 20–23% of children with nonaccidental burns (*Table 6*). As in other forms of child abuse, there is often a delay in seeking medical treatment and it is common for a nonoffending family member or caregiver to bring the child in for a medical evaluation. When parents do seek treatment, they often report that the event was unwitnessed, was caused by a sibling, or give a history inconsistent with the patient's injury.

Table 3 **Classification of burns**

DEGREE	APPEARANCE	SKIN LAYERS	PAIN	PERMANENT DAMAGE
First	Erythema/swelling	Epidermis	Min/mod	None
Second	Vesicles/blisters, weeping exudate	Partial thickness: Entire epidermis and variable portion of dermis	Extremely painful, viable nerve endings exposed	May scar
Third	Dry and leathery	Destruction of entire epidermis and dermis	Minimal, due to destruction of nerves	Grafting needed, permanent scarring

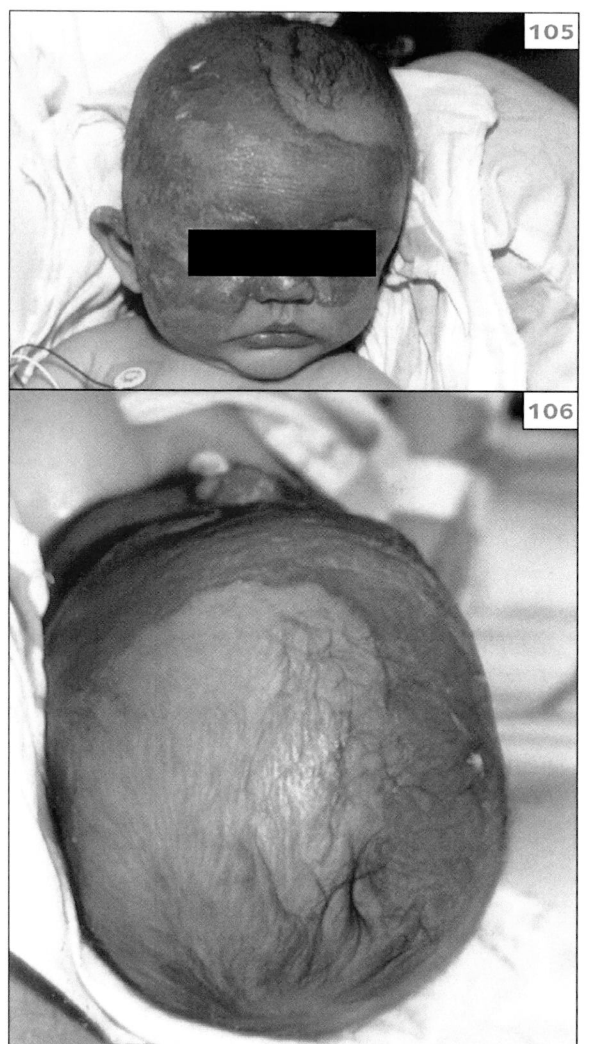

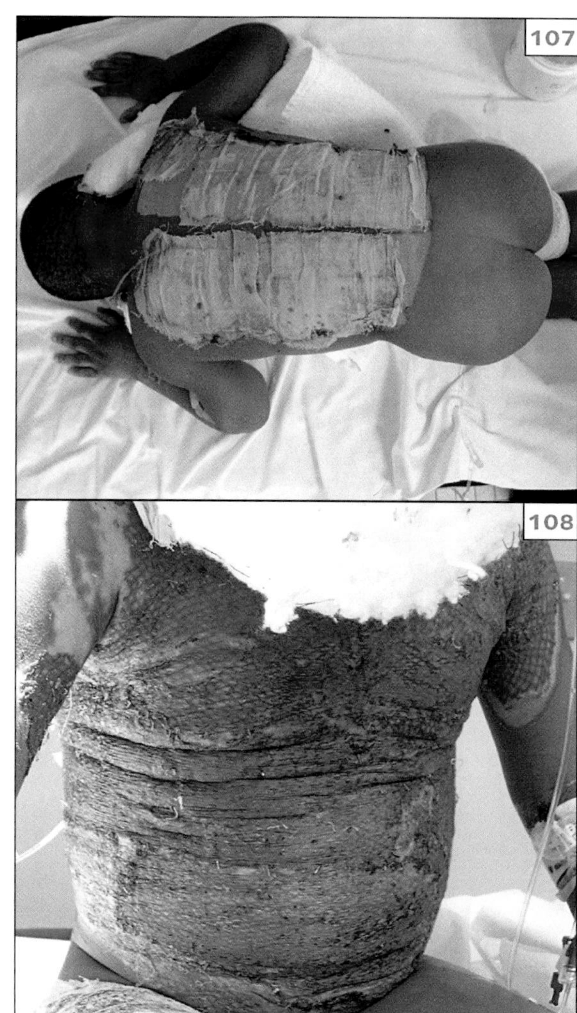

105, 106 A 3-month-old child who was reportedly sitting in a high chair. There was a bowl of hot soup on the table and the child's face and head fell into the soup. The injury is not consistent with the history. There is a well-defined area of burned skin and an absence of splash marks. Based on the reported mechanism, one would expect only the front of the child's face to be burned, but the top of the head is also burned. The child suffered second-degree burns, severe scarring, and was removed from the home.

107, 108 A split thickness skin graft was harvested from the patient's back and used to treat burns of the patient's chest and abdomen. The graft site heals by granulation and is dressed with a semipermeable dressing. Wound contracture leads to the irregularity of the skin. It is not uncommon for grafts to heal with differences in color and texture.

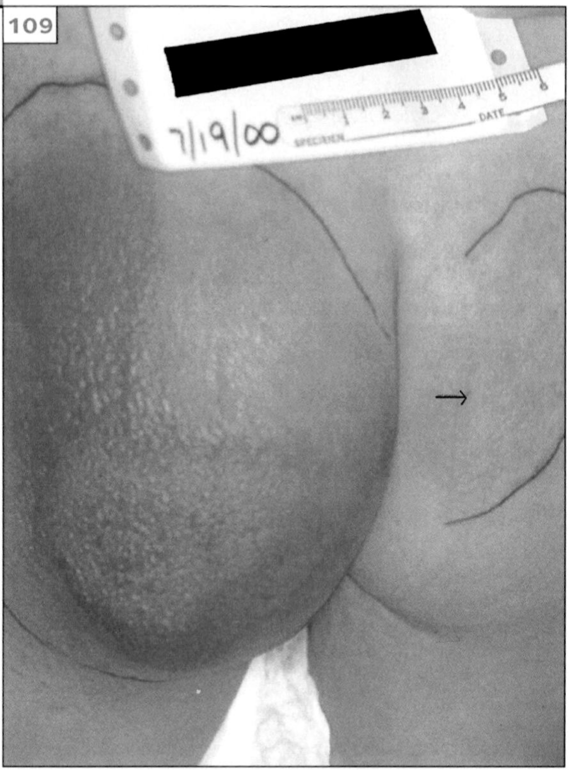

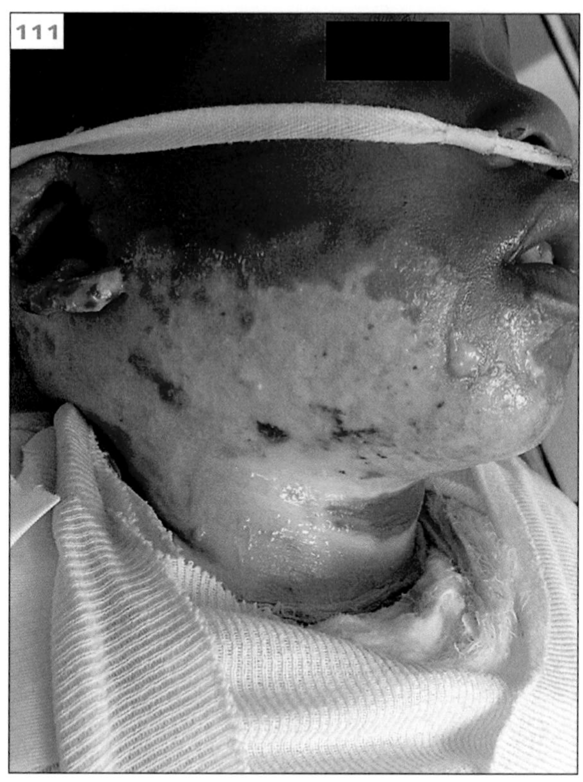

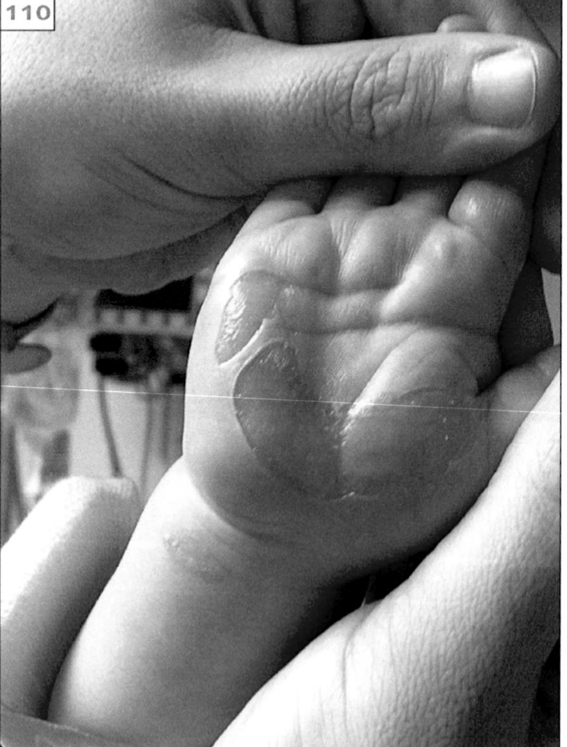

109 First-degree burn seen on the right buttock. There is erythema of the skin (epidermis only) without breakdown of the tissue. The left buttock has evidence of a second-degree burn and the white tissue discoloration may be an evolving third-degree burn.

110 Second-degree burn; the blister that was present has ruptured, leaving a clear exudate. This involves the entire epidermis and variable portions of the dermis.

111 Third-degree burn which involves the entire epidermis and dermis. The skin appears white, dry, and leathery.

Table 4 **Characteristics of families with abusive burns**[1,3,12]
1. Single parent/lack of support
2. Poorly educated
3. Responsible for many children
4. Victims of abuse/neglect themselves
5. Low income
6. Substance abuse
7. Mental illness
8. Poor impulse control
9. Expectations inconsistent with child development
10. May be hostile to hospital staff
11. Lack of concern for the injury
12. Previous child protective services involvement
13. Lack of responsibility for after-burn care

Table 5 **Characteristics of child victims of inflicted burns**[12]
1. Ages 1–4 years
2. Youngest child in home
3. Signs of previous abuse
4. Toilet training accidents
5. Developmental delay
6. Child may be withdrawn and tolerant of painful procedures

Table 6 **Characteristics of abusive burn event**
1. Reported as unwitnessed
2. Sibling blamed
3. Delay in seeking medical care
4. Nonoffending person brings child in for treatment
5. Inconsistent history
6. History not consistent with child's development
7. Other injuries (49% of patients)[4,16,19]

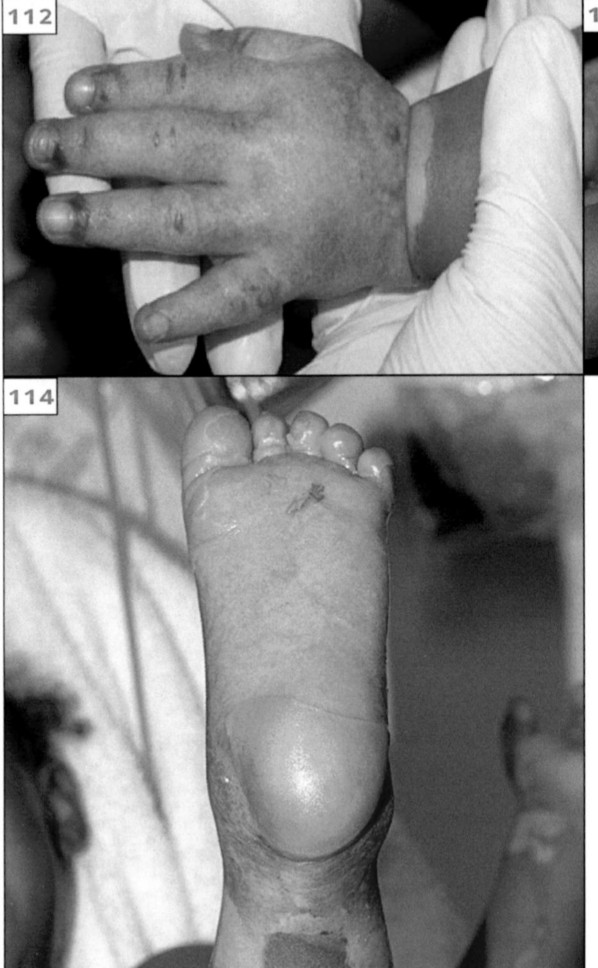

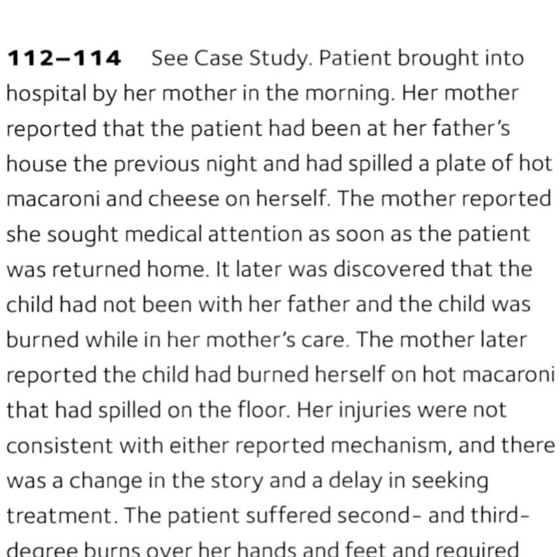

112–114 See Case Study. Patient brought into hospital by her mother in the morning. Her mother reported that the patient had been at her father's house the previous night and had spilled a plate of hot macaroni and cheese on herself. The mother reported she sought medical attention as soon as the patient was returned home. It later was discovered that the child had not been with her father and the child was burned while in her mother's care. The mother later reported the child had burned herself on hot macaroni that had spilled on the floor. Her injuries were not consistent with either reported mechanism, and there was a change in the story and a delay in seeking treatment. The patient suffered second- and third-degree burns over her hands and feet and required skin grafting. The child was placed in foster care.

Case study

The patient (**112–114**) was brought to the emergency room by her mother who reported that the patient had spilled a plate of hot macaroni and cheese on herself while at her father's home the night prior. The mother reported she sought medical care as soon the child returned home. It was later discovered that the child's father was not involved with her care (she was never at his home) and the child was burned while with her mother. The mother later stated the child had burned herself on macaroni that had spilled on the floor. The patient's injuries demonstrate a 'stocking-glove' pattern with sparing of the palm of the hand and partial sparing of the sole of the foot. Neither of the stories reported is consistent with the burn pattern. One would expect a burn to the face, chest, or thighs if the patient had spilled food on herself or a burn to the sole of the foot if the patient had stepped on hot food. The patient suffered second- and third-degree burns over her hands and feet and required skin grafting. This case demonstrates many of the characteristics seen with abusive burns: a single parent, child is 2 years of age, inconsistent and changing history, and delay in seeking treatment. The child was placed in foster care.

How are children burned?

There are many different burn mechanisms, including scalds/immersion, contact, friction, electrical, flame, chemical, and ultraviolet light. Scalds, immersions, and contact burns are the most common burns seen in both accidental and nonaccidental injuries. It can be difficult to distinguish accidental from abusive burns, but there are characteristics that help differentiate between the two.

Accidental burns

Accidental burns are often superficial because a child's automatic response is to withdraw from the painful stimulus. Movement gives the burn an irregular pattern and splash marks are generally present with scalds. Accidental burns usually occur from brief contact with a hot object or hot liquid on areas of the body that are exposed during daily activities: face, palms, and chest. Most accidental burns are witnessed and the parent and the patient are very clear about how the injury occurred. These children are brought to medical attention by their caregivers shortly after the injury (*Table 7*).

Case study

The patient (**115, 116**), a 22-month-old male was brought to the hospital by ambulance. He was accompanied by both parents who reported that the patient accidentally pulled a pan of hot grease off the stovetop at home. Both parents and other family members witnessed the event. Hot grease splashed the patient's face, chest, abdomen, and both arms

Table 7 **Characteristics of accidental burns**
1. Splash marks
2. Superficial
3. Object not well defined
4. Location: palms, soles of feet, anterior chest wall, face
5. Irregular borders
6. Good history of event
7. Caregivers promptly medical care

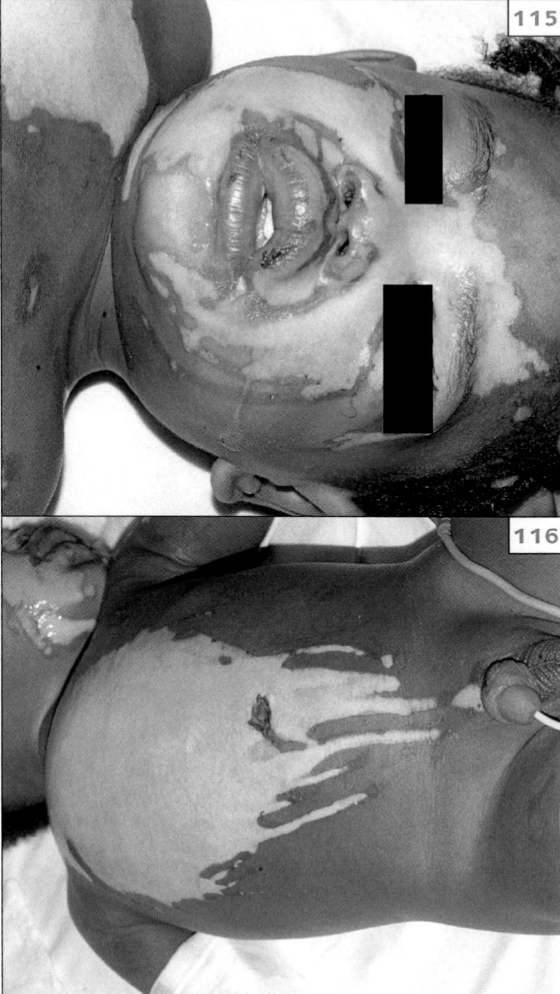

115, 116 See Case Study. A 22-month-old was brought into hospital by ambulance accompanied by both parents who reported that the patient accidentally pulled a pan of hot grease off the kitchen stovetop. Both parents were at home and witnessed the injury. Other family members were also present at the time of the injury. Hot fat splashed on the patient's face, chest, abdomen, and both arms and feet. The child was taken to the hospital immediately. The burn pattern is consistent with the history (notice the splash and drip marks).

Table 8 **Characteristics of abusive scald burns**

1. Absence of splash marks
2. Deep
3. Well-defined outline of object
4. Dorsae of hands and feet, face, buttocks, back of arms, and legs
5. Well-defined borders (stocking-glove)
6. Poor history of event/unwitnessed
7. Delay in seeking treatment

Table 9 **Time to produce full-thickness scald burns in adults[15]**

WATER TEMPERATURE		TIME
°C	°F	
49	120	5–10 minutes
52	125	2 minutes
54	130	30 seconds
57	135	10 seconds
60	140	5 seconds
63	145	3 seconds
66	150	1–5 seconds
68	155	1 second or less
70	158	<1 second

and feet. Medical attention was sought immediately. The patient's pattern of injury is consistent with the history. His face and trunk are burned, which is expected when children pull hot liquid onto themselves. There are splash marks and the injury is most severe on the face and chest which is the initial point of contact. There was no delay in seeking treatment and the injury was witnessed by the family.

Abusive burns

Abusive burns are characteristically deeper than accidental burns. This is because of forced and prolonged contact with the offending liquid or object. Enforced restraint leads to fewer or no splash marks and creates a more uniform depth of the burn. Abusive burns are often seen on both extremities and on areas of the body typically protected by clothing, genitalia, buttocks, backs of the arms and legs, and the dorsae of the hands and feet (**117, 118**) (*Table* 8).

Scalds

Although scald injuries account for the majority of childhood burns, only 7–17% of accidental scalds result in hospitalization, whereas 87% of intentional scalds victims are hospitalized[14]. The severity of scald injuries depends on the liquid's temperature, time of exposure, and skin characteristics. The data correlating water temperature, exposure time, and severity of burns was gathered in the 1950s from human adult volunteers and from guinea pigs. This information was extrapolated to children. Children's skin is thinner than adult skin, resulting in a more severe burn in a shorter period of time (**119–124**). Many American homes have their water heater set at 140°F (60°C), a temperature that can cause a third-degree burn in 5 seconds. The American Academy of Pediatrics recommends that all homes have their water heaters set at 120°F (49°C). As a point of reference, comfortable bath water is 101°F (38°C) and hot bathwater is 104–108°F (40–42°C).

When investigating scald injuries, it is important that investigators check not only the water heater temperature in the home, but the water temperature where the injury occurred and the time it takes for the running water to get to the maximum temperature. This information helps determine if the explanation for the injury is plausible (**125–132**).

Stocking and glove patterned injuries are virtually pathognomonic for abusive burns (*Table* 9). They are often bilateral and are caused when a child's feet or hands are forcibly held in hot water (**133–139**). Forced immersion burns of the buttocks, genitalia, and lower extremities are frequently seen as punishment for toilet training accidents (**140**). When children are restrained in hot water, there will often be well-defined areas of unburned skin in the flexion creases. Areas that are often spared are seen around the hips, knees, and lower part of the abdomen. Children who are intentionally burned may take on a defensive position out of fear or pain with their knees bent and drawn toward their chest. This position leads to skin-to-skin contact which protects these areas from being burned (**141, 142**).

Skin sparing is also seen when there is direct skin contact with the bottom of the bathtub (often seen on the bottom of the feet or the buttocks). Sparing of the central area of the buttocks is sometimes referred to as a 'doughnut burn'. This is seen when a child is forcibly immersed in hot water with the buttocks held against the bottom of the bathtub, which is cooler than the surrounding water. It is important when evaluating a burn victim to try to move them into the position they were in when they were burned. 'Burn patterns can be used to reconstruct the child's position in the water. The key to recognition of abusive burns is the burn-pattern evidence of restraint.'[14]

Bath immersion injuries are often assumed to be abusive in nature. However, a study by Allasio and Fischer found that 35% of children aged 10–18 months were able to climb into a bath unassisted[15]. A quarter of these children climbed in head first and the remainder sideways. The ability to climb into a tub filled with hot water could lead to an immersion injury of the head, hands, and legs. There would be a difference in burn pattern between children who climbed into a bath of hot water compared with those who had been forcibly immersed. Children who climb or fall into a tub of hot water might present with immersion injuries to their hands and feet, but they would also have irregular burn patterns and splash marks. In all burn cases, it is important to assess the child's developmental abilities when trying to determine the mechanism of injury.

Scald injuries not only occur in the bathroom, but also are seen when children pull hot liquids onto themselves or when scalding liquid is poured or thrown at them. Water follows the pull of gravity and it cools as it flows downward. The point of contact is where the burn is most intense. These types of scald injuries often show the 'arrow sign,' with the most severe injury at the point of contact and less severe injury seen as the water flows downward. An imaginary arrow is formed in the direction the water flows (**143, 144**). A child who accidentally pulls hot liquids onto himself will often burn his chin (if looking up), face, shoulder, and anterior trunk (**145–147**). In contrast when hot liquid is thrown or poured on a victim, the chin is spared[14] and the posterior aspect of the body or the trunk is burned (**148–150**).

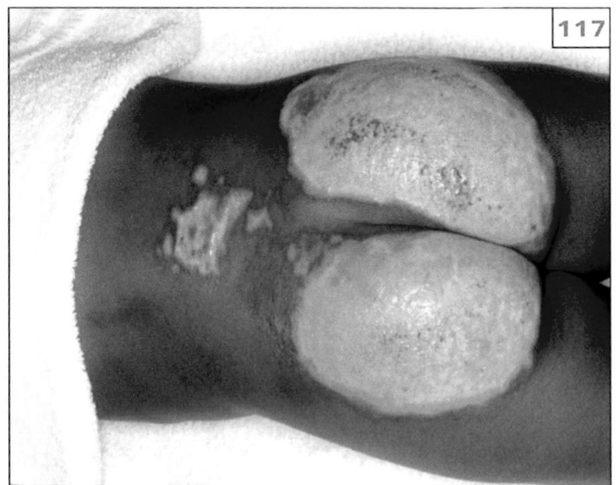

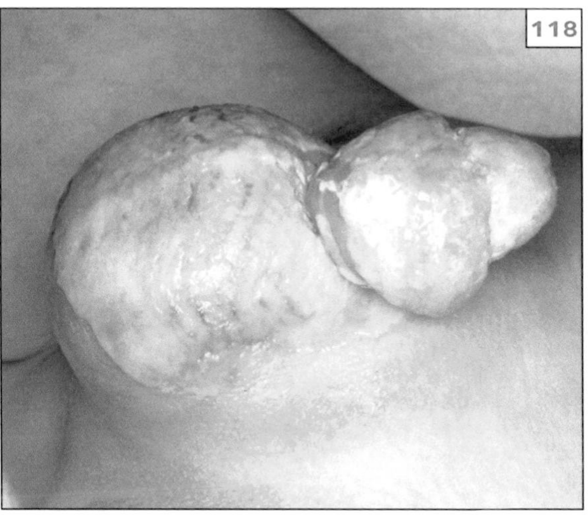

117 An isolated burn to the buttocks is pathognomonic for abuse. There are no splash marks and the surrounding skin is not burned. This child was held in a jack-knife position and his bottom was placed in scalding water.

118 An isolated burn to the penis without surrounding splash marks consistent with child abuse.

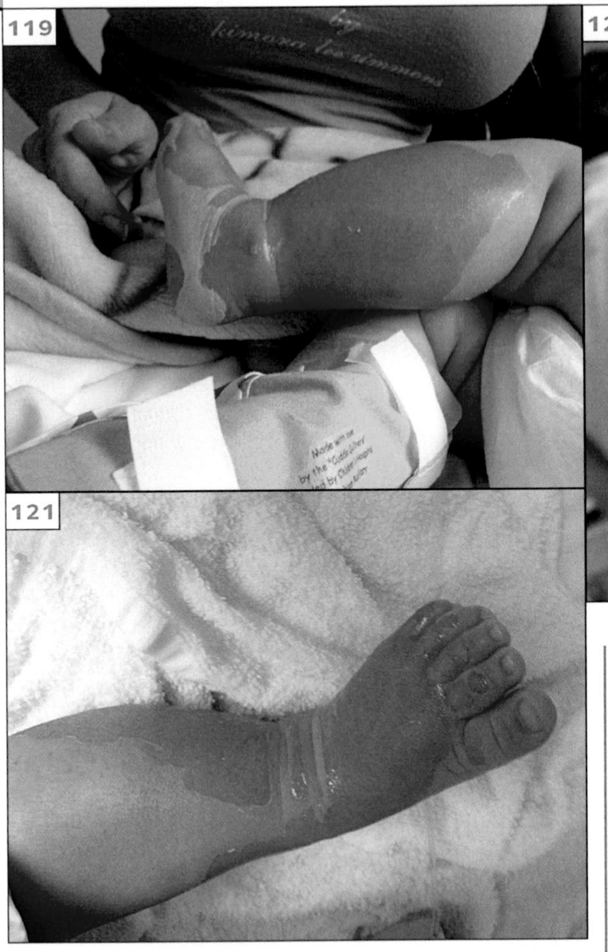

120

119–121 A 6-month-old child was placed in the bath with the water running. The patient's leg was under the running water. Mother did not realize how hot. The patient was removed from the water as soon as she started crying and was brought to medical attention immediately. She still suffered 5% burn to the right leg; the water temperature was well above 120°F (49°C). Notice the splash marks and uneven areas of burn. There is not a clear line of demarcation. There is some skin sparing where the ankle was dorsiflexed.

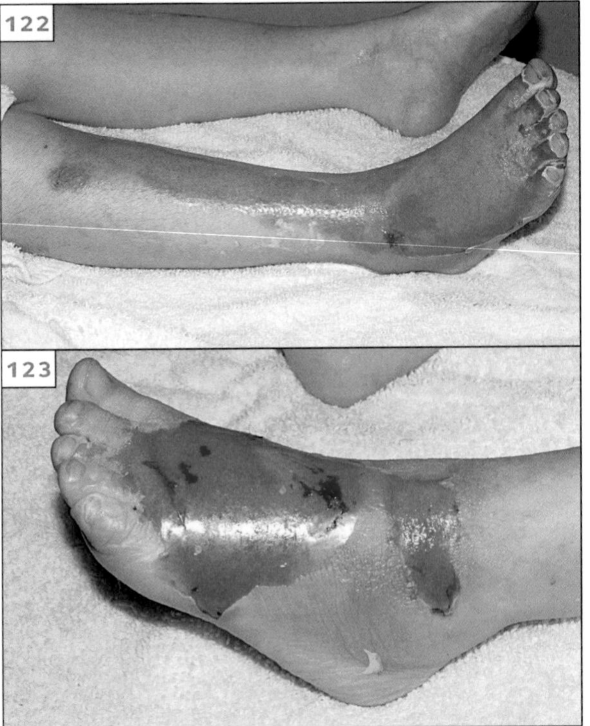

122, 123 The patient was in the bath with her sister. Her sister turned off the cold water and the patient suffered a second-degree burn to her leg and foot. There are splash marks and the area of burn is not well defined. It was felt that the patient's sister was developmentally capable of turning the water on and off. There was concern for lack of supervision and child protective services were contacted for neglect.

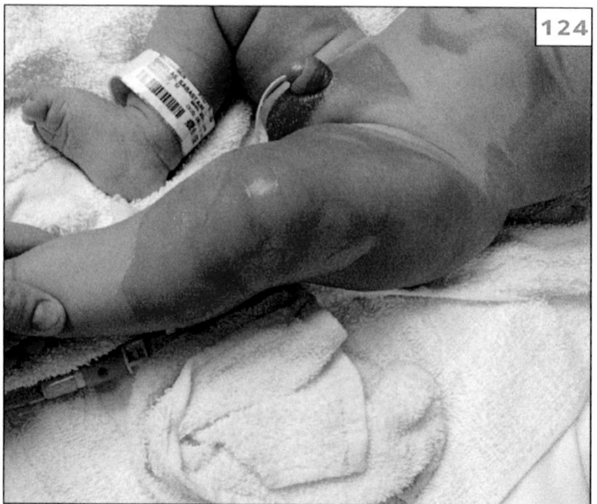

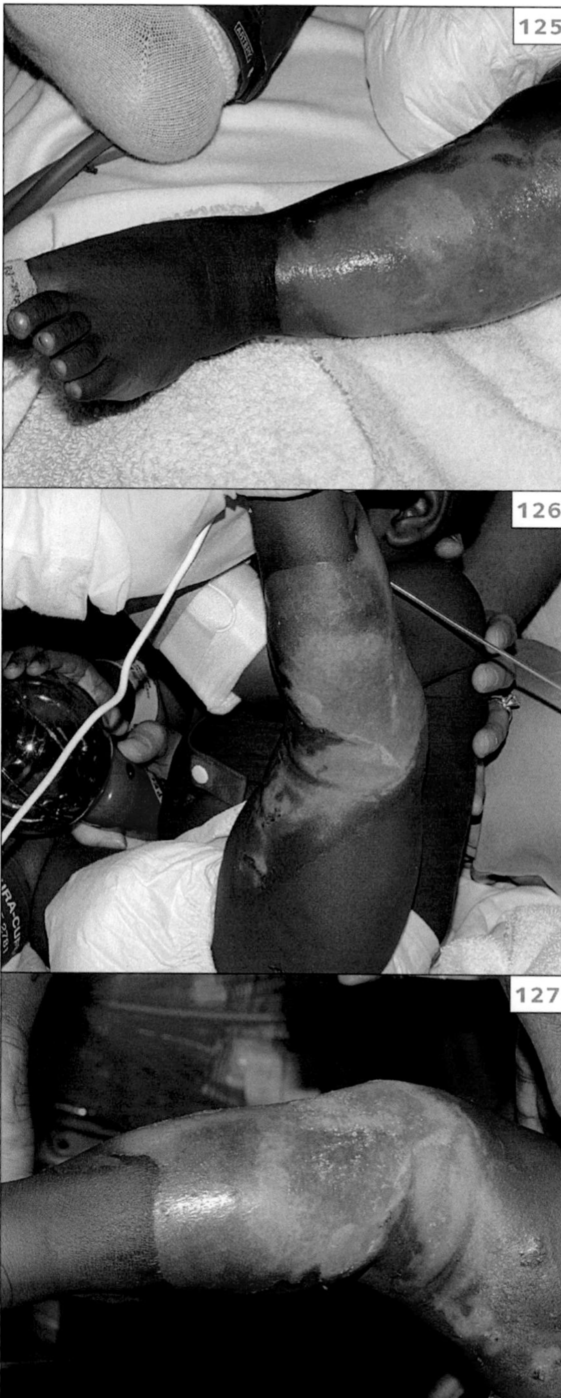

124 The patient was being bathed by a babysitter in the sink. The child was removed from the water as soon as the caregiver realized how hot the running water was. The child was brought to the hospital immediately by the parents and the babysitter. Notice skin sparing of the abdomen where the leg was drawn up. The pattern of the burn on the leg is irregular.

125–127 A 10-month-old was being given a bath by an aunt with the water running. The baby turned off the cold water with his foot and was burned. The patient was brought in 3 days later with second-degree burns. The burn area was uneven and there were splash marks. There was skin sparing around the popliteal fossa and posterior part of the leg. The injury was consistent with the reported mechanism, but there was a delay in seeking treatment. A report was made for neglect.

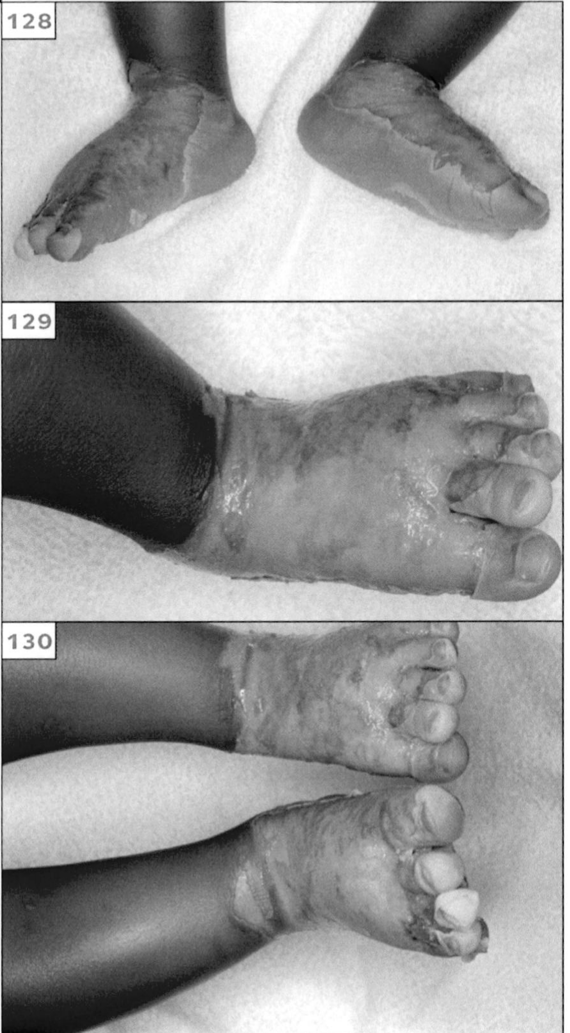

128–130 Burns to the bilateral feet in a 'stocking' pattern. This type of injury is pathognomonic for child abuse and occurs when the feet are forcibly held in scalding water. The skin on the sole of the foot is spared by being in contact with the bottom of the bathtub. This child suffered second-degree burns to both feet.

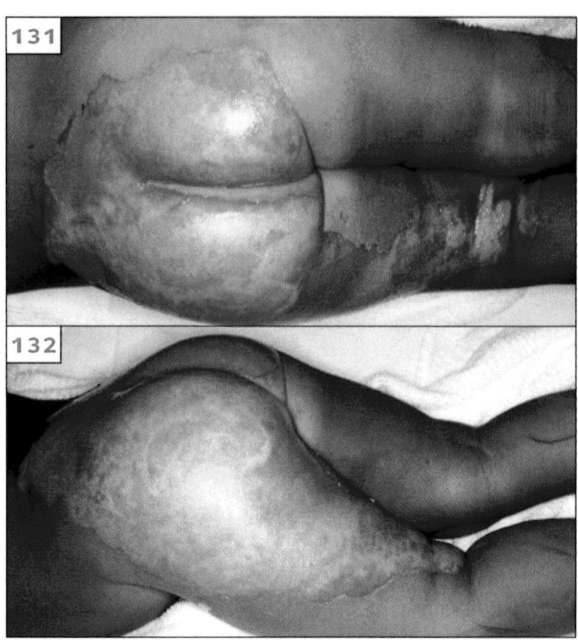

131, 132 Isolated burn to the buttocks of a child that was forcibly held in scalding water for a toilet training accident. The area of burn was well demarcated and the skin appeared evenly burned. There were no surrounding splash marks. Loop marks were also evident on both of the child's legs.

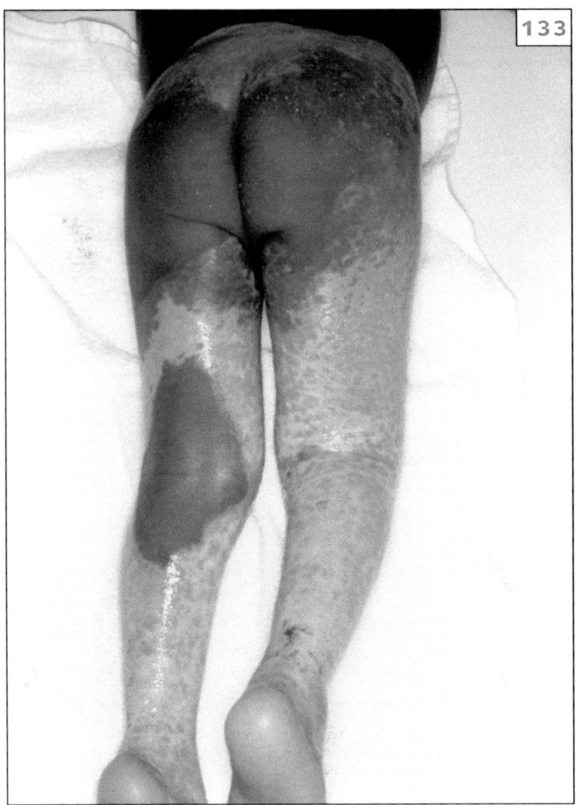

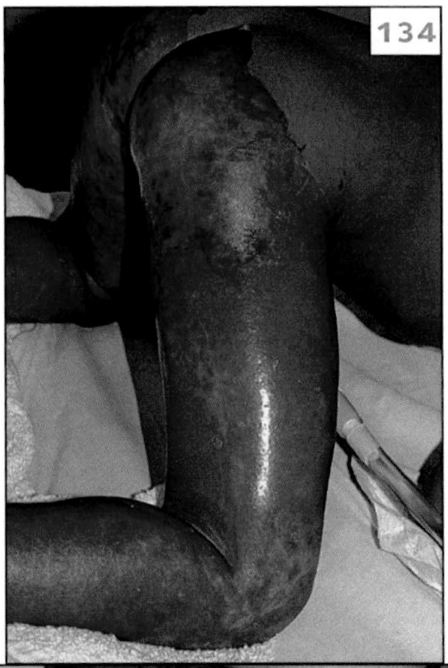

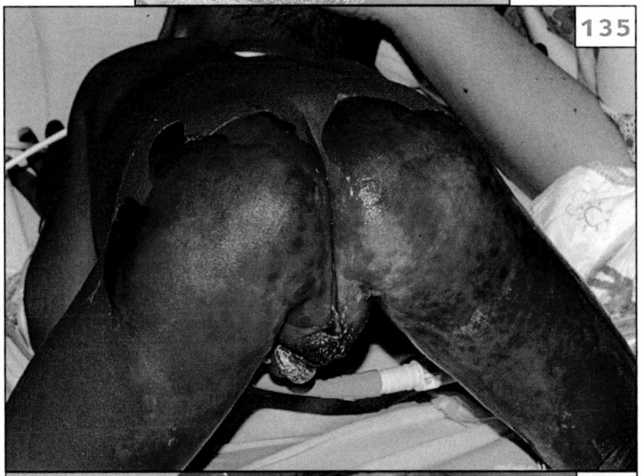

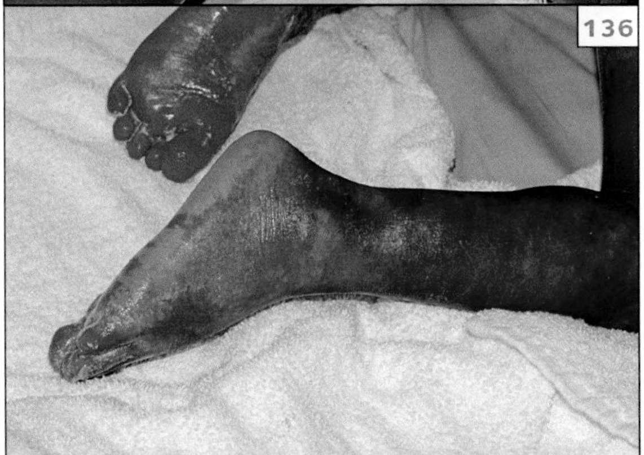

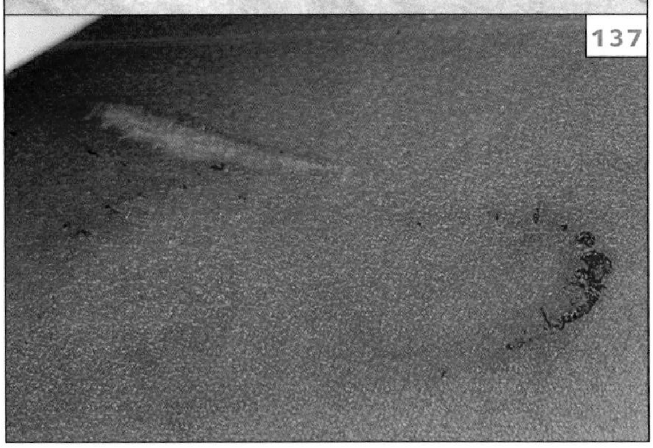

133 Doughnut-shaped burn to the buttocks of a child who was forcibly held in scalding water. The central area of the buttocks is spared as the bathtub surface is cooler than the surrounding water. This type of burn is pathognomonic for child abuse. There is sparing of the popliteal fossa where the patient's leg was bent.

134–137 A 3-year-old male brought in by his mother for burns to his lower extremities. The mother reported she was running hot water for a bath and the child jumped into the bath with his underwear and T-shirt on. She stated that she quickly pulled the child out, but he had already sustained a burn. She admitted to 'whipping' the child earlier in the day for a toilet training accident. The injury was not consistent with the history given as there were no splash marks, the burn was isolated to the genital area and lower legs, there was a well-defined area between burned and unburned skin, and the mother admitted she had whipped the child for a toilet training accident that day. The patient was hospitalized for 23 days for skin grafting and burn care and was removed from the mother's care.

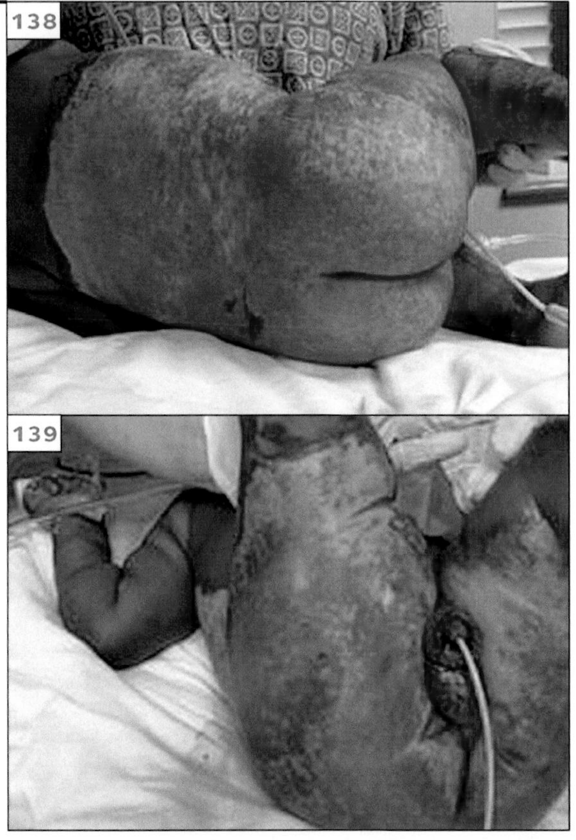

138

139

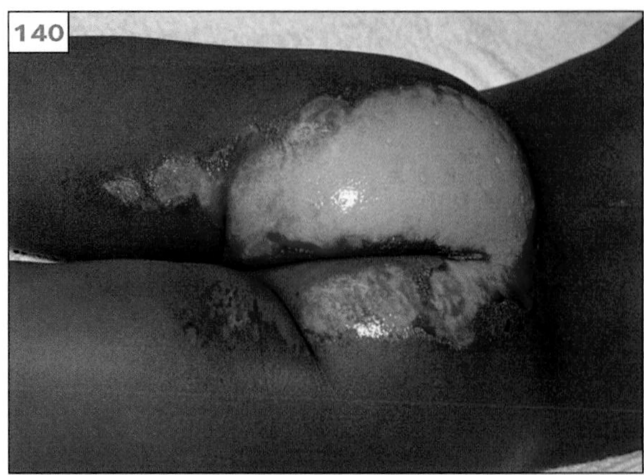

140

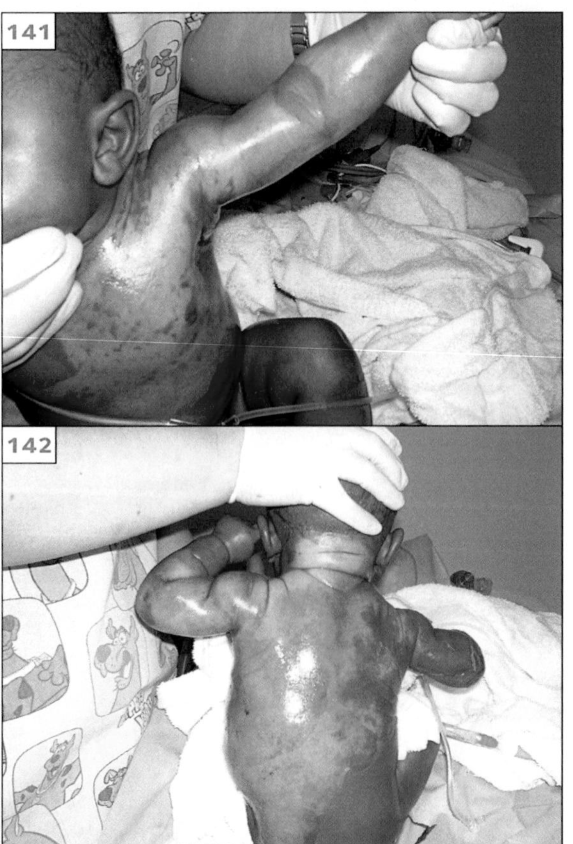

141

142

138, 139 The patient is an 18-month-old male. The mother reported that she had filled the bathtub with boiling water from the stove as her hot water heater was not working. She left the patient and his 4-year-old brother in the bathroom alone and then heard screaming and found the patient in the bath. The history was inconsistent with the injury, no splash marks, clearly demarcated area between the burned and unburned skin. Mother later admitted to the police that the patient's father had burned the patient. The patient and his sibling were removed from the home.

140 The patient is a 3.5-year-old who reportedly had had a toilet training accident 2 days prior to being seen. The patient's father stated that he had attempted to wash the stool off the patient's buttocks with warm water and a cloth, but underestimated the temperature of the water. Treatment was sought after the mother became aware of the injury. The injury was inconsistent with the history and there was a delay in seeking medical treatment.

141, 142 The patient suffered second-degree burns over 40% body surface area (BSA). The father reported that he left the 5-month-old child in the bath with a hand-held shower running. The water was reported to be cold when he left the room. Father went to answer the phone, when he returned child was lying in the bath and there was hot water coming from the showerhead. There is clear line of demarcation between burned and unburned skin and no splash marks. This injury is consistent with the child being immersed in hot water.

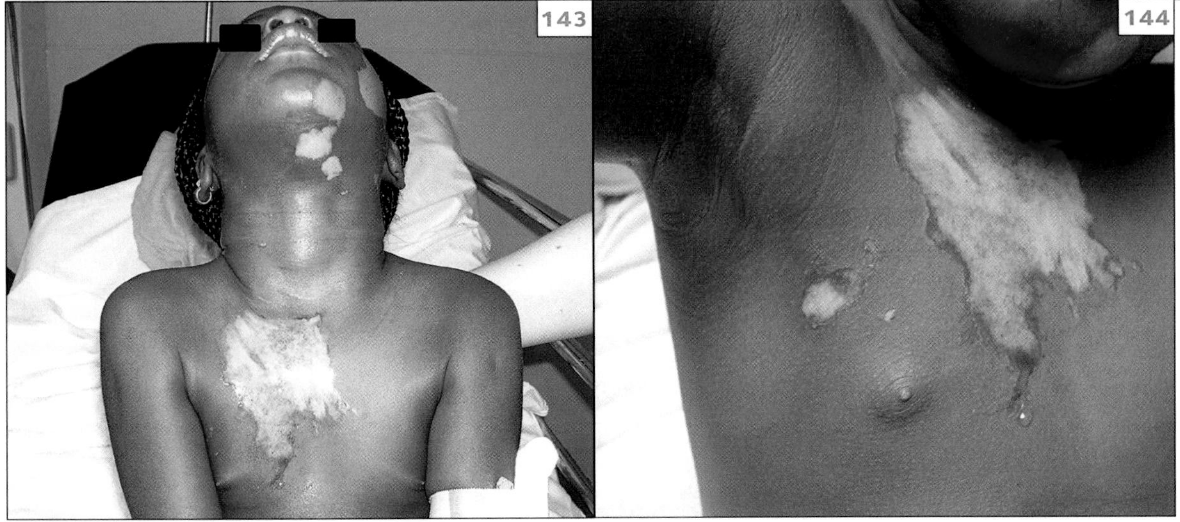

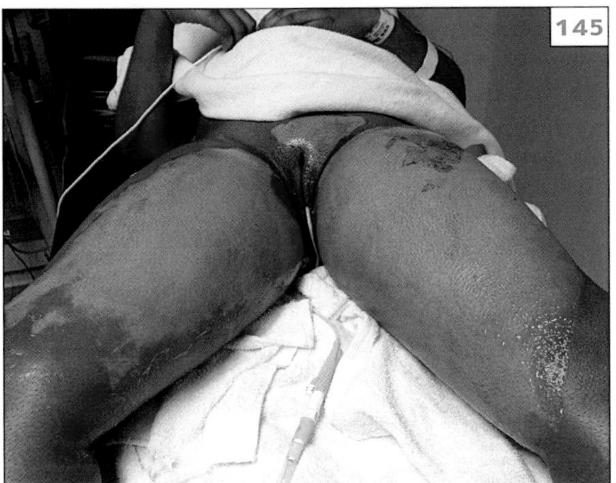

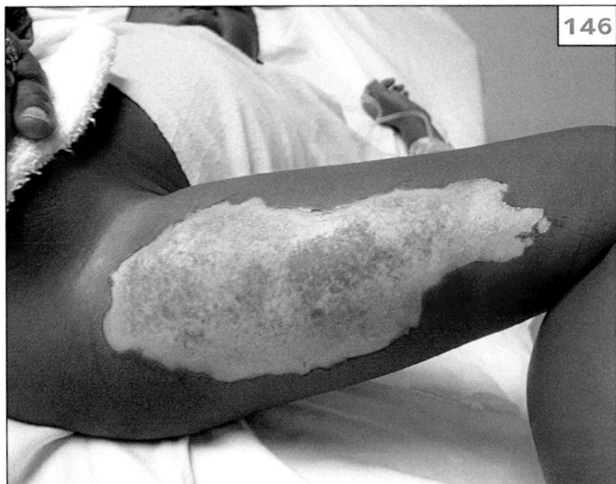

143, 144 The patient pulled hot water from a work surface down onto herself. She was brought immediately to the emergency room by her mother. Her chin and anterior trunk was burned which is expected in this type of injury. Note the 'arrow sign'. Burn decreases in severity as the water flows downward.

145 A 12-year-old spilled hot water onto her lap while making tea, suffering second-degree burns to 12% of her body surface area.

146 The patient spilled hot noodle soup onto his lap, suffering second- and third-degree burns to his left inner thigh.

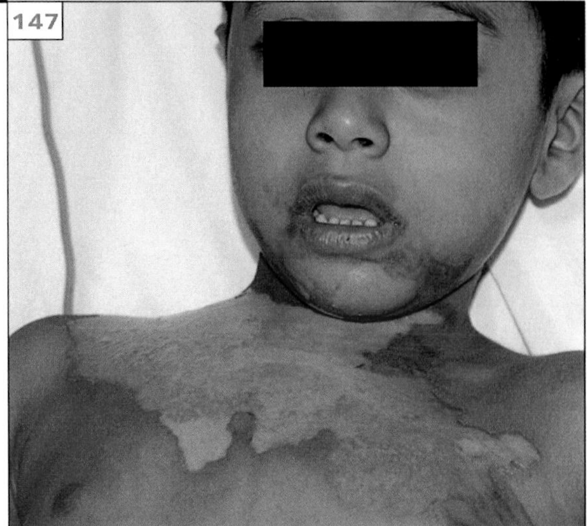

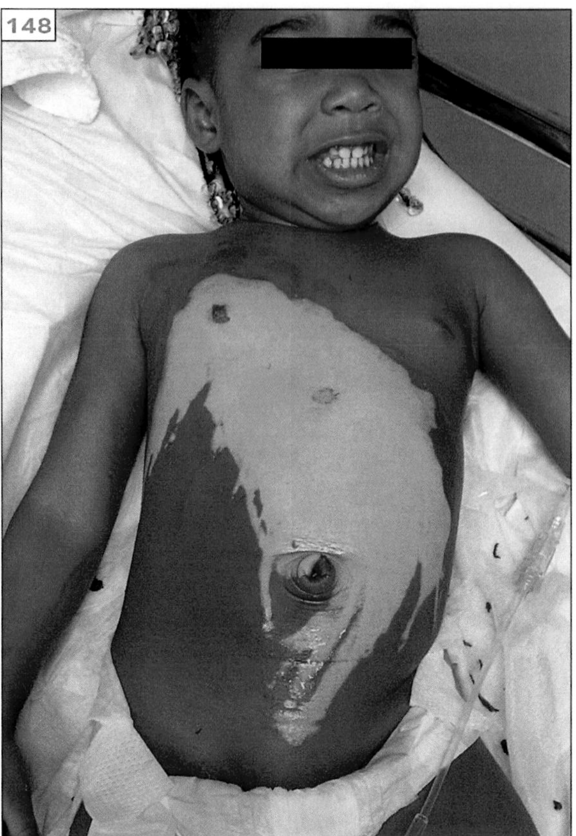

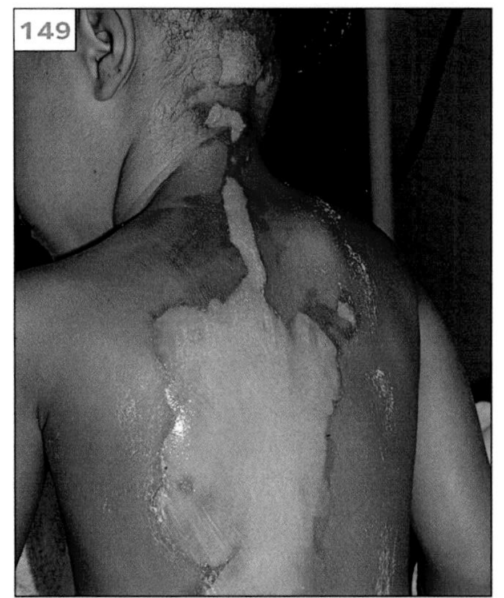

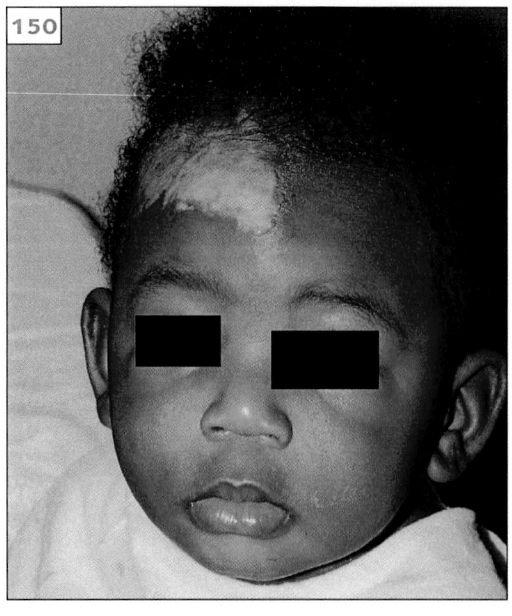

147 The child pulled a cup of hot tea off the work surface burning his anterior trunk and chin.

148 The patient pulled a cup of hot coffee off the work surface burning her anterior trunk. There are clear drip marks. The arrow sign is appreciated as the water cools and the 'stream' narrows as it flows downward and decreases in severity from the point of initial contact.

149 Injuries sustained by a 2-year-old who reportedly pulled a cup of hot water off a table and onto herself, burning the back of her neck and back. This is not the pattern of injury you would expect with this history. You would expect a burn to the anterior, not posterior, aspect of the body. You can easily see the direction the water flowed as the injury becomes less severe down her back (arrow sign). She suffered second-degree burns to 4% of her body surface area.

150 The parents reported that coffee was accidentally spilled on the patient's forehead. This is a well-localized burn without any drip marks. Given the location and the history, there was concern for abuse.

Contact burns

Accidental contact burns often involve the palms of the hands and the soles of the feet. These injuries are caused by a child accidentally grabbing or stepping on a hot object. Children also pull hot objects off elevated surfaces resulting in contact burns on their face and anterior trunk (**151, 152**). Intentional contact burns will involve the back of the body, the buttocks, and the dorsae of the hands and feet. Objects commonly used in abusive burns include metal heating grates, cigarette lighters, hair dryers, curling irons, clothes irons, and heated silverware. Forced contact burns will leave a well-demarcated burn pattern and the object used can often be identified from the burn pattern (**153–165**).

Cigarette burns are a common abusive injury, but are infrequently brought in for medical attention. Although cigarettes generally burn a small surface area, they burn at a temperature of over 400°F (204°C). Intentional cigarette burns are often multiple, usually found on areas protected by clothing. They leave a deep clear circular imprint about 8 mm in diameter. Once healed, they resemble a smallpox vaccination scar. Unintentional cigarette burns are superficial and usually involve the face or arm. These burns may have a more linear appearance caused by the cigarette accidentally brushing against the child's skin (**166, 167**).

Other less common causes of burn injuries include flame burns, electrical injuries, chemical burns, and exposure. Flame burns are seen in house fires, firework injuries, and when flammable substances ignite (gasoline/petrol and alcohol). It is not uncommon to see these injuries in families who are using their stoves or ovens to heat the house (**168–178**). 'Electrical injuries are caused by electricity passing through the body. Tissue's resistance to current generates thermal energy and results in tissue damage[6].' Low voltage (<1000 V) injuries are seen when children chew on electrics cords (**179, 180**). High voltage (>1000 V) injuries are seen with high-tension wire injuries. Chemical burns can be caused by numerous household products including certain foods, cleaning products, drain openers, detergents, pesticides, and gasoline/petrol (**181–183**). The degree of injury depends on the substance, the duration of contact, and the surface area of the body exposed. Exposure injuries are seen when children get severe sunburns; they may be accidental, nonaccidental, or due to neglect.

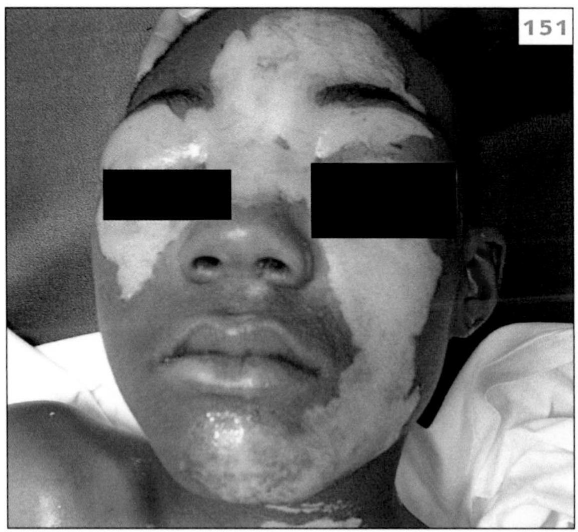

151 This patient sustained injuries when eggs from the microwave exploded in the patient's face.

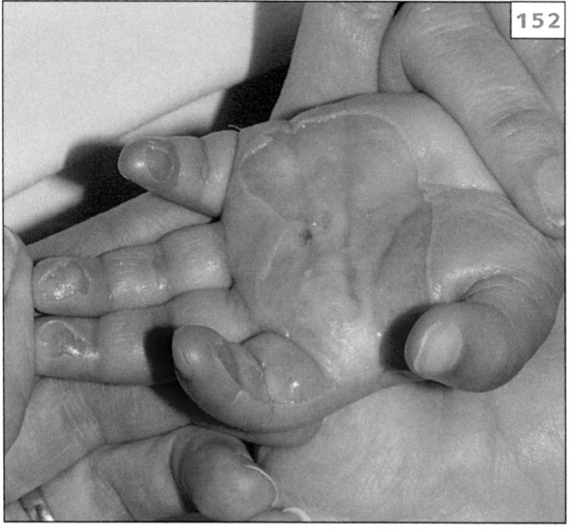

152 The patient's hand was placed on a hot fireplace screen.

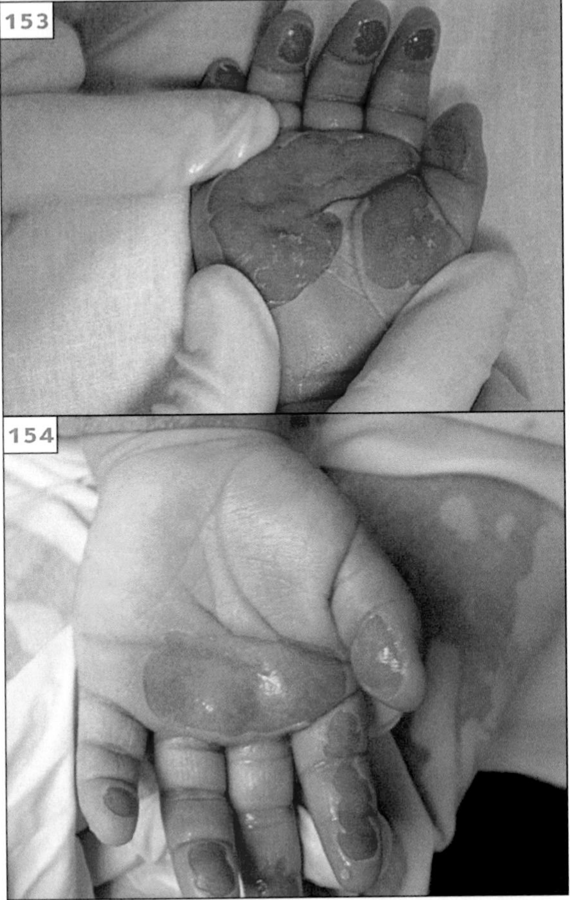

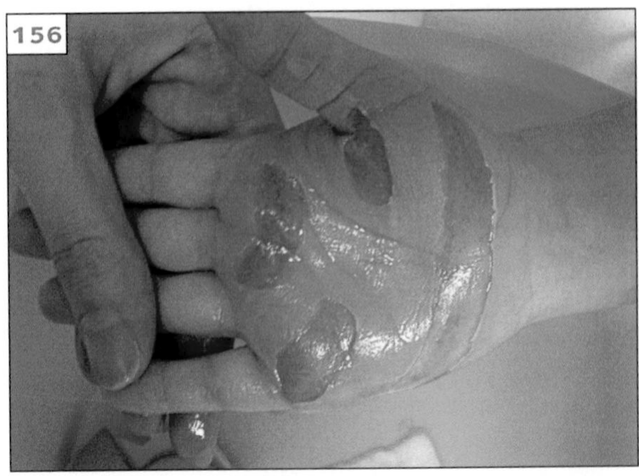

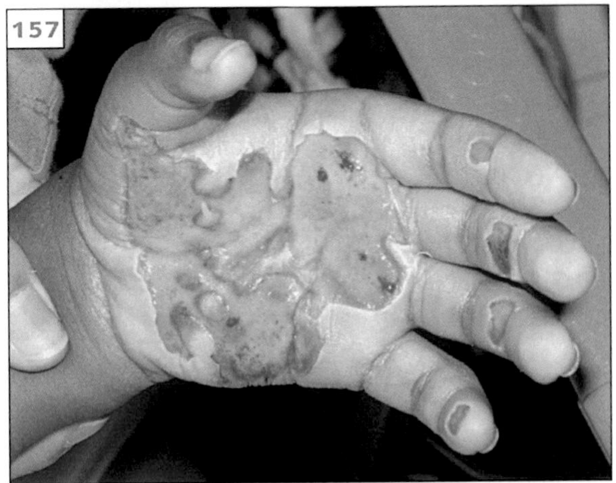

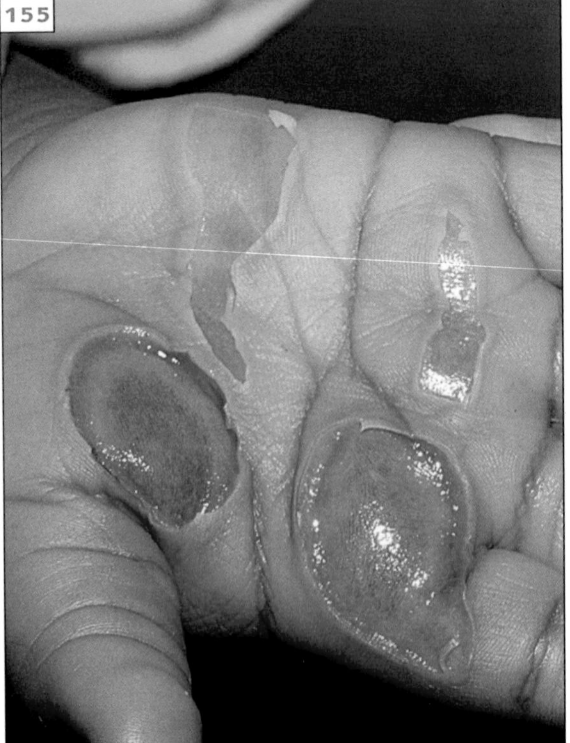

153, 154 A 10-month-old child who was learning to walk. The patient was sitting in the kitchen and used the oven door to help stand up. Second-degree burns were sustained to both palms (1% of the body surface area). Both parents were present and the patient was brought to the hospital immediately.

155 The patient suffered burns while grabbing a hot curling iron. There was sparing of the middle of the palm where the skin was in contact with the unheated portion of the curling iron.

156 The patient was helping his mother cook and put his hand onto the hot stove burner. The outline of the burner can be clearly seen.

157 The patient tried to catch a hot iron that fell off the ironing board. Careful inspection revealed circular sparing consistent with the circles on an iron soleplate.

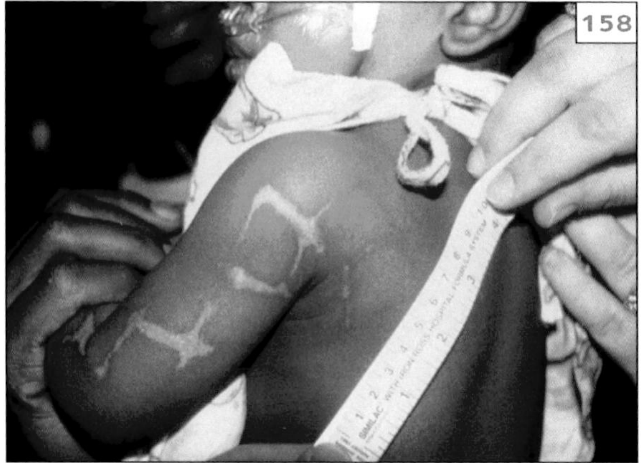

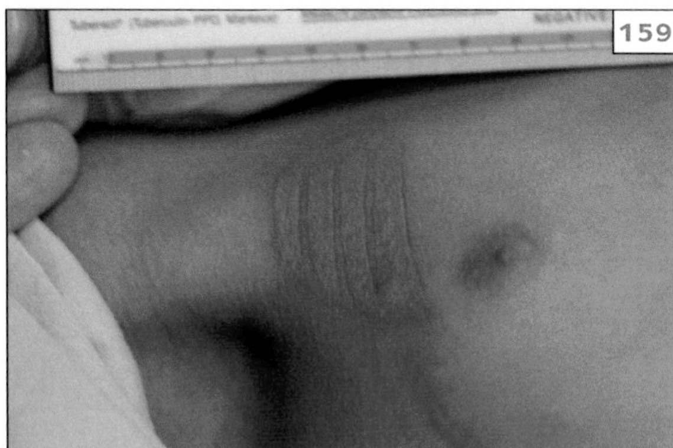

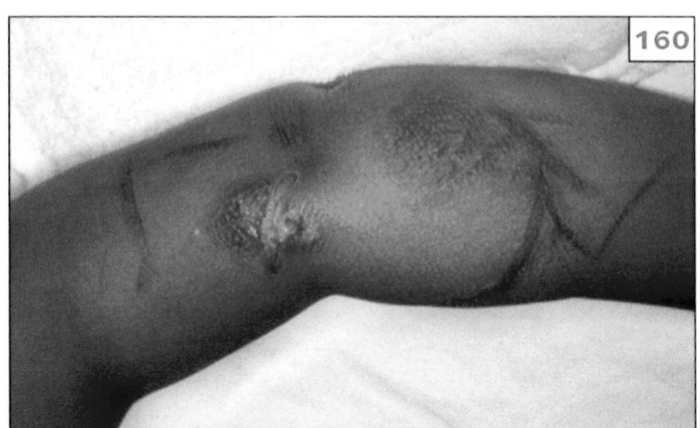

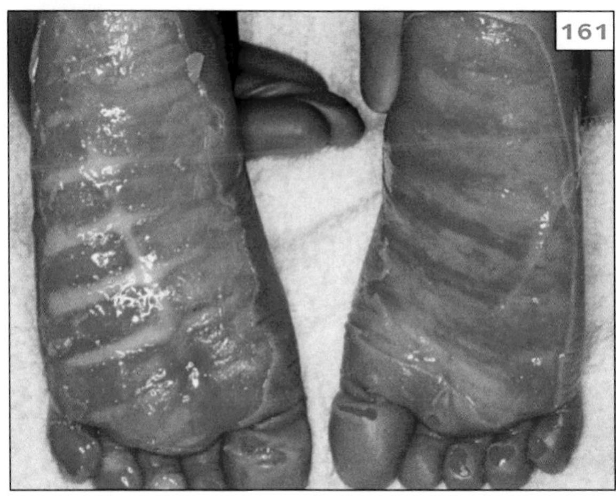

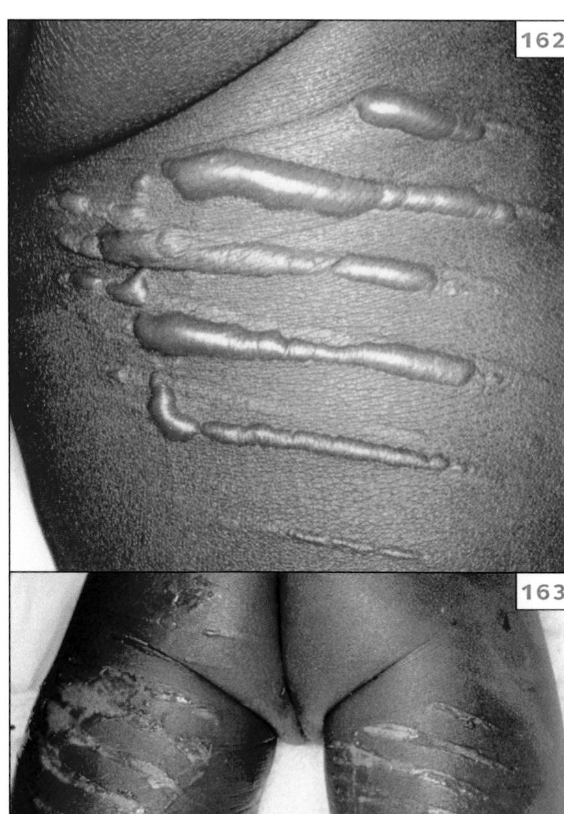

158 Child was admitted for a respiratory illness and, when undressed, was found to have scars consistent with a previous burn. The outline of the object can be seen, however, the instrument used was never identified.

159 A fork was heated and placed on the child's skin as punishment. The outline of the fork is identifiable.

160 Cross-shaped burn to the arm surrounded by linear whip marks.

161 A young patient was forced to stand on a hot metal grate as punishment for fighting with his sibling. The outline of the grate is easily visible.

162, 163 12-year-old child forced to sit on a hot metal heating grate. Photographs of the grate matched patient's injuries exactly. Photographs taken at different stages of healing.

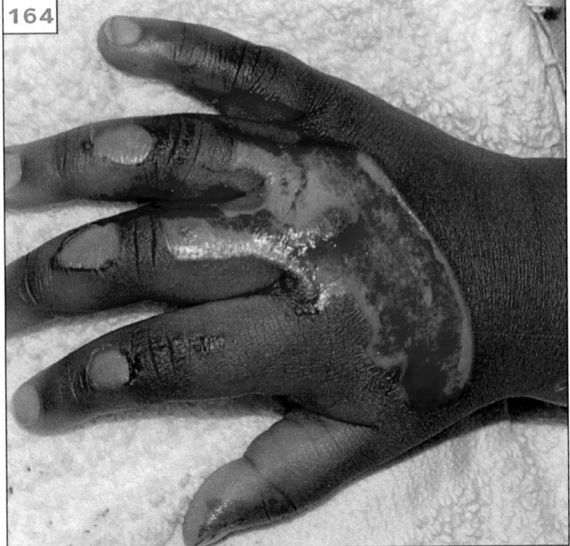

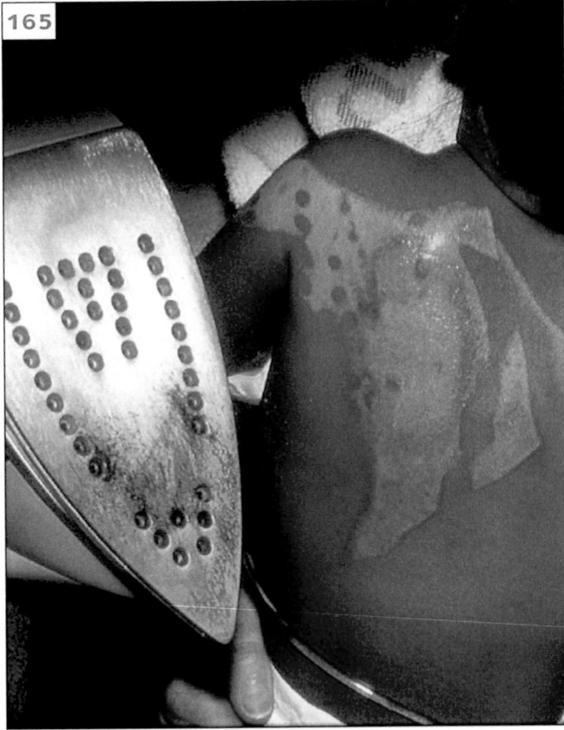

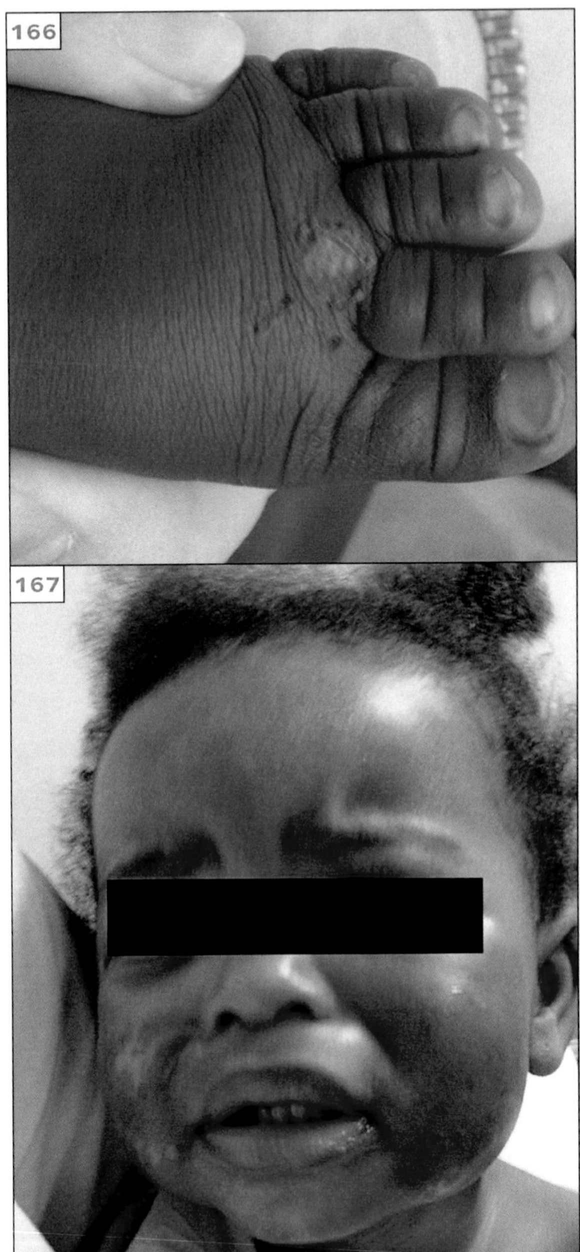

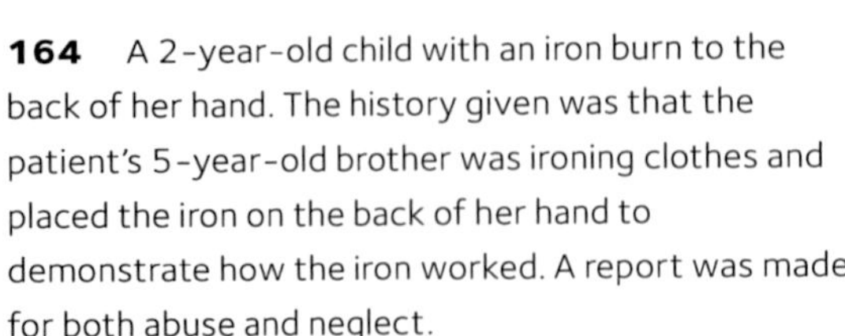

164 A 2-year-old child with an iron burn to the back of her hand. The history given was that the patient's 5-year-old brother was ironing clothes and placed the iron on the back of her hand to demonstrate how the iron worked. A report was made for both abuse and neglect.

165 Injuries sustained to a child who was branded by an iron. The patient's mother was mentally ill.

166, 167 A 16-month-old who was picked up from the father's house and found to have a well-circumscribed cigarette burn to the dorsum of her foot (166). The patient also had facial swelling, multiple bruises, excoriation of the cheek and peri-anal area, and posterior parietal skull fracture (167).

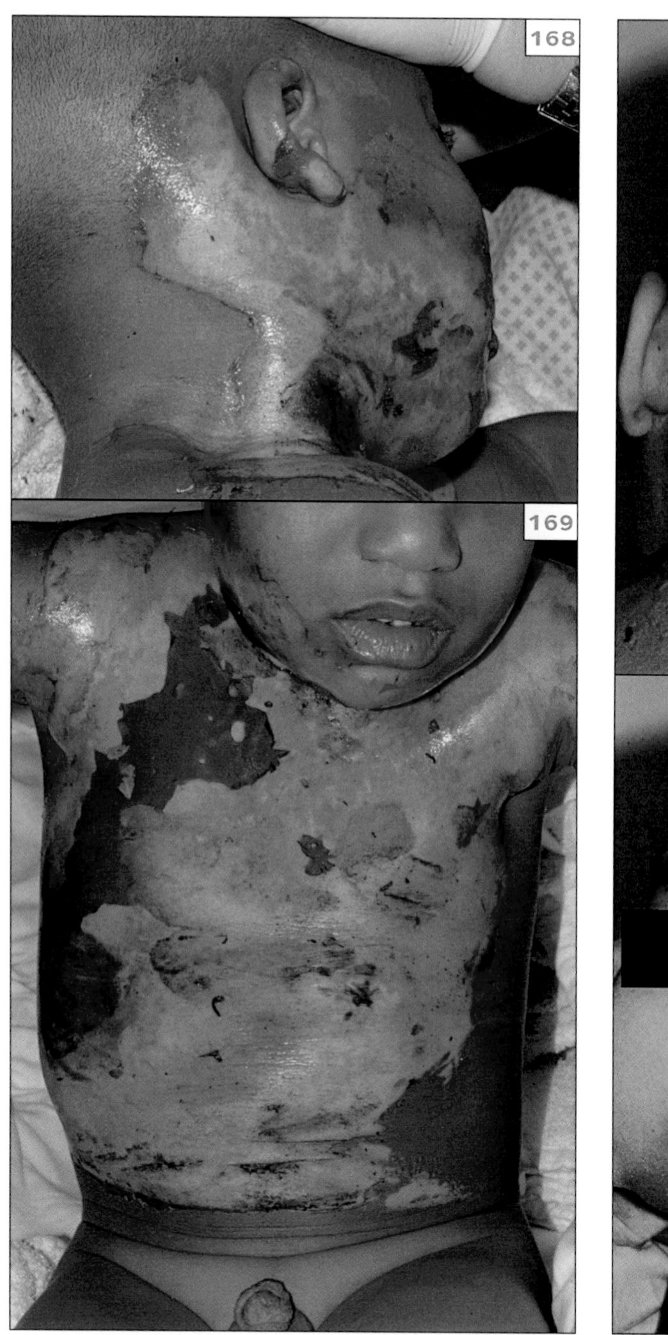

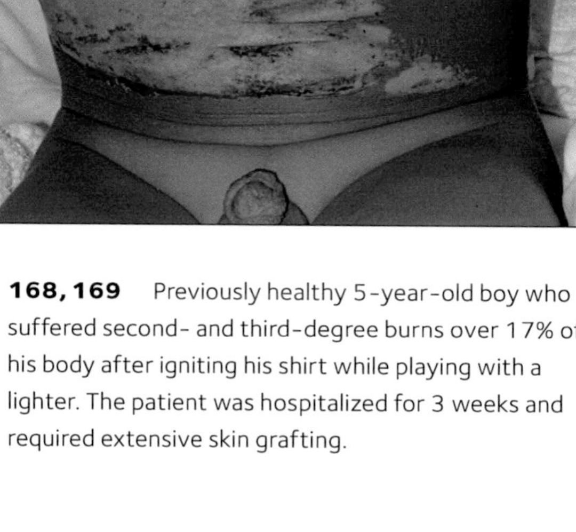

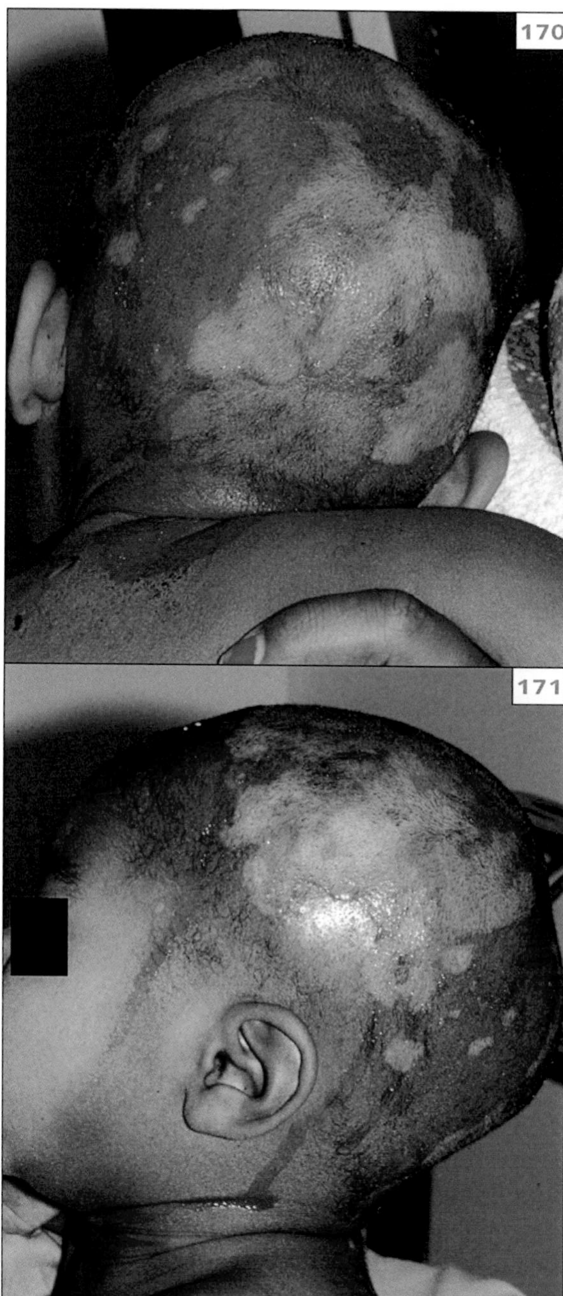

168, 169 Previously healthy 5-year-old boy who suffered second- and third-degree burns over 17% of his body after igniting his shirt while playing with a lighter. The patient was hospitalized for 3 weeks and required extensive skin grafting.

170, 171 Injuries sustained to a 2-year-old whose 7-year-old brother was playing with a lighter and set her hair on fire. She suffered second-degree burns to 5% of her body surface area. The sibling was removed from the home.

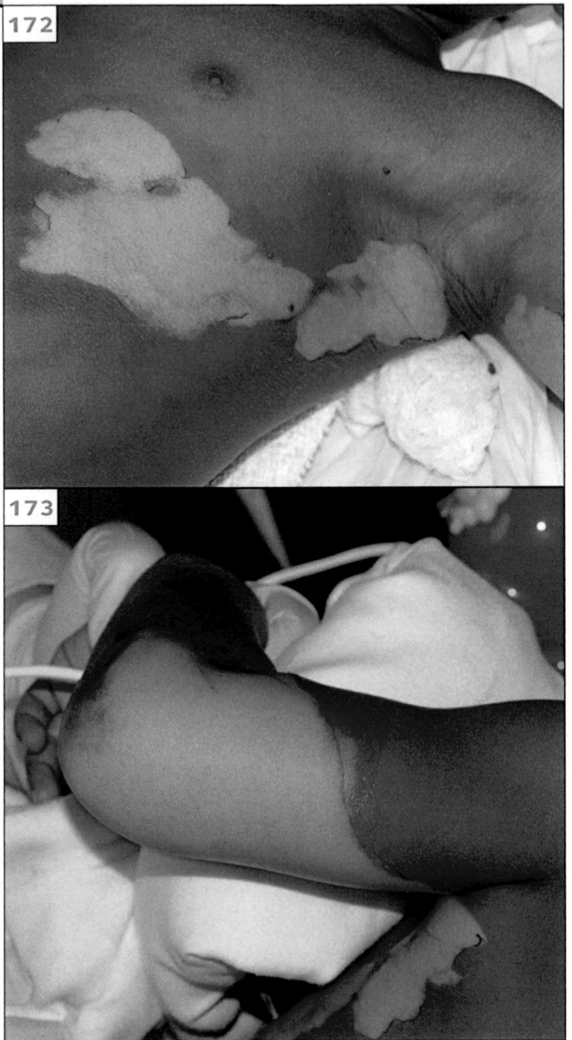

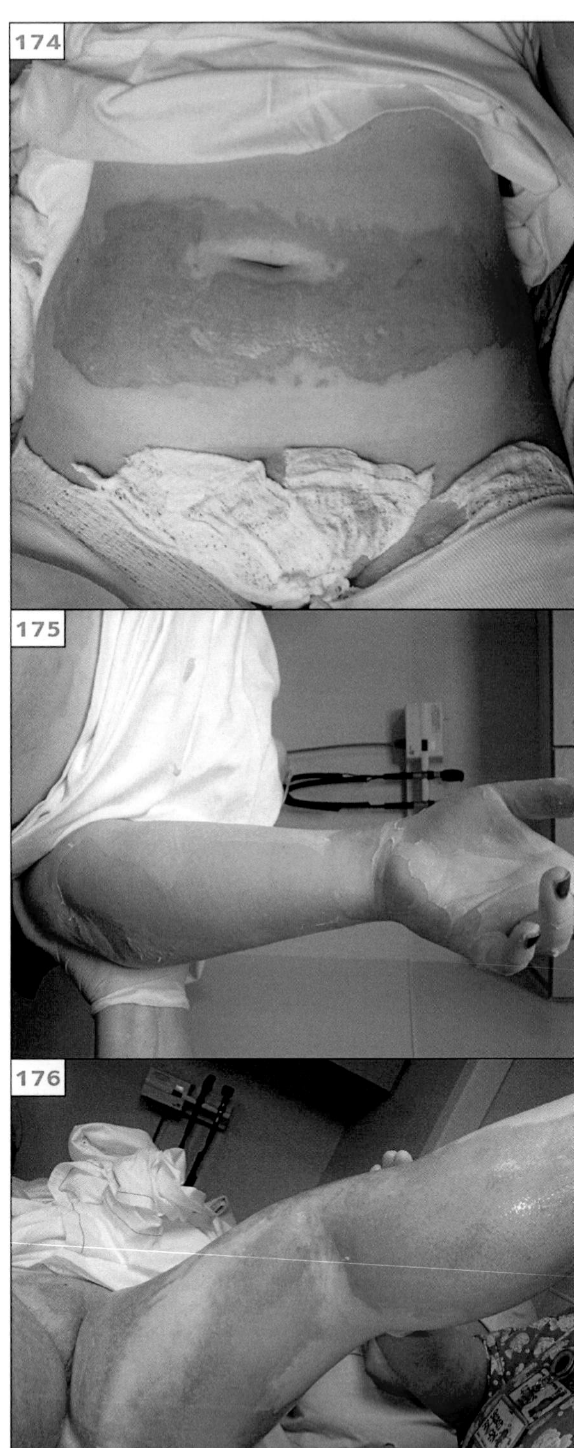

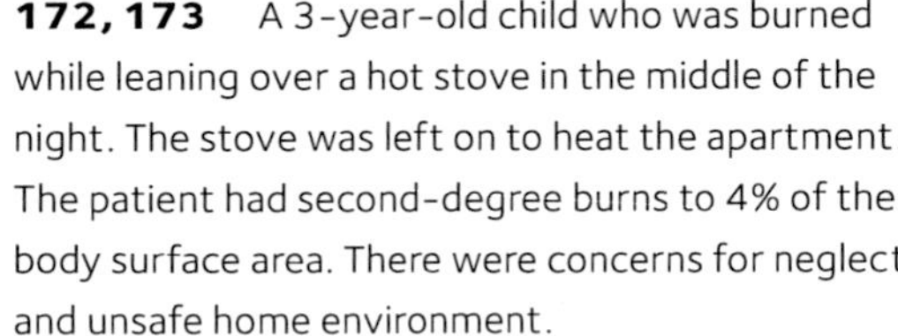

172, 173 A 3-year-old child who was burned while leaning over a hot stove in the middle of the night. The stove was left on to heat the apartment. The patient had second-degree burns to 4% of the body surface area. There were concerns for neglect and unsafe home environment.

174–176 Burns occurred after the patient accidentally spilled rubbing alcohol onto herself and then lit a cigarette. Her clothes caught on fire leaving her with second- and third-degree burns to 37% of her body surface area.

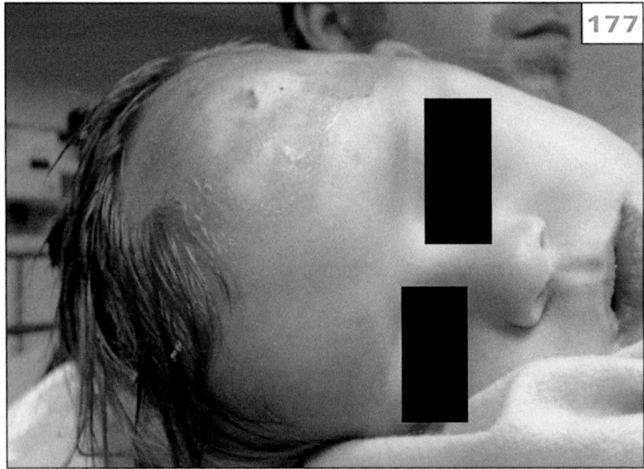

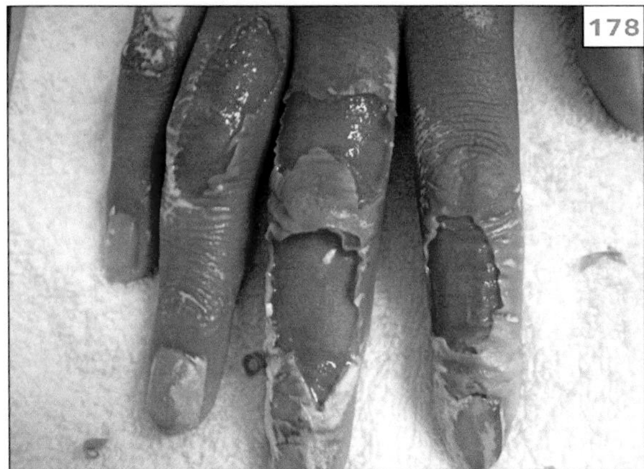

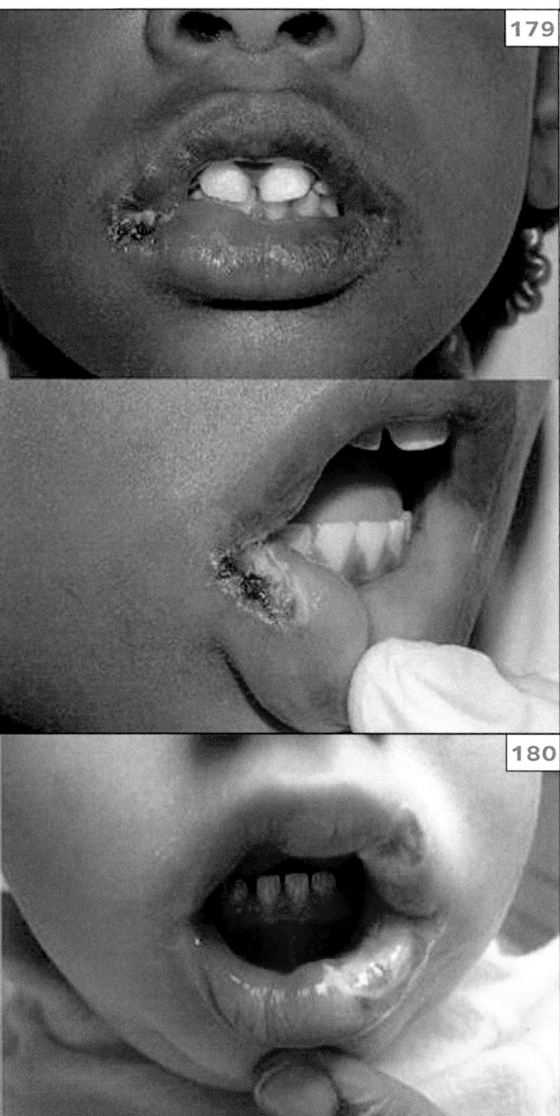

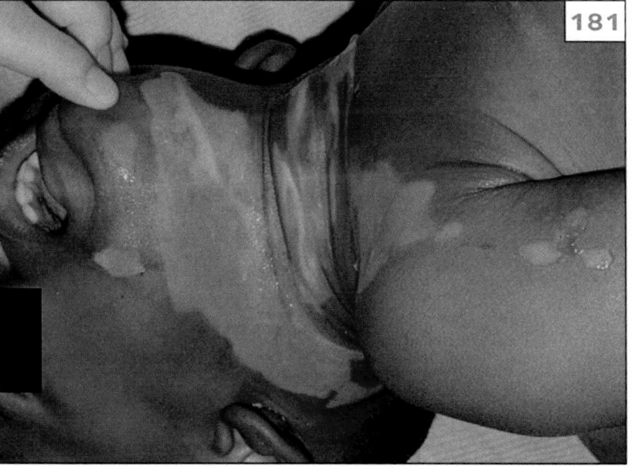

177 3-year-old whose hair caught on fire when she leaned over a lit candle. She suffered second-degree burns to her face.

178 Injuries were sustained to this patient when he was in a chemistry class at school and a test tube with chemicals exploded in his hand.

179, 180 Both patients chewed on electric cords and suffered a low voltage injury to the corner of the mouth.

181 The patient had a cold, and the grandmother heated a vapor rub in a microwave and placed it in front of patient to inhale. The patient suffered a steam burn to his face and neck.

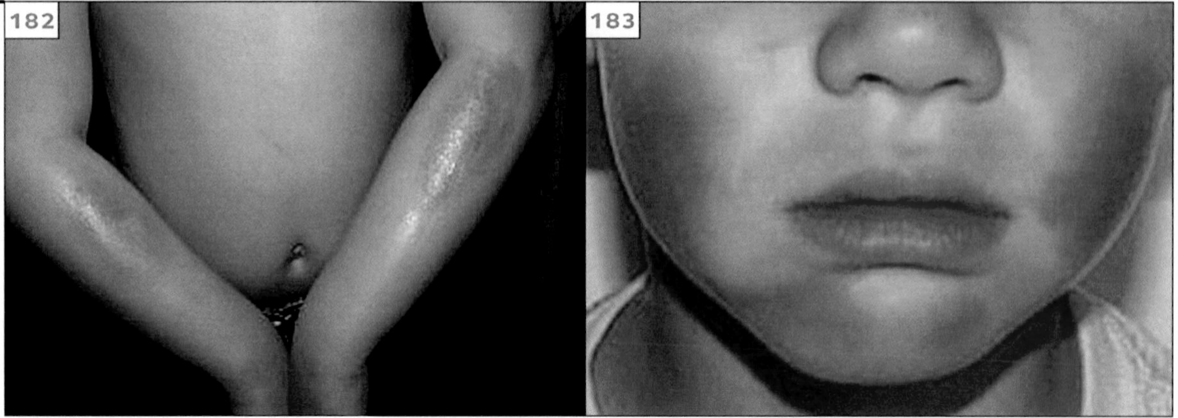

182, 183 A 5-year-old child was using a 'magic eraser sponge' to remove crayon from the wall. The patient rubbed the sponge against his arms and face and was chemically burned. Many of these products contain an alkaline agent that can cause significant burns and skin irritation. There were no warnings on the package about the potential danger of this product.

Assessment

When assessing a burn, physicians not only need to think about intentional injuries, but neglect as well. 'Neglect is the omission by the caregiver to take minimal precautions for the proper supervision of the child's health, thus failing to protect the child from injury.'[12] As Greenbaum *et al.*[11] put it, 'Infants need supervision in almost everything. If McDonald's can be sued for serving hot coffee to its adult customers, it is time that parents bear serious responsibility when their infants suffer scalds at home… burns from negligence can be prevented.'

A study undertaken by Chester *et al.*[16] in the United Kingdom found burns from neglect to be more prevalent than intentional burns in their patient population. They also found that victims of neglect have burn distributions and patterns akin to those of accidental burns, but their social histories are similar to those of victims of abusive burns. The similarities between these groups can make recognizing neglect victims difficult. A mutidisciplinary approach is critical in evaluating these cases. Neglect should always be considered when evaluating burn patients, because victims of neglect are at risk for further neglect, abuse, or even death (**184–188**).

The assessment of children with nonaccidental burns must be undertaken in a thorough and systematic manner. The initial investigation is medical and is the responsibility of the medical team. The subsequent management is a team approach with the combined efforts of the medical team, social work, protective services, and police. The physician's role is not to give a personal opinion of the caregiver, but to use his or her medical knowledge and experience to help determine how an injury may or may not have occurred. It is also the physician's duty to identify children at risk and document and record their history and physical findings.[12] When a pattern of injury is suspicious for abuse and the circumstances surrounding the event are consistent with abuse, reporting is mandatory.[17] Abusive burns should always be considered when the burn pattern is not compatible with the reported mechanism of injury or the patient's developmental capabilities, the child has other injuries or signs and symptoms of neglect, and there is delay in seeking medical treatment. The physical examination will often reveal well-demarcated burns with an absence of splash marks, a stocking-glove pattern of injury, isolated burns to the buttocks and genitalia, burns on the posterior aspect of the body, and, with contact burns, a well-defined outline of an object.

The medical documentation of a child's injuries should be thorough and complete. The depth and full extent of the burn may be difficult to determine

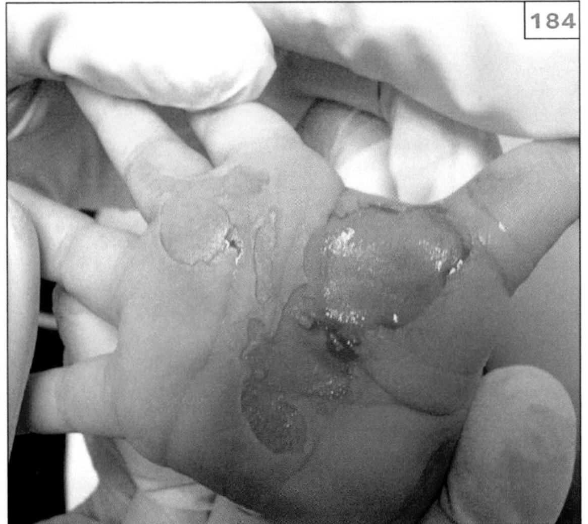

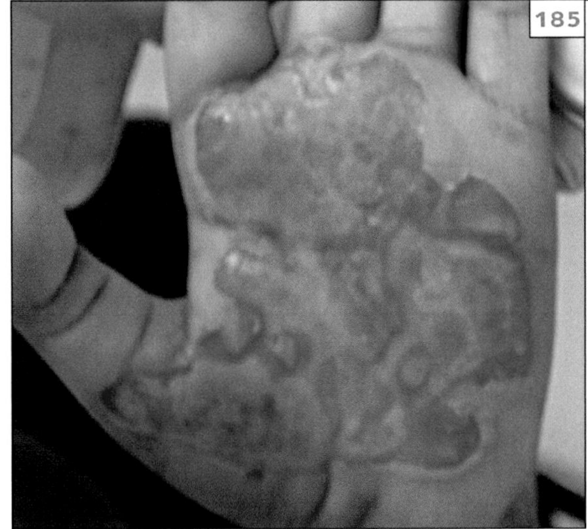

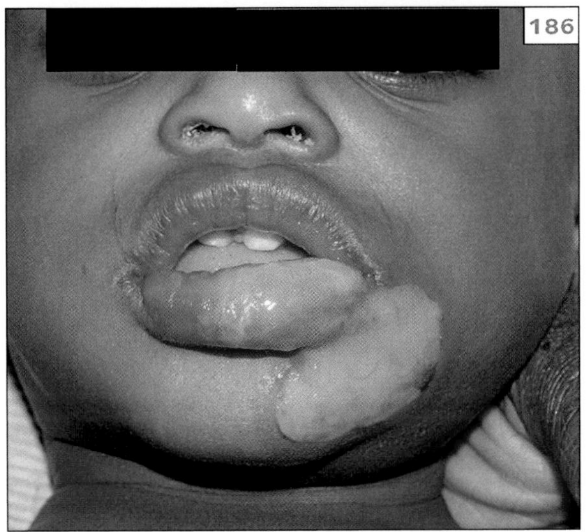

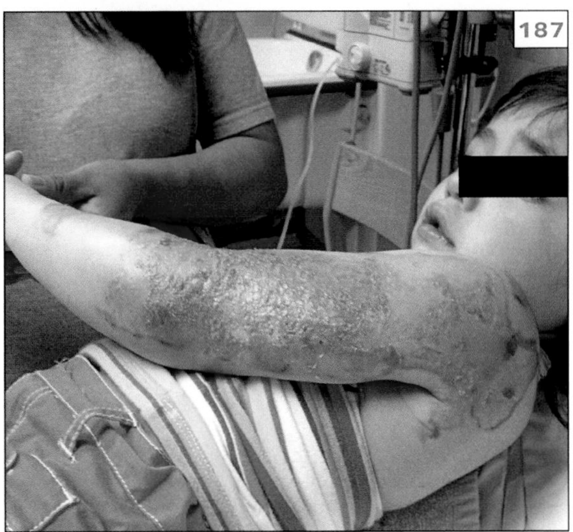

184 The patient grabbed an exposed heater in the house. This injury has physical characteristics consistent with an accidental injury; however, on further investigation, it was found that the family had had multiple referrals to the child protective services. There was concern for neglect and a new report was filed.

185 The patient had caught a hot iron 2 days before presenting for treatment. The patient's mother had been dressing the wound at home and did not seek medical treatment. There were concerns for neglect.

186 The patient was given oatmeal that was too hot and suffered a second-degree burn to the side of her mouth.

187 Family members could not provide the prescribed outpatient treatment for this burn. The injury was neither cleaned nor properly cared for and a report was filed for medical neglect.

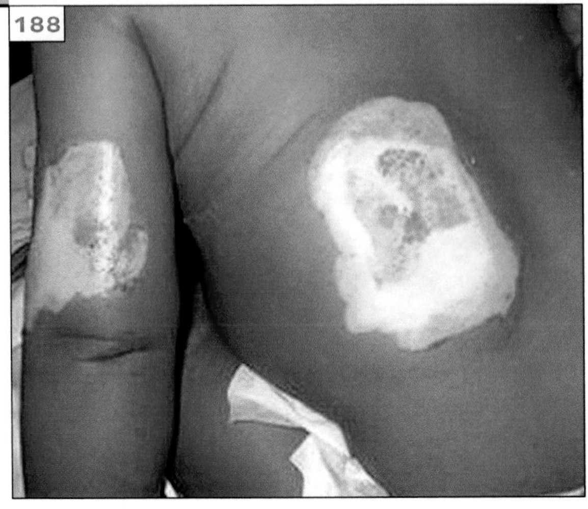

188 Patient and family were staying in the basement of their home to be near the water heater as they did not have central heating. The patient became wedged between the water heater and the mattress in the basement.

in the first 24 hours, and the injury will need to be re-examined daily. Photographs of the injury should be taken by a medical photographer (if available) as soon as the patient is stabilized and should be taken at various stages of healing, at different angles, and with the child in different positions. Measurements of the injuries should be taken and it is helpful to place a ruler next to the injury in photographs. Photographs can help determine water height and the position of the child when the injury occurred.[12] Recording these injuries is 'fundamental to the competent care of these patients'[11].

Teaching points

- Abusive burning occurs all too frequently, and physicians caring for children need to be able to identify risk factors in the family and characteristics of burn injuries which can help differentiate abusive from accidental burns.
- Through examination, documentation, and scene investigation are important in determining the potential cause of burns in children.
- There is overlap in some of the patterns, but abusive burns tend to be deeper, require more treatment, and affect different parts of the body than do accidental burns.
- While a developmentally consistent or accidental cause may be likely in some cases, physicians should also consider the degree of supervision and the potential for neglect when assessing the causation of burn injuries.

Acknowledgments

The author would like to thank Heather Schaewe RN, BSN, CPN, trauma/burn nurse clinician at Children's Hospital of Michigan and David Allasio, LMSW, clinical social worker at Children's Hospital of Michigan Burn Unit for their contributions to this chapter. They are both dedicated members of the burn team and work to ensure the health and safety of children on a daily basis. Thank you for your help and for all you do.

Chapter 4

CUTANEOUS CONDITIONS MIMICKING CHILD ABUSE

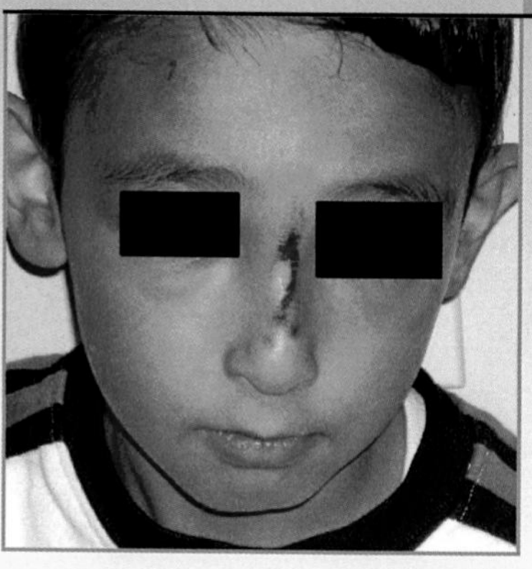

Dena Nazer MD and
Mary Smyth MD

Introduction

Cutaneous lesions are the most common presenting manifestation of child abuse[1]. Many diseases affecting the skin may be mistaken for child abuse. Such misdiagnoses may be due to an unusual presentation of a disease, the presence of a rare disorder, or because of the physician's unfamiliarity with the disease. A high-risk social situation may also lead to the misdiagnosis of abuse[2]. Thus, it is of vital importance to become familiar with a number of skin conditions that mimic child abuse and the features that differentiate them from true child abuse. A thorough medical history and physical examination in addition to laboratory testing in certain conditions are the most important skills used to differentiate such conditions. However, it is important to remember that children with conditions mimicking child abuse may also be victims of abuse.

In this chapter, the skin conditions mistaken for abuse are divided into those mistaken for bruises and those mistaken for burns. A few conditions may be mistaken for both bruises and burns depending on the stage of the lesion. We will focus on the characteristic features that differentiate these conditions from abuse.

Skin conditions mistaken for abusive bruising

Accidental injuries

Trauma resulting in the appearance of bruises may be accidental in nature and play-related in active children. These bruises are typically small and nonspecific in configuration. Important 'mimics' of abusive bruises are those caused by accidents (see Chapter 2, Bruises) (**189**). It is important to remember that abusive bruises differ from accidental bruises in that accidental bruises are generally located on bony prominences: the shins, knees, hips, spinous process of the vertebral column, chin, forehead, elbows, and extensor surfaces of the forearms[2,3] (**190–192**). Some accidental injuries may be patterned or simulate child abuse (**193**). However, these injuries usually have a mechanism of causation that is consistent with the clinical findings. In addition, bruises, abrasions, and sometimes bullae resulting from tight clothing, socks, or friction marks from shoes and sandals are other findings that may mimic physical abuse (**194–197**). Abrasions resulting from shoes and sandals may be mistaken for burns (**198**). A thorough history of how the injury occurred and having the caregiver bring in the clothing in question are necessary to establish the diagnosis (**199**).

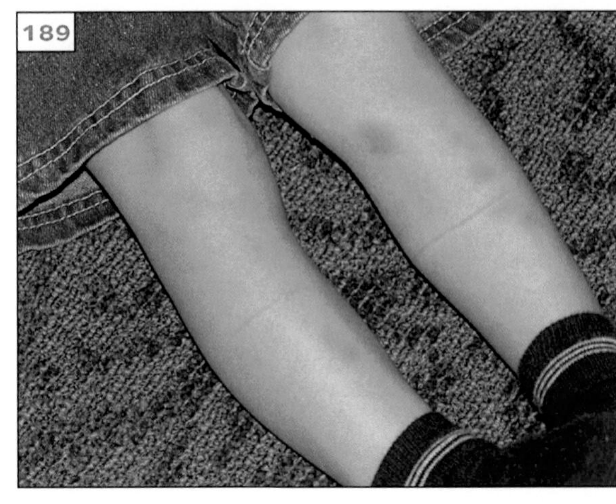

189 Accidental bruises in an active 3-year-old boy. Notice the nonspecific, nonpatterned bruises on bony prominences (both shins). Photograph courtesy of Earl R. Hartwig.

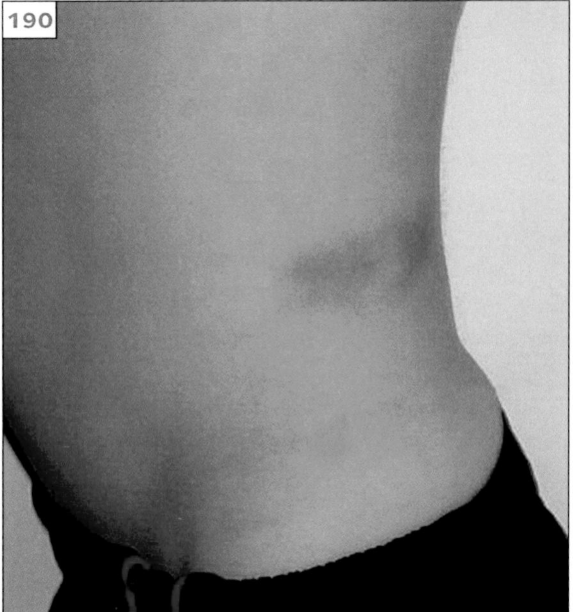

190 An active 4-year-old child with bruising over his left hip and a history of falling in the playground. The diagnosis was accidental trauma. The bruising is consistent with the fall and is located over a bony prominence. Photograph courtesy of Dena Nazer.

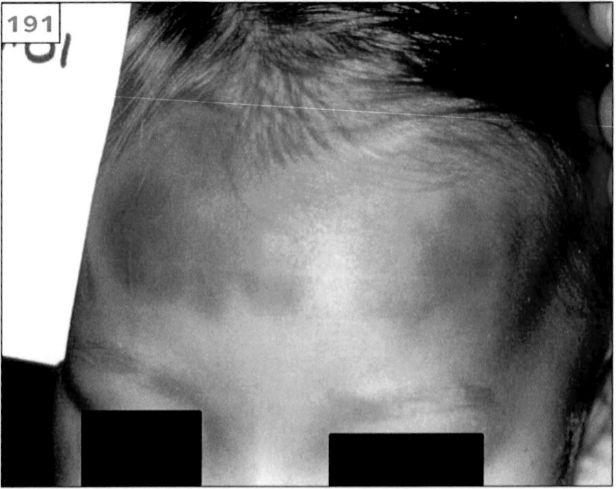

191 A child with bruising of her forehead. The diagnosis was head banging. Photograph courtesy of Mary E. Smyth.

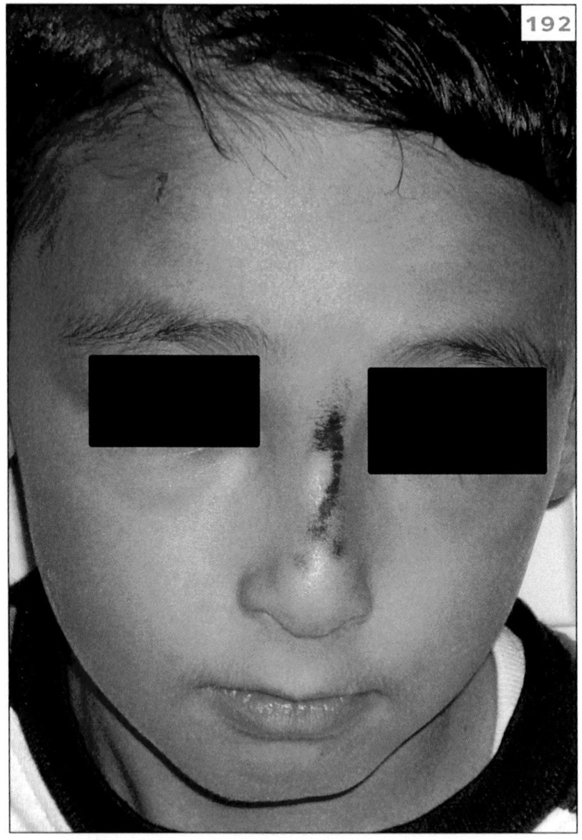

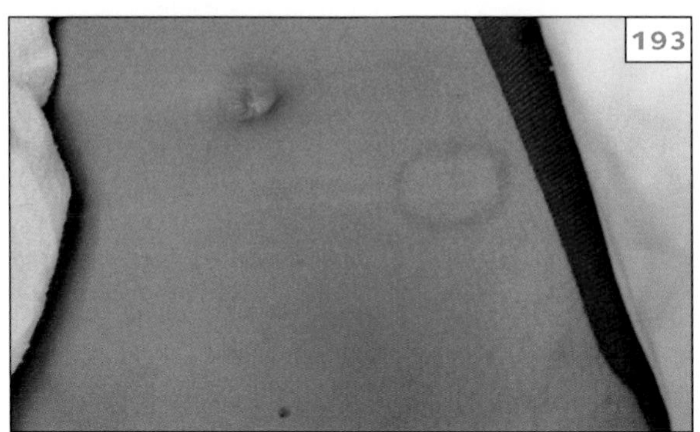

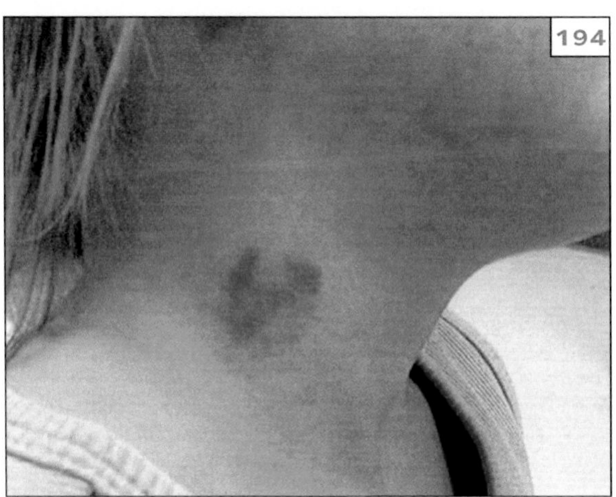

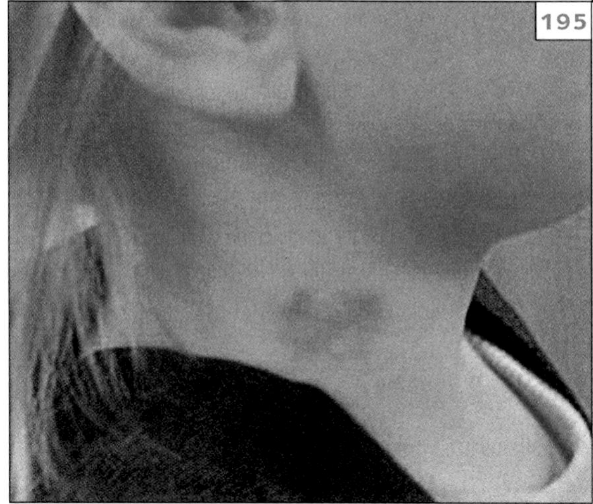

192 A 4-year-old boy with a nose abrasion sustained when he fell while playing on a carpeted floor. Photograph courtesy of Dena Nazer.

193 A patient with a lesion resembling a bite mark. Further history revealed he fell off his bicycle and the handle of his bicycle caused the bruising. Photograph courtesy of Earl R. Hartwig.

194 A 6-year-old girl referred by protective services for evaluation of sexual abuse due to suspected suction marks noticed on her neck. Reproduced with permission from *Consultant for Pediatricians*, photograph courtesy of Stephen Messner.

195 The same child as described in 194. Notice how the straps from the backpack aligned perfectly with the lesions. When the child walked, the straps rubbed against her neck. The diagnosis was friction-induced petechiae. Reproduced with permission from *Consultant for Pediatricians*, photograph courtesy of Stephen Messner.

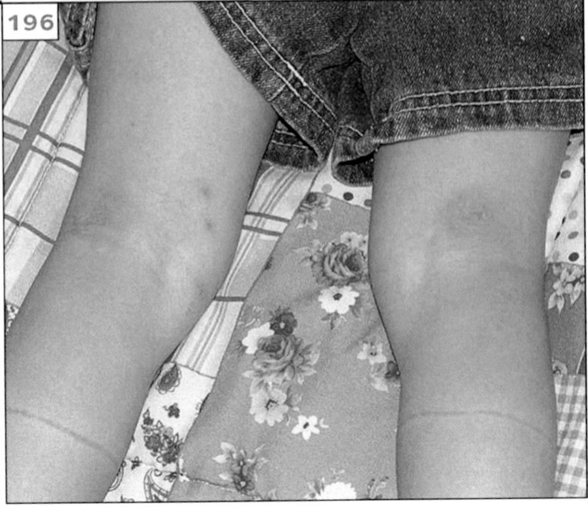

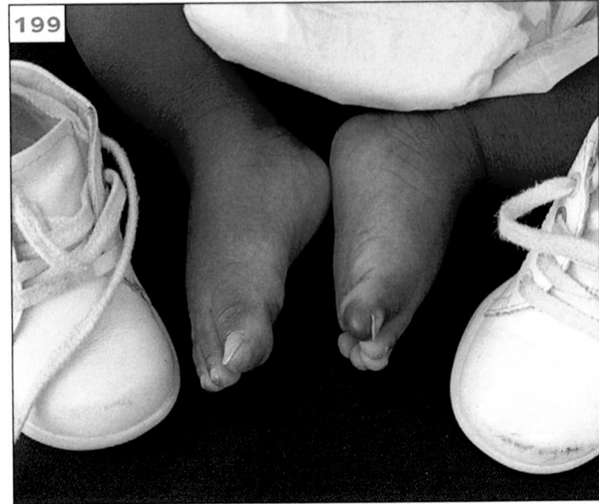

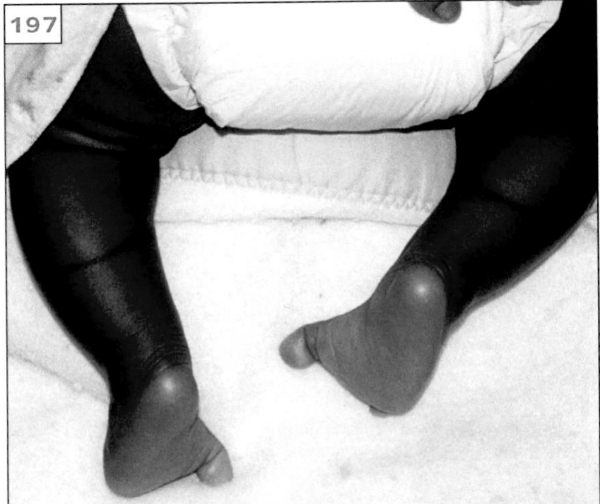

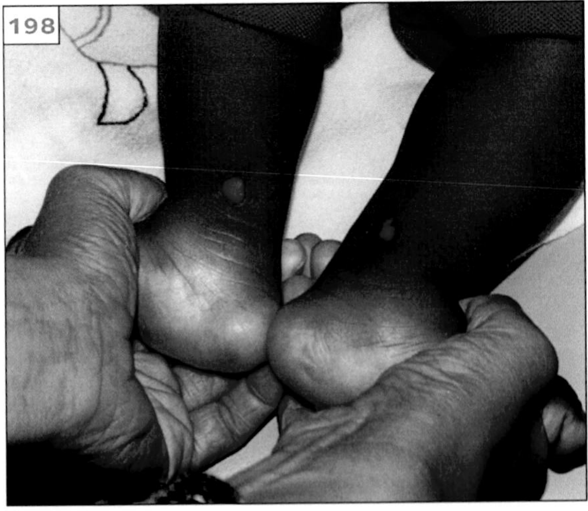

196 A 4-year-old child with constriction marks from tight elastic in his socks. Photograph courtesy of Earl R. Hartwig.

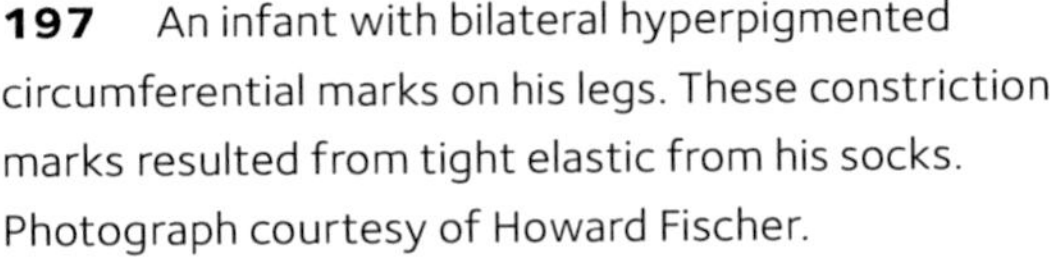

197 An infant with bilateral hyperpigmented circumferential marks on his legs. These constriction marks resulted from tight elastic from his socks. Photograph courtesy of Howard Fischer.

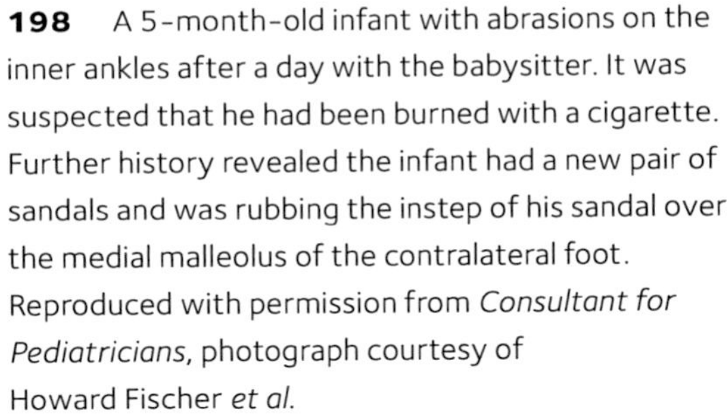

198 A 5-month-old infant with abrasions on the inner ankles after a day with the babysitter. It was suspected that he had been burned with a cigarette. Further history revealed the infant had a new pair of sandals and was rubbing the instep of his sandal over the medial malleolus of the contralateral foot. Reproduced with permission from *Consultant for Pediatricians*, photograph courtesy of Howard Fischer *et al.*

199 An infant with bilateral pressure bullae on his big toes from shoes. Photograph courtesy of Tor A Shwayder.

Mongolian spots

Mongolian spots are gray or blue-gray hyperpigmented macules of irregular shape and size[1]. They are most often located on the back, buttocks, and sacral region, but can be seen virtually anywhere on the body (**200–202**). They are caused by a relative overabundance of melanocytes in the skin in these locations. Mongolian spots can be mistaken for bruises due to their gray-blue color and their distribution on the lower back and buttocks, a common area of abuse. Distinguishing features in the history include their presence at birth. On physical examination, they are nontender and do not evolve in color, in contrast to bruises which are tender and evolve over days. They usually disappear by 4 to 5 years of age. On occasion, they may persist into adulthood[3,4]. If physical abuse is still a concern, the child can be re-examined in 7–10 days. Mongolian spots will still be present; bruises should be resolving or resolved by that time. If the lesions are extensive or in unusual locations, document the findings in the child's record and obtain photographs. This may spare parents future accusations.

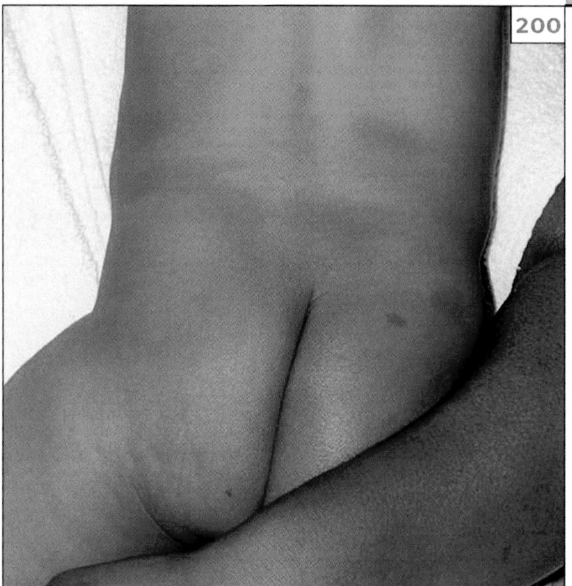

200 A 6-month-old baby girl brought for examination by child protective services due to bruising noted at a child care facility. Further history revealed the lesions noted were present from birth. Examination reveals numerous large areas of hyperpigmentation to the buttocks and lower back, as well as extremities. There was no swelling or tenderness noted and the edges exhibited a 'soft margin' which gradually blended with surrounding skin. No other lesions were noted. The diagnosis was Mongolian spots. Photograph courtesy of Earl R. Hartwig.

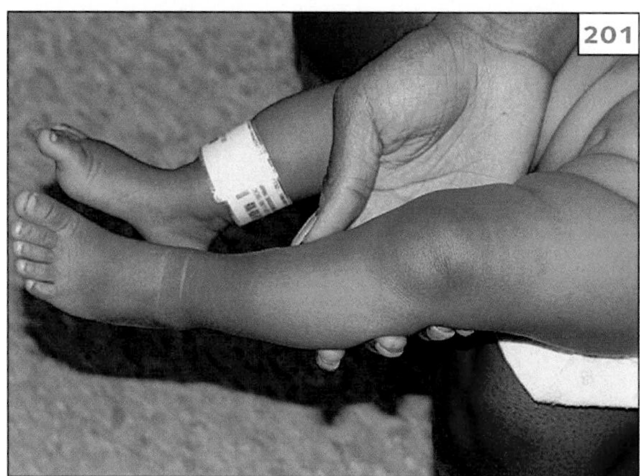

201 The same infant as described in 200. Notice the hyperpigmentation around the ankle. The diagnosis was Mongolian spots. Photograph courtesy of Earl R. Hartwig.

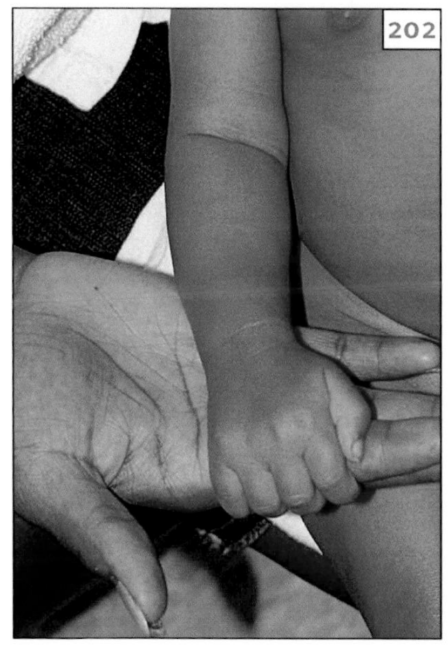

202 The same infant as described in 200. Notice the hyperpigmentation around the wrist. Photograph courtesy of Earl R. Hartwig.

Vasculitis

Henoch–Schönlein purpura (HSP) is a small-vessel vasculitis resulting in a characteristic purpuric rash and may involve multiple organ systems[5]. There may be a prodrome of fever, headache, and malaise lasting a few days. A rash typically located on the legs and buttocks follows and may occur in crops. Patients may also have abdominal pain and arthritis. The illness can last from one to several weeks and there may be recurrences. The most notable physical examination finding in HSP is the classic purpuric rash. It begins with pink or red macules and papules, which become purpuric over time, with the color changing to purple and brown as the lesions fade. The rash typically begins on the lower extremities and buttocks, but subsequent crops may involve other areas of the body. There may be accentuation of the rash in dependent areas, such as the scrotum, or over pressure points, such as the feet, wrists, and ankles giving an appearance suggestive of bruises, and may be confused with those resulting from physical restraints (**203–205**). The diagnosis of HSP is clinical. Differentiation from physical abuse is made primarily through the history and clinical presentation and the associated systemic involvement in HSP.

Erythema multiforme is a self-limited erythema thought to be due to a skin reaction to infectious agents, such as herpes simplex and mycoplasma, or drugs, such as penicillin and sulfonamides[3]. There may be a history of cold sores. The child may have systemic findings in the form of low-grade fever and myalgia. Skin lesions are erythematous, symmetric, and fixed papules that darken. They are predominantly acral, but may develop in any area of the body and evolve into the characteristic target lesions (**206**). Severity ranges from a minor self-limited form to a major form (Stevens–Johnson syndrome), which involves mucous membranes and has serious systemic consequences. The sudden appearance of these ecchymotic lesions with no history of trauma leads to the misdiagnosis of child abuse[3].

Disorders of blood vessels

Hemangiomas are vascular malformations. They may be mistaken for bruises. The lesions grow rapidly during the first 6 months of life, plateau in growth rate for the next 6–12 months, then regress. Maximum regression is usually reached between 5 and 10 years of age.

Common locations include the scalp, head, neck, and facial structures, such as the eyelids and lips. Less commonly they are seen on the sacrum, vulva, clitoris, and hymen[6]. Bleeding lesions on areas such as the lip have been mistaken for lesions produced by trauma associated with physical abuse (**207–209**). Hemangiomas on the genital area have also been confused with bruising, raising a suspicion of sexual abuse (**210, 211**). Any lesion that might be confused with a lesion produced by abuse should be documented in the child's primary medical record and followed on subsequent physical examinations.

Coagulation disorders

Bruising or persistent bleeding may result from coagulation disorders. These disorders include congenital disorders, e.g. von Willebrand disease, hemophilia, and acquired disorders, such as immune thrombocytopenic purpura (ITP) and vitamin K deficiency[2]. The resulting bruises and bleeding may be diagnosed as nonaccidental in nature. These lesions can be differentiated from abuse by a thorough history, physical examination, and laboratory evaluation. Children with coagulation defects may have a personal and a family history of easy bruising. Some patients with hemophilia may have a history of prolonged bleeding at circumcision or at cord separation. Those with von Willebrand disease have mild to moderate bleeding tendencies resulting in easy bruising, nose bleeds, and prolonged bleeding after dental procedures. On physical examination, petechiae may be present in addition to bruises in patients with ITP (**212–214**). The configuration, but not the severity, of bruising is consistent with the mechanism of injury in patients with clotting factor deficiencies (**215**). Laboratory studies include a complete blood count, platelet count, prothrombin time, and partial thromboplastin time. In certain cases where a clotting factor deficiency is suspected, a full coagulation profile and additional studies may be needed.

Malignancies

Neuroblastoma is a malignancy of the peripheral sympathetic nervous system. Many infants and children present with a mass, often in the chest or abdomen, frequently with metastases to lymph nodes or other sites. Abdominal pain may be the chief complaint. Symptoms related to metastases include fatigue, fever, weight loss, irritability, bone pain, subcutaneous blue nodules, peri-orbital ecchymoses, and proptosis. Patients who present with peri-orbital ecchymoses and swelling, especially if no mass is easily identified, have been mistaken for victims of child abuse (**216**). Associated symptoms of neuroblastoma, physical examination, laboratory and imaging studies help differentiate it from abuse. Leukemia and other oncologic conditions resulting in thrombocytopenia may also present with petechiae, ecchymoses, and bleeding after minor trauma. Clinical presentation, physical examination, and a complete blood count assist in initial evaluation.

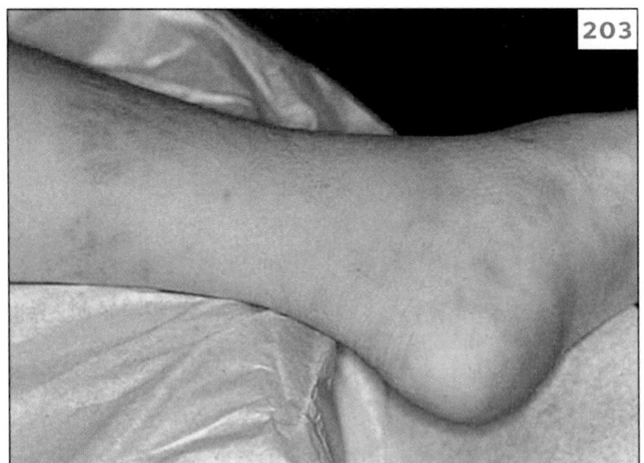

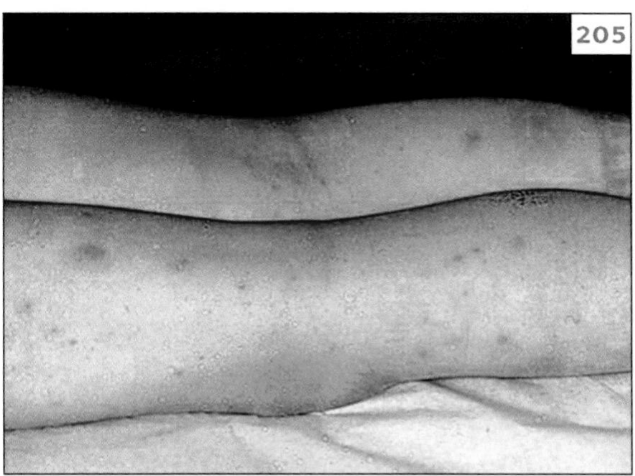

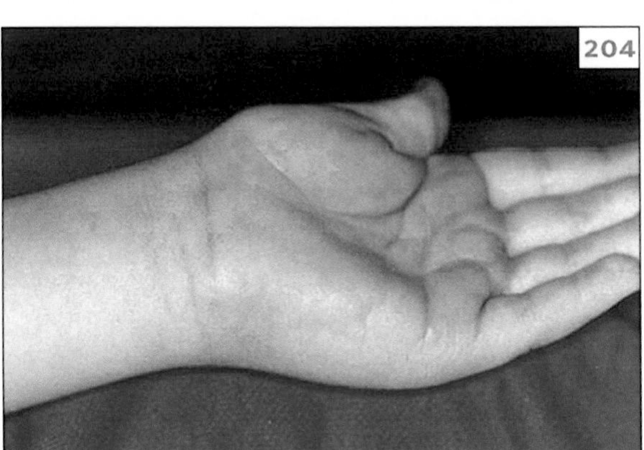

203 A child referred to the child protection team for suspicion of physical abuse and ligature marks around the wrists and ankles. The diagnosis was Henoch–Schönlein purpura (HSP) with bruising around constriction marks from the clothes as a result of vasculitis. Photograph courtesy of Mary E. Smyth.

204 The same child as described in 203 with bruising around the wrists. The diagnosis was Henoch–Schönlein purpura (HSP). Photograph courtesy of Mary E. Smyth.

205 The same child as described in 204. Once the child was undressed, the purpuric rash was visible over the posterior thighs and buttocks. The diagnosis was Henoch–Schönlein purpura (HSP). Photograph courtesy of Mary E. Smyth.

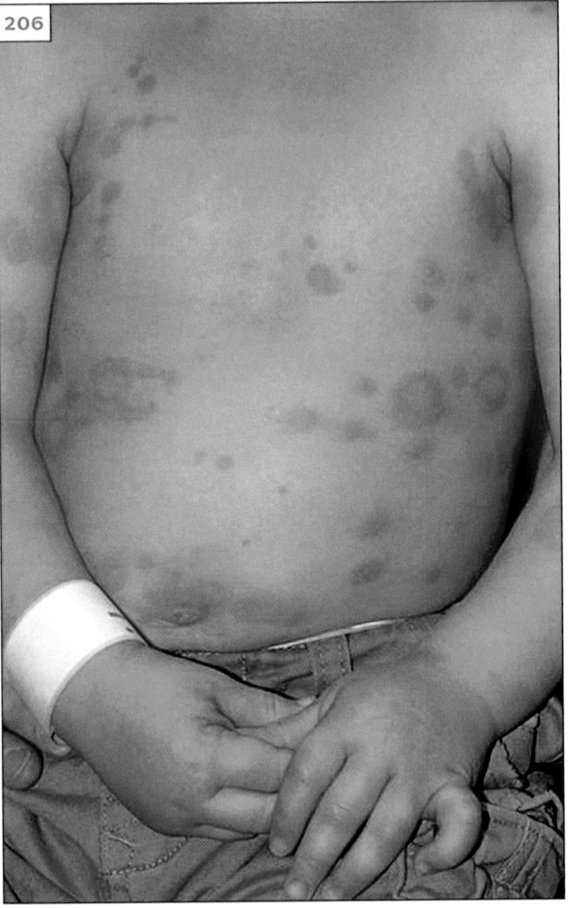

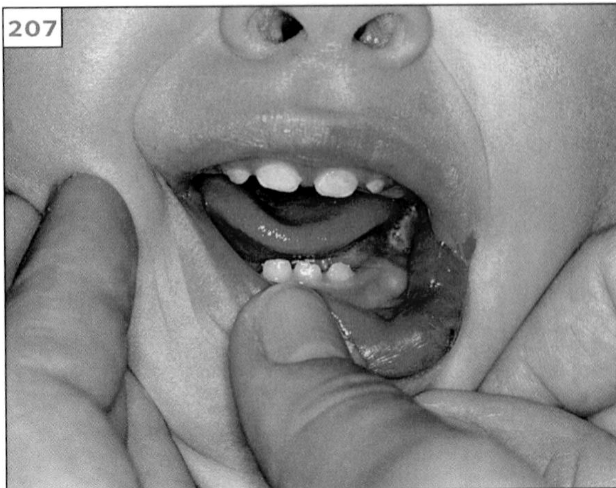

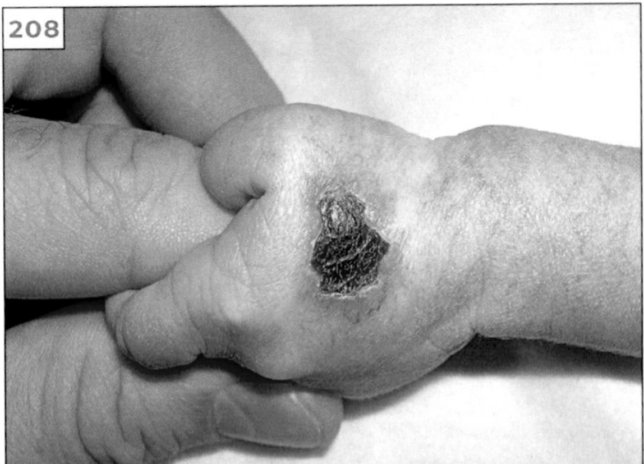

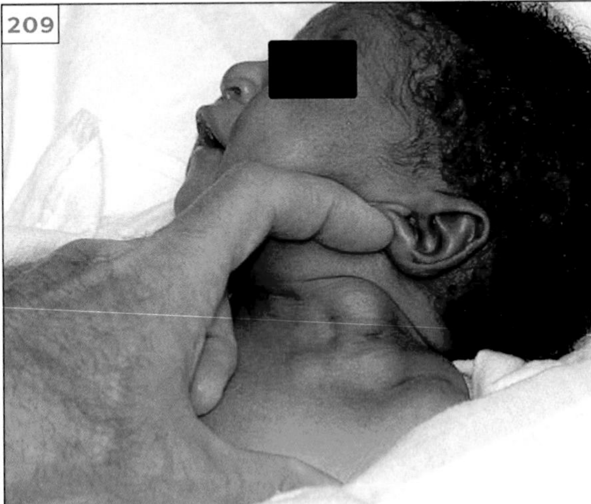

206 A child who presented with fever and a rash. The diagnosis was erythema multiforme. Notice the characteristic target lesions. Photograph courtesy of Earl R. Hartwig.

207 A child who presented with bleeding and suspected oral trauma. Further history and examination revealed a hemangioma of the lower lip which was friable and bled easily. Photograph courtesy of Mary E. Smyth.

208 A 4-day-old baby with an ulcerated hemangioma on his hand. Photograph courtesy of Tor A. Shwayder.

209 An infant with a vascular malformation. Photograph courtesy of Earl R. Hartwig.

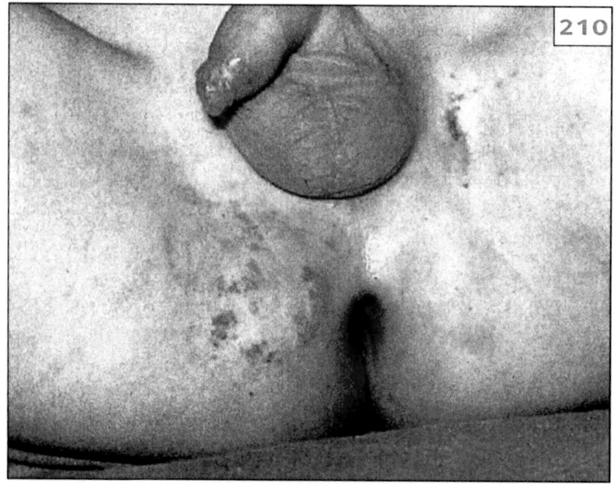

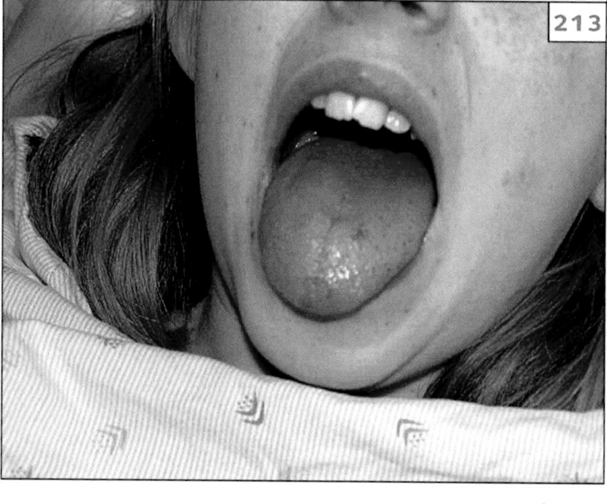

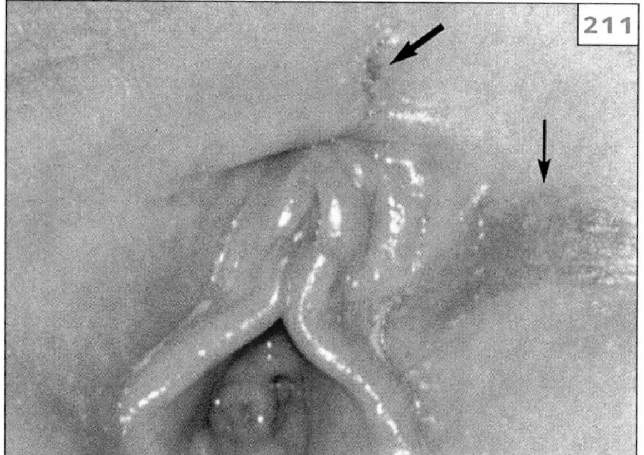

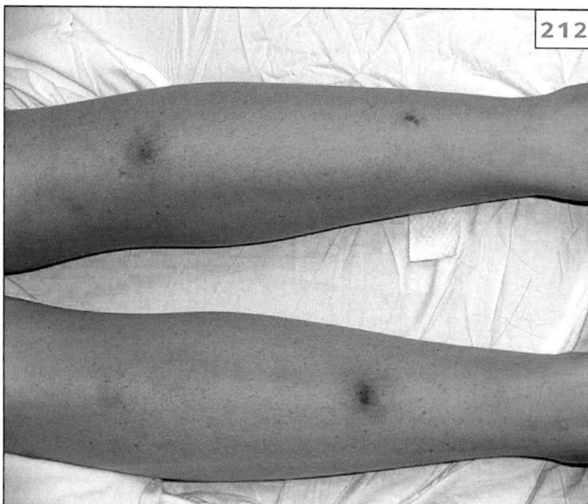

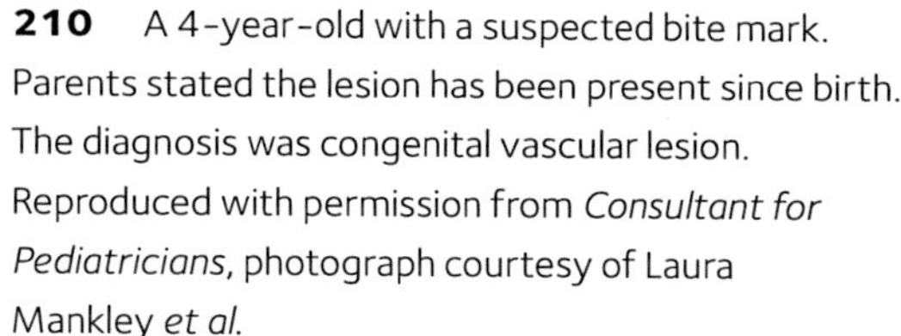

210 A 4-year-old with a suspected bite mark. Parents stated the lesion has been present since birth. The diagnosis was congenital vascular lesion. Reproduced with permission from *Consultant for Pediatricians*, photograph courtesy of Laura Mankley *et al.*

211 A 12-month-old with a suspected genital abrasion referred to child protective services. Further history revealed the lesion has been present since birth. The diagnosis was hemangioma. The thick arrow points to a small anterior commissure fissure probably created by traction during the examination. Reproduced with permission from *Consultant for Pediatricians*, photograph courtesy of Laura Mankley *et al.*

212 An 11-year-old girl with petechiae and bruises. Laboratory studies revealed thrombocytopenia. The diagnosis was immune thrombocytopenic purpura (ITP). Photograph courtesy of Earl R. Hartwig.

213 The same child as described in 212. Notice the petechiae on her tongue. The diagnosis was immune thrombocytopenic purpura (ITP). Photograph courtesy of Earl R. Hartwig.

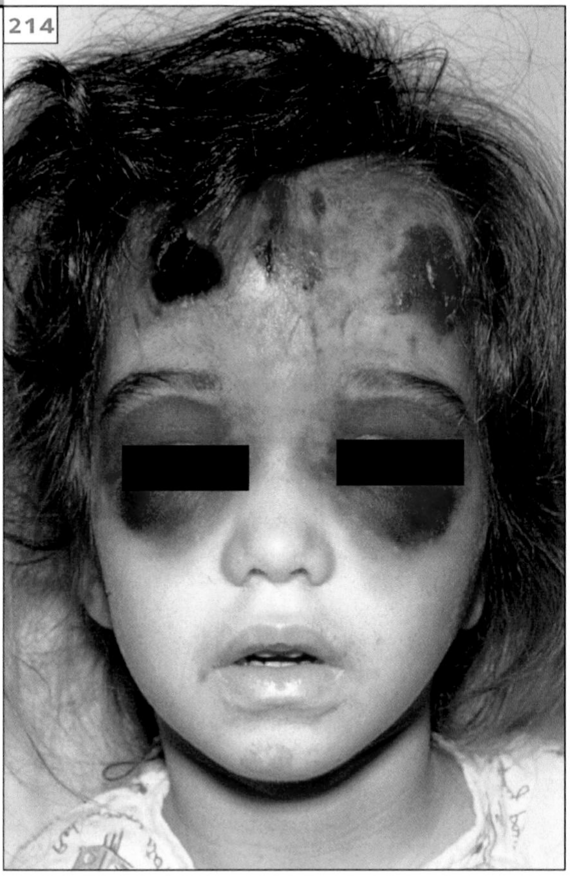

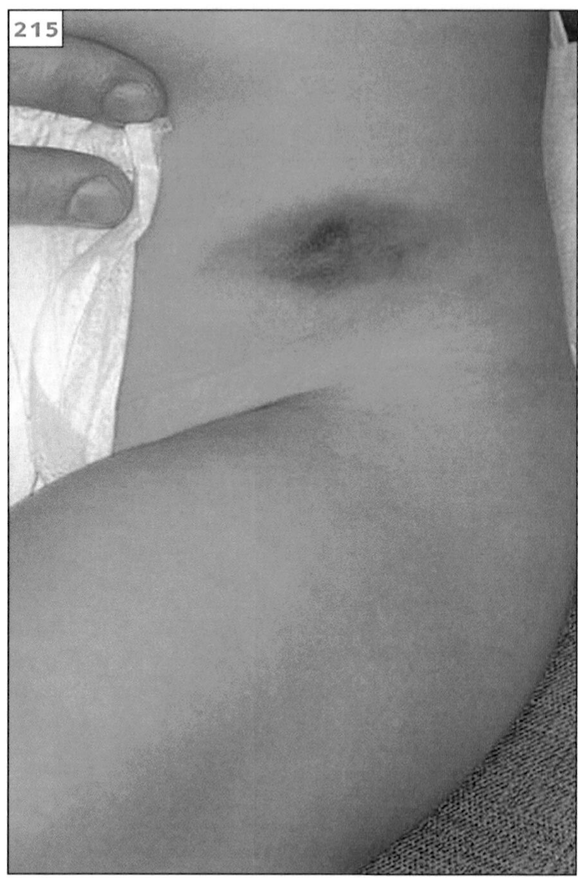

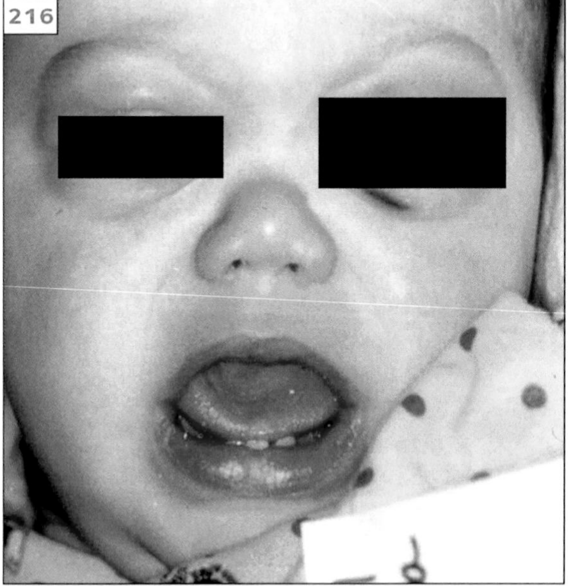

214 A child with immune thrombocytopenic purpura (ITP) and history of trauma to her face when she walked through revolving doors. Photograph courtesy of Earl R. Hartwig.

215 An 11-month-old baby with a bruise overlying his anterior superior iliac crest after he started crawling. The diagnosis was hemophilia B. Notice how even with minor trauma the bruises still occurred in typical locations over the bony prominences. Photograph courtesy of Earl R. Hartwig.

216 An infant presented with bilateral peri-orbital swelling and ecchymoses. The diagnosis was neuroblastoma. Photograph courtesy of Mary E. Smyth.

Collagen synthesis defects

Ehlers–Danlos syndrome is a rare connective tissue disease associated with skin lesions that may mimic physical abuse[2]. Patients with this syndrome have skin hyperelasticity, easy bruisability, and joint hypermobility (**217, 218**). The skin after minor injury and healing is described as 'cigarette paper thin'. The skin of children affected with this syndrome is hyperelastic, velvety, and fragile. Children with Ehlers–Danlos syndrome may present with gaping scars and a history of multiple lacerations with poor healing resulting from minor trauma[1]. Recurrent joint dislocation may result from the joint hypermobility. A detailed family history and physical examination may help differentiate this condition from abuse. Osteogenesis imperfecta (OI) is a heterogeneous disorder characterized by abnormality in quantity or quality of type 1 collagen synthesis. Type 1 OI is associated with easy bruising, blue sclerae, hearing impairment, and osteopenia (**219**). Child abuse may be suspected due to the bruising and the fractures, especially when caused by minor trauma[7–9].

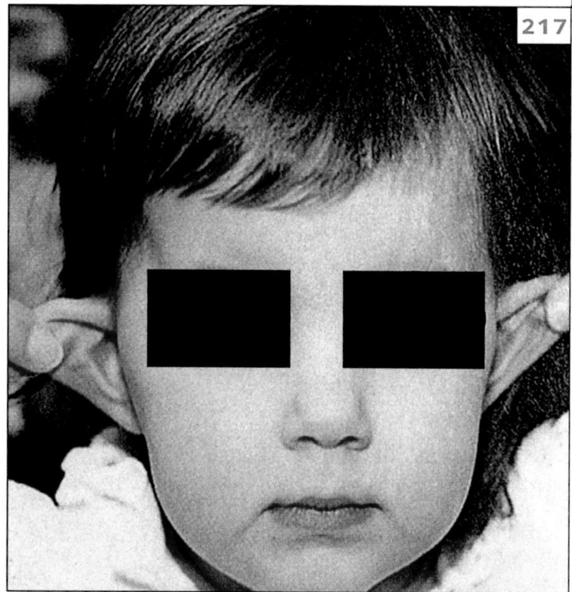

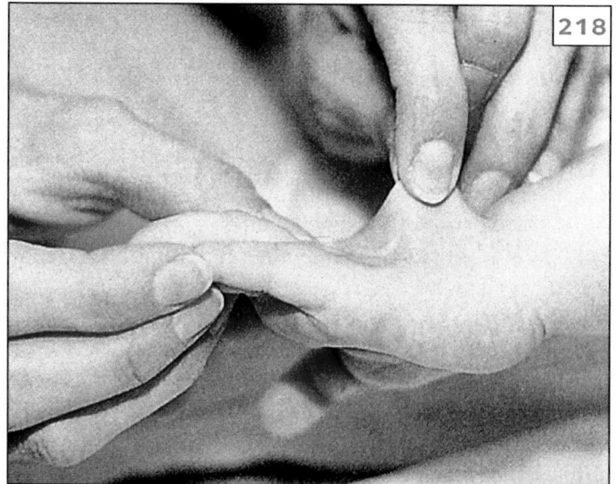

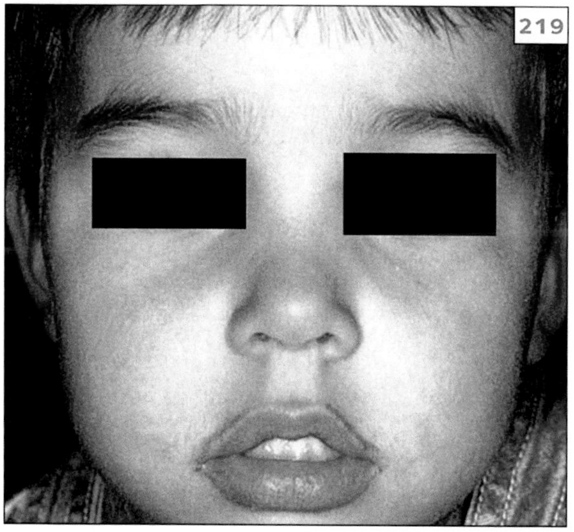

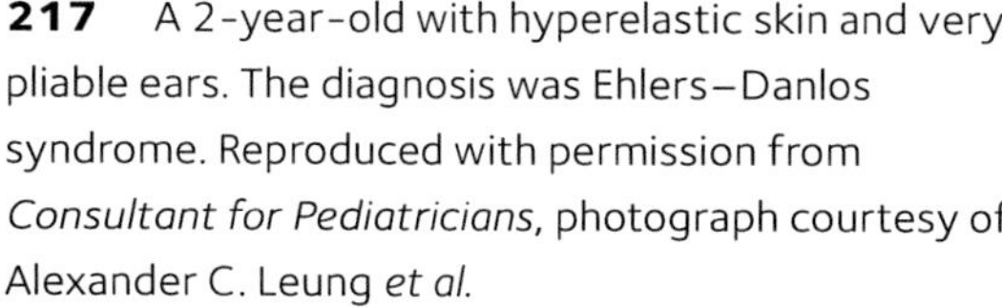

217 A 2-year-old with hyperelastic skin and very pliable ears. The diagnosis was Ehlers–Danlos syndrome. Reproduced with permission from *Consultant for Pediatricians*, photograph courtesy of Alexander C. Leung *et al.*

218 A 2-year-old with hyperelastic skin and hyperextensible joints. The diagnosis was Ehlers–Danlos syndrome. Reproduced with permission from *Consultant for Pediatricians*, photograph courtesy of Alexander C. Leung *et al.*

219 A 3-year-old boy who presents with blue sclera, a history of tibial fracture following a short fall, and easy bruisability. The diagnosis was osteogenesis imperfecta type 1B. Reproduced with permission from *Consultant for Pediatricians*, photograph courtesy of Daniele Pacaud *et al.*

Cultural practices

There are several cultural practices that one must be aware of because they may produce findings confused with child abuse. While these practices are not intentionally abusive, they may result in skin conditions mimicking bruises or burns. It is important, however, to be sensitive to cultural practices and ask the parents about such practices in a nonjudgmental way to obtain the needed history[10–12]. Coining is a southeast Asian cultural remedy[11]. It is used to treat a variety of symptoms including fever, headaches, seizures, and vomiting. The edge of a coin or other object is rubbed over oiled skin resulting in ecchymoses and petechiae from the rubbing and stroking. Ecchymoses are usually linear due to the downward linear way the coin is rubbed on the skin. Spooning, similar to coining, is another folk remedy resulting in bruising. Water is applied to the neck, shoulders, back, chest, or forehead. The area is then pinched or massaged until it reddens and is then rubbed with a porcelain spoon until ecchymotic lesions appear. Cupping is an Eastern European, Latin American, and Asian cultural remedy. It is used to treat various symptoms, for example, fever, pain, and poor appetite[10]. A glass is heated to create a vacuum and applied to the skin. A circular bruise or a cluster of petechiae result from the suction created by the vacuum. Burns may also result from this practice.

Other conditions

Systemic infections may be associated with ecchymoses and petechiae that may mimic child abuse. A careful history of associated symptoms, systemic symptoms, and laboratory tests help point towards an infectious etiology of such lesions. Dermatitis may result in pigmented lesions resembling bruises or healed burns. It may be subdivided into different types based on etiology: photocontact dermatitis, irritant contact dermatitis, contact urticaria, allergic contact dermatitis, and reactions to pharmacologically active agents.

Phytophotodermatitis is an exogenous chemical phototoxic reaction resulting from the activation of certain plants' furocoumarin (psoralen) by sun exposure after the plants or their products contact the skin.[13–19] Causative plants include lime, lemon, figs, parsnip, and celery[13]. Phytophotodermatitis typically results in hyperpigmented lesions as a chronic reaction, but may initially result in bullae and visible inflammation mistaken for burns. Lesions may be streaky with hyperpigmentation in the shape of a hand and may be mistaken for bruises (**220, 221**). In suspected cases, a history of exposure to a psoralen-containing plant followed by sun exposure may assist in diagnosis. Lesions are also uniformly deep-brown in color in contrast to the multiple hues in healing bruises[13]. Redness develops within the first 24 hours followed by development of vesicles that coalesce into bullae over subsequent days. They lack the color variations of bruises. In cases where lesions blister, they may be confused with abusive burns especially when no history is elicited[14–19]. Because these lesions mimic burns and occur with no reported history of injury, a diagnosis of nonaccidental burn may be incorrectly made.

Irritant contact dermatitis is a condition caused by direct injury of the skin. An irritant is any agent that is capable of producing cell damage in any individual if applied for sufficient time and in sufficient concentration. Allergic contact dermatitis is a type IV hypersensitivity reaction only affecting previously sensitized individuals. An example of allergic contact dermatitis is the allergic reaction to plants, such as poison ivy, poison sumac, and poison oak.

Popsicle (ice lolly) panniculitis is a benign cold-induced subcutaneous fat necrosis of the cheeks. It occurs in young children as a result of sucking on frozen confections[20, 21]. It may also be caused by ice packs or cold air. It appears as red, painless, indurated nodules or plaques on one or both cheeks. Similar lesions may develop on any skin surface. The lesions may be confused with bruises, especially with the lesions usually appearing 1–3 days after the cold exposure. Parents may not correlate the cold etiology with the lesions (**222**). A careful history of exposure to cold, asking about cold remedies for teething, and a diet history may help establish the diagnosis. In addition, the color variation of bruises differentiates physical abuse. It is best to re-examine the child if doubt still exists. Discoloration of a child's skin may mimic bruises, especially when resulting from dye from fabric, such as denim. Diagnosis is made by a history of contact with a dyed fabric that became wet and 'ran'. Patients may present with self-inflicted injuries such as tattoos, burns, scratch marks, and scars (**223**).

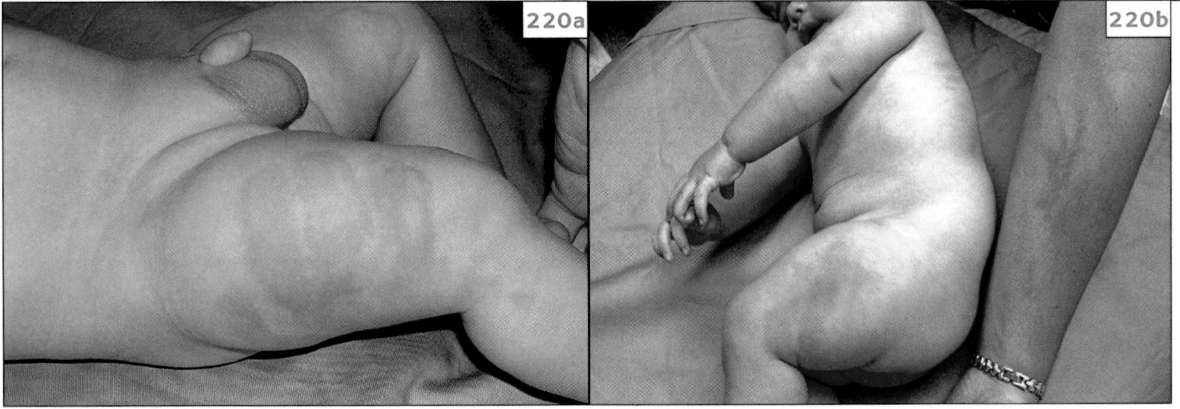

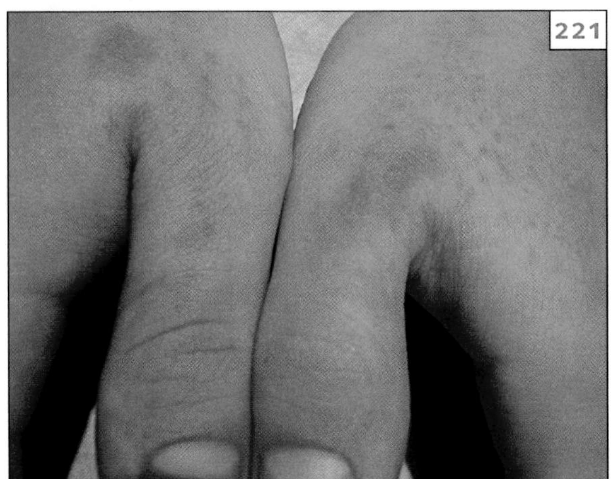

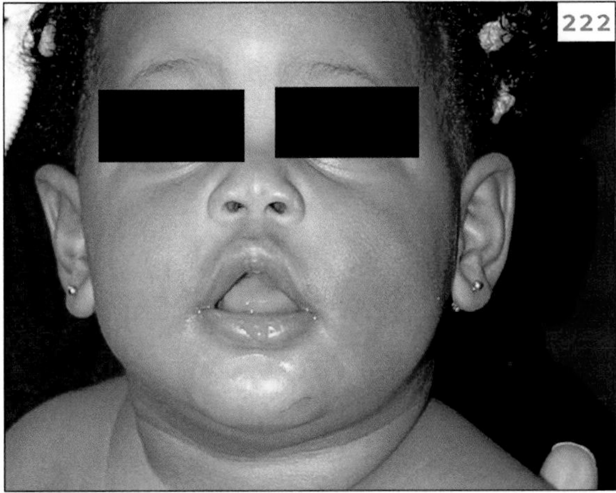

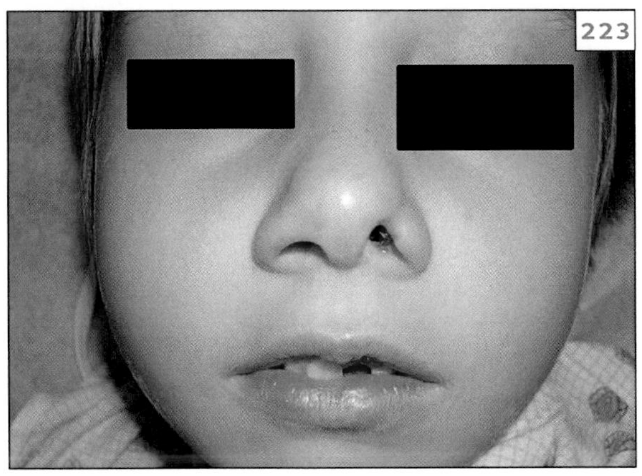

220a, b A child with phytophotodermatitis. Notice how the marks resemble handprints after the baby was held by his mother (220a). His mother also had similar lesions (220b). Photographs courtesy of Tor A. Shwayder.

221 This teenager had rapidly developing dark spots over her hands after handling limes and lemons while preparing 'Margaritas.' She then went to the beach. The lesions lasted 3 weeks and slowly faded without treatment. They could easily be confused with small burns, insect bites or inflammatory/ pigmentation disorders had the history not been obtained regarding the exposures.

222 A 7-month-old who came to her mother's custody after a visit to her father. Her mother was concerned about a bruise on her left cheek. Further history revealed a history of eating popsicles (ice lollies) while at the father's house. The diagnosis was popsicle panniculitis. Photograph courtesy of Earl R. Hartwig.

223 A child with deformity of his nose as a result of nose picking. Photograph courtesy of Tor A. Shwayder.

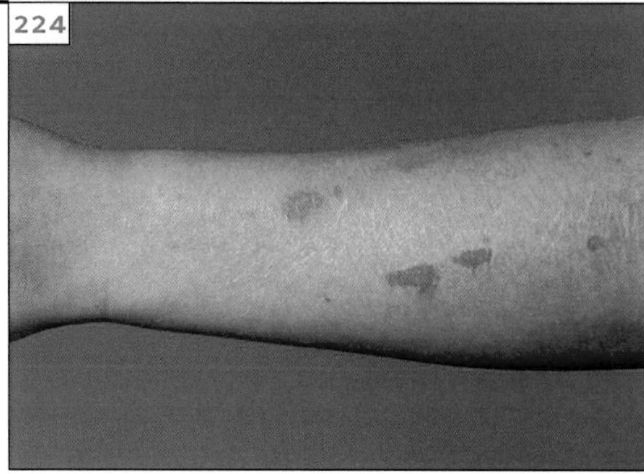

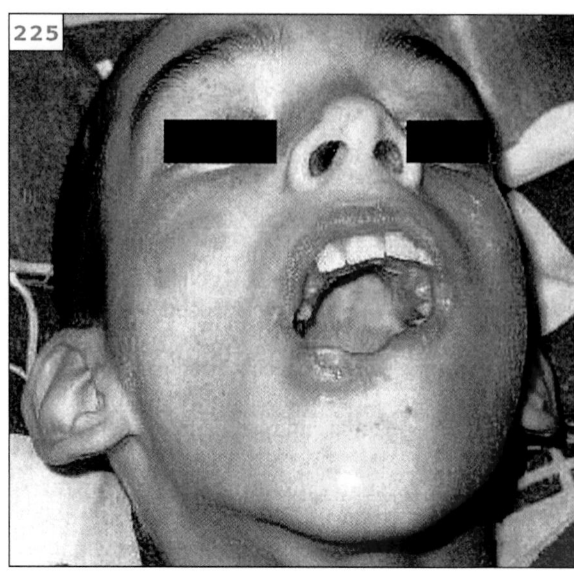

Dermatitis artefacta is the deliberate and conscious production of self-inflicted skin lesions to satisfy an unconscious psychological or emotional need (**224**). Patients are most commonly adolescents or young adults. They may have associated chronic dermatologic conditions, such as acne. History usually reveals stress, family history of psychiatric illness, and patients may disclose a childhood history of abuse or neglect. On physical examination, lesions are in areas accessible to the patient and have bizarre and variable presentations, depending on the mechanism of injury. Patients with certain diseases and syndromes may also exhibit self-injury, e.g. Lesch–Nyhan syndrome (**225**).

224 Self-inflicted scratch marks in a teenager. The diagnosis was dermatitis artefacta. Photograph courtesy of Tor A. Shwayder.

225 A 14-year-old boy with Lesch–Nyhan syndrome and chronic scarring of the lip as a result of self-mutilating behavior that characterizes this syndrome. Reproduced with permission from *Consultant for Pediatricians*, photograph courtesy of Deepak Kamat.

Skin conditions mistaken for burns

It is important to differentiate burns from other disorders that can mimic them. Conditions that may be mistaken for burns include impetigo, staphylococcal scalded skin syndrome, and epidermolysis bullosa.

Skin disorders

Blisters resulting from several dermatologic conditions may mimic burns and lead to the suspicion of physical abuse. Cellulitis results in erythema and sometimes bullae and may mimic burns (**226, 227**). Atopic dermatitis may mimic burns if superinfected and extensive (**228**). Other infections may result in blisters mimicking burns. Epidermolysis bullosa has different subtypes with various presentations. The resulting blisters may be mistaken for those of burns (**229–231**). Toxic epidermal necrolyis may also result in blisters mimicking burns (**232, 233**). Mastocytomas (urticaria pigmentosa) appear early in childhood and may appear anywhere on the skin. Rubbing may cause them to redden, swell, and sometimes blister as their histamine is released (**234**).

Diaper/nappy dermatitis may mimic burns from child abuse, especially when severe. Rashes resulting form infections with *Candida* species are intensely erythematous with sharp margins and satellite lesions. Contact diaper dermatitis usually begins as acute erythema on the convex skin surfaces of the pubis and buttocks. The skin folds are characteristically spared. Impetigo is a superficial bacterial skin infection affecting infants and children. Impetigo lesions are irregular, crusted, superficial, and heal without scarring. It is commonly seen on the face, trunk, and extremities (**235**). Impetigo is usually caused by *Staphylococcus aureus*. Group A beta-hemolytic *Streptococcus* is a frequent secondary invader. There are two types: bullous and nonbullous impetigo, which is the more common type. In nonbullous impetigo, lesions start as a macular erythema evolving into pink erosions with straw-colored fluid and subsequently crusted erosions with golden-yellow crusts. In bullous impetigo, the macular erythema vesiculates and expands into fragile bullae that break, leaving a collarette of scales surrounding the normal skin (**236**). Most cases require treatment with topical or oral antibiotics. When blisters rupture, they may leave a shallow circular ulcer that may appear like a burn[2,3]. Bullous impetigo may resemble an infected cigarette burn; however, it is more superficial and heals completely with antibiotic therapy. Both may occur in crops. Cigarette burns are usually in crops and occur commonly on the face, hands, and feet. They are usually deep, well-demarcated lesions with a central crater and they heal with scarring. Lesions are 7–10 mm in diameter. Frostbite from improper use of icepacks and cold therapy may present with swelling, pain, and discoloration of the affected area (**237**).

Xeroderma pigmentosa is a rare autosomal recessive condition characterized by decreased ability to repair DNA. Patients present with history of severe sunburn following minimal sun exposure (**238**). Burns resulting from this condition may mimic inflicted burns, especially when the history of sun exposure is minimal and there is no documented mechanism of injury (**239**). Hair tourniquet or thread tourniquet syndrome occurs when thread or hair wraps tightly around an infant's digit[1]. The area of the digit distal to the constriction becomes painful, edematous, and discolored (**240**). This may result in this condition being misdiagnosed as a nonaccidental burn. This condition is relatively common and involves the fingers, toes, or external genitalia and may mimic burns, cellulitis, or trauma. It is important when suspecting a hair tourniquet syndrome to carefully examine the area for the constricting material.

Lesions from spider bites may have characteristics simulating burns, but, unlike burns, victims report minimal discomfort immediately after the bite[22]. The bite will appear red, and a central punctum or vesicle may be seen (**241, 242**). Within a few hours, the bite site will become painful. In 12–24 hours, as the reaction to the toxin progresses through vasodilatation, vasoconstriction, and thrombosis, the lesion demonstrates the 'red, white, and blue sign' of color changes. Severe lesions may progress to cellulitis and frank necrosis (**243**). Because clinical laboratory tests are not readily available, the diagnosis of spider bites is often presumptive.

A geographic tongue may appear to be a burn but is simply nontraumatic loss of filiform papillae on the tongue. Lesions appear as reddish plaques surrounded by an irregular white border, commonly on the lateral sides and dorsum of the anterior two-thirds of the tongue[23]. Most patients are asymptomatic, although they may occasionally have a burning sensation in the tongue or sensitivity to hot and spicy food. Lesions of a geographic tongue may be mistaken for burns, especially if the condition is not recognized by the physician (**244**). This condition runs in families. The tongue findings are migratory and lack the eschar and tissue coagulation of a burn.

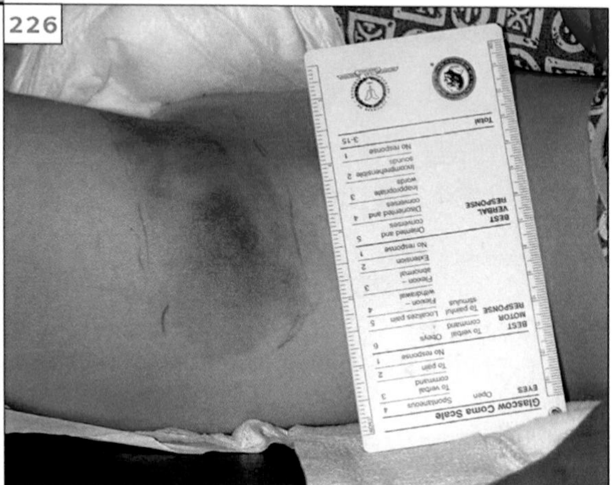

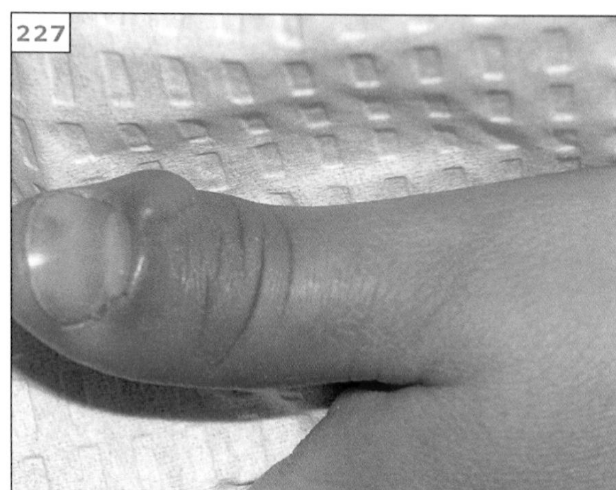

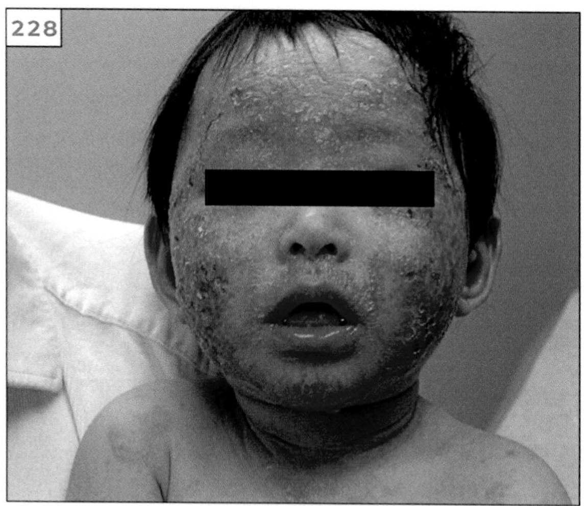

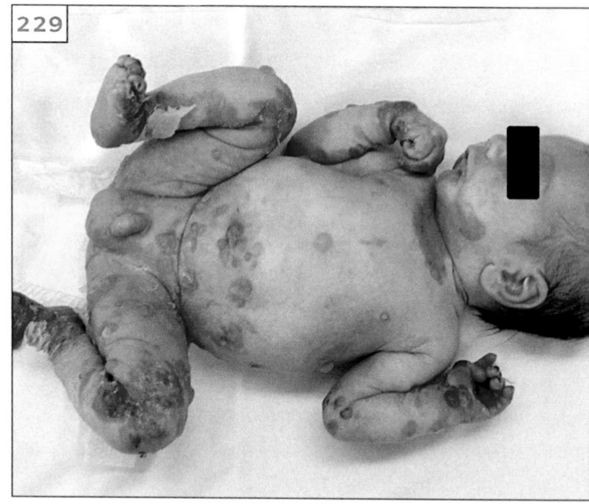

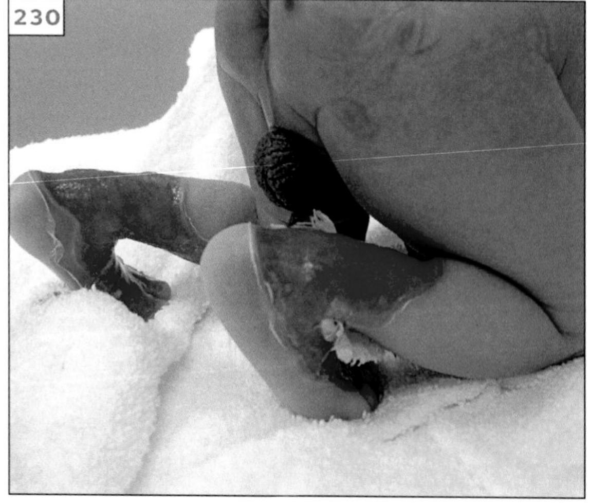

226 A patient with fever and painful erythema of her proximal thigh. The lesion is warm to touch and exquisitely tender, erythematous, and nonblanching. The diagnosis was cellulitis with suspected necrotizing fascitiitis. Photograph courtesy of Earl R. Hartwig.

227 A 5-year-old boy with blistering dactylitits. Photograph courtesy of Tor A. Shwayder.

228 A child with infected atopic dermatitis. Photograph courtesy of Tor A. Shwayder.

229 An infant with epidermolysis bullosa simplex. Photograph courtesy of Tor A. Shwayder.

230 An infant with junctional epidermolyis bullosa. Photograph courtesy of Tor A. Shwayder.

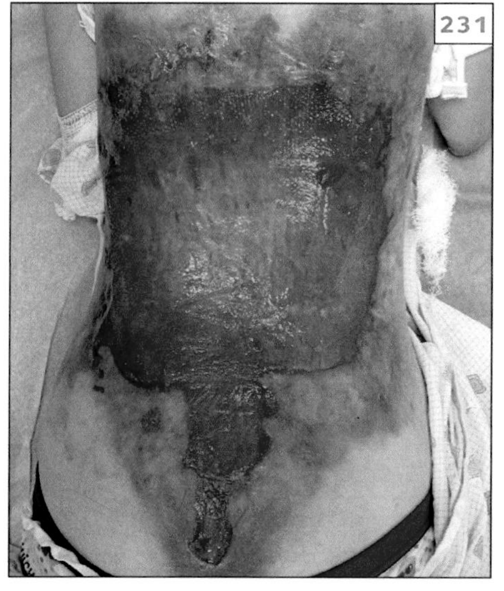

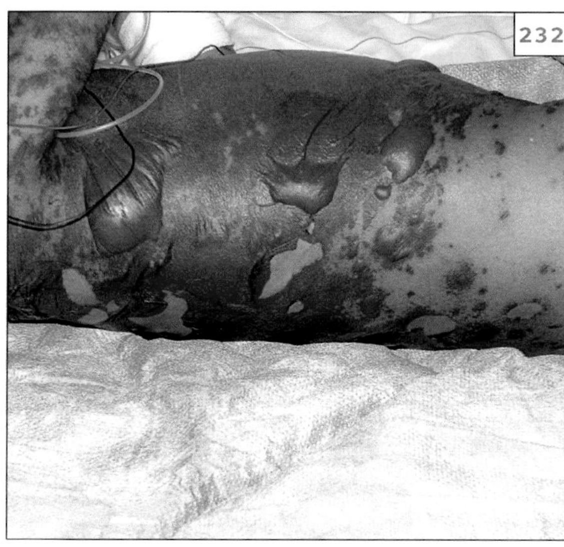

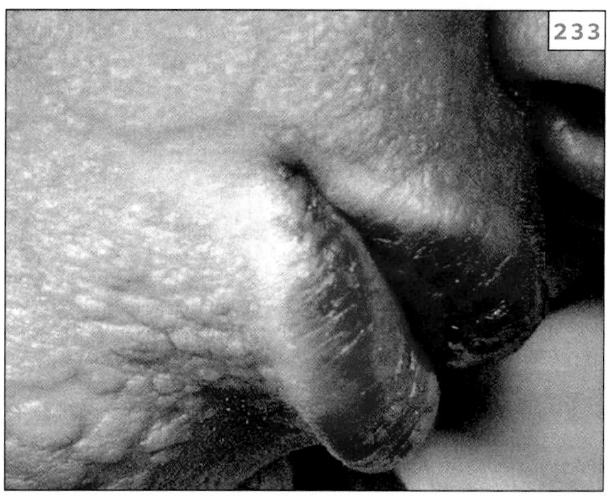

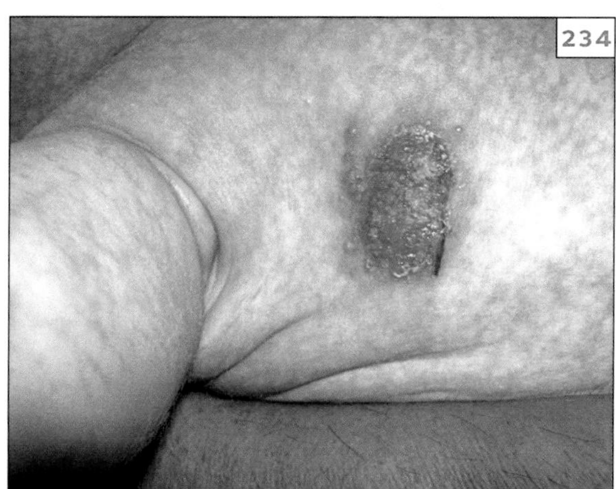

231 A 17-year-old with epidermolysis bullosa. Photograph courtesy of Tor A. Shwayder.

232 Toxic epidermal necrolyis. Photograph courtesy of Tor A. Shwayder.

233 A 15-year-old girl with an erythematous vesicular rash on the face 2 months after she started taking lamotrigine for a seizure disorder. The diagnosis was toxic epidermal necrolyis. Reproduced with permisison from *Consultant for Pediatricians*, photograph courtesy of Waldo Nelson Henriquez Barraza.

234 A 7-week-old with a blistering mastocytoma. Photograph courtesy of Tor A. Shwayder.

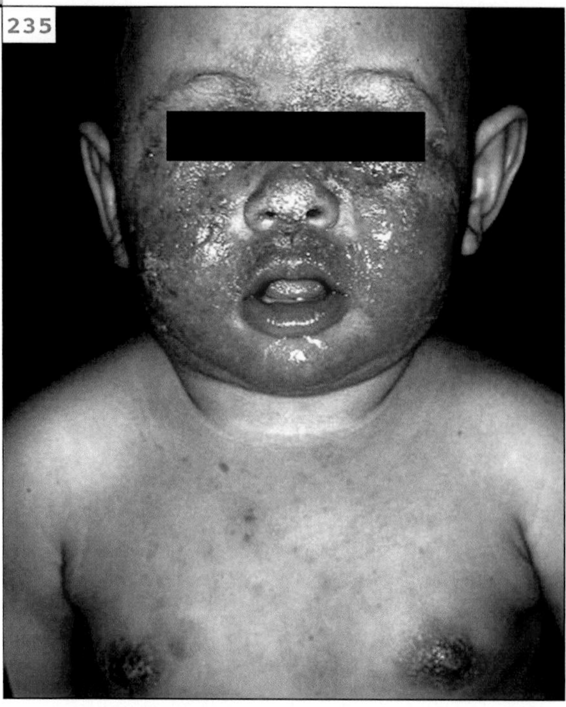

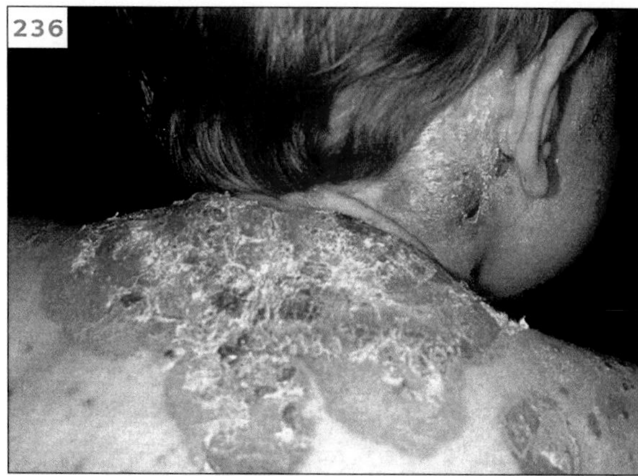

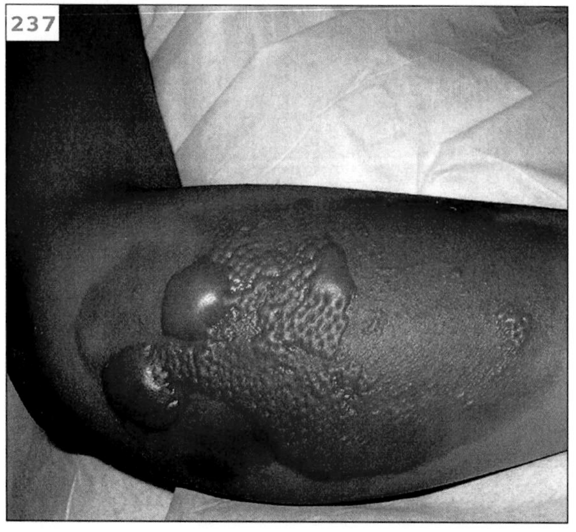

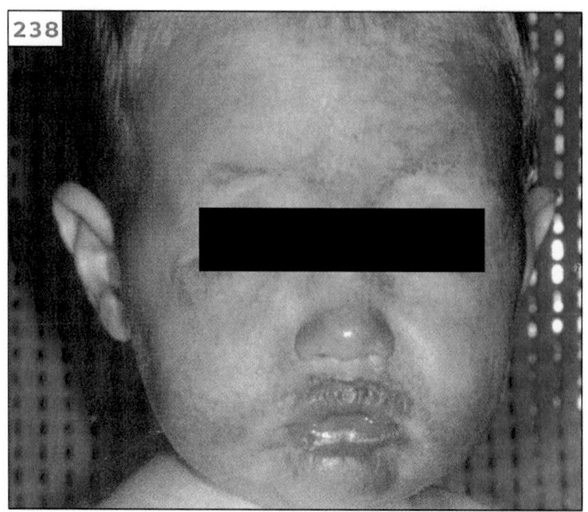

235 An infant with atopic dermatitis complicated by impetigo. Photograph courtesy of Tor A. Shwayder.

236 A 3-year-old boy with superficial blistering of his skin over the previous 3–4 months with scaling and crusting. The diagnosis was bullous impetigo. Reproduced with permission from *Consultant for Pediatricians*, photograph courtesy of Kirk Barber.

237 A 6-year-old boy who presented with increased pain, swelling, and skin discoloration. The child had a history of fall on the right arm and had fallen asleep with an icepack on his forearm. The diagnosis was frostbite. Reproduced with permission from *Consultant for Pediatricians*, photograph courtesy of Abu Khan *et al.*

238 An infant who presented with a blistering sunburn, conjunctivitis, and photophobia. He was in the shade of a large umbrella for a few minutes. The diagnosis was xeroderma pigmentosa. Reproduced with permission from *Consultant for Pediatricians*, photograph courtesy of Kirk Barber.

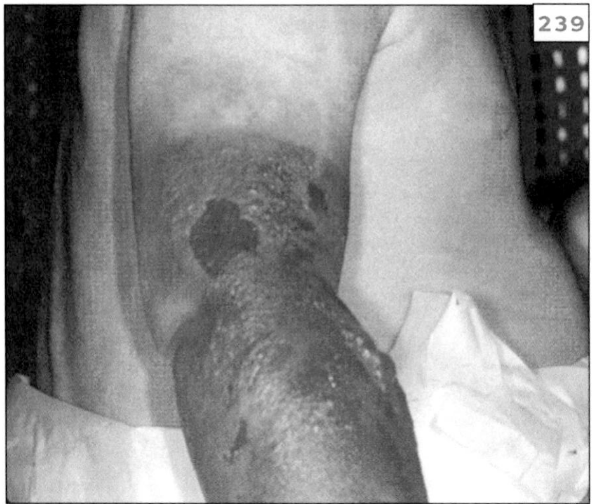

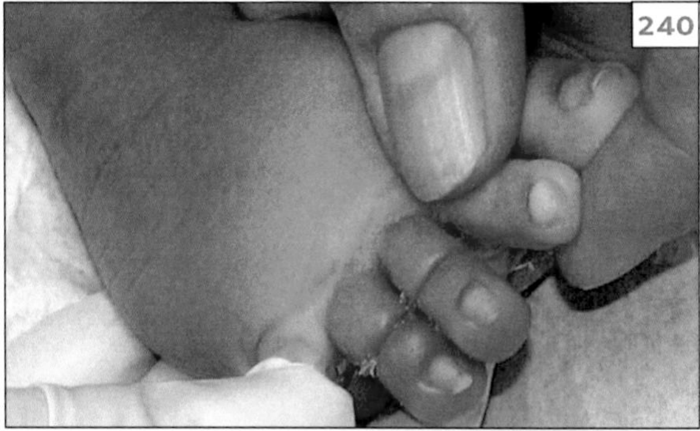

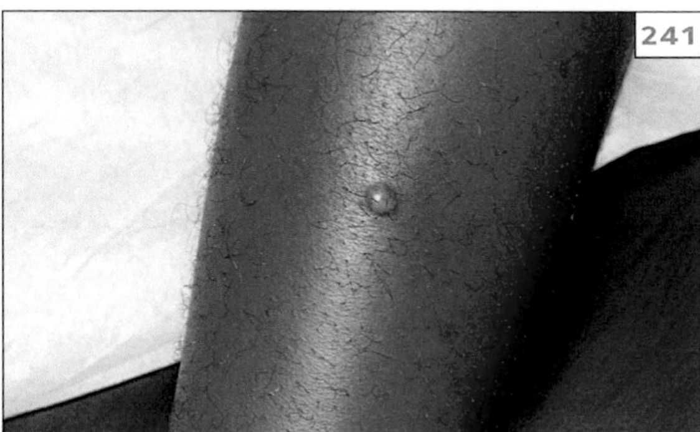

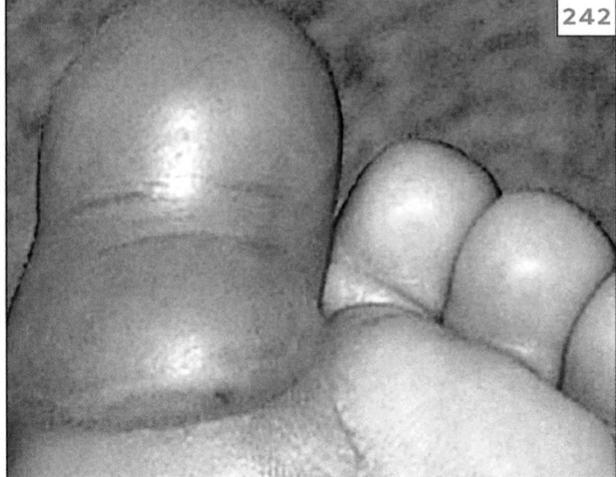

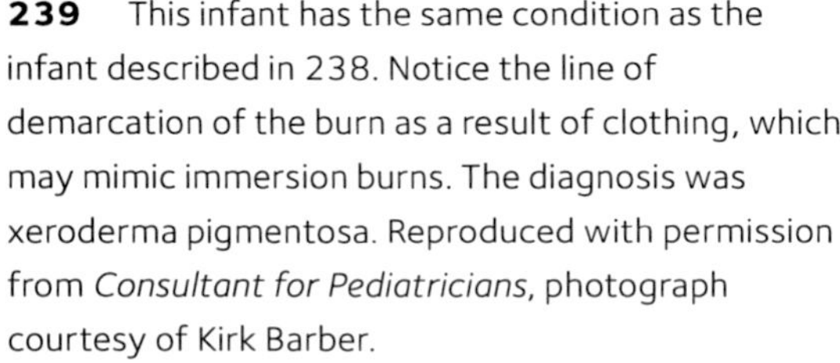

239 This infant has the same condition as the infant described in 238. Notice the line of demarcation of the burn as a result of clothing, which may mimic immersion burns. The diagnosis was xeroderma pigmentosa. Reproduced with permission from *Consultant for Pediatricians*, photograph courtesy of Kirk Barber.

240 An infant who presented with swelling and redness of the third and fourth toes. The diagnosis was hair tourniquet syndrome. Photograph courtesy of Earl R. Hartwig.

241 A patient who presented with erythema after a presumptive insect bite. The diagnosis was cellulitis. Photograph courtesy of Earl R. Hartwig.

242 A female who presented with painful swelling of her toe. The diagnosis was presumptive spider bite. Photograph courtesy of Mary E. Smyth.

Cultural practices

Cupping and coining are discussed above. 'Maquas' are burns that are inflicted with hot metal spits or coals near an area of illness or pain. It is part of Bedouin (Arabic), Russian, and Druse cultural practices (**245–247**). Moxibustion is an Asian cultural practice that involves the application of heat to the skin, most commonly with a burning object, such as incense[24]. Moxa is an aged form of mugwort, *Arsensia vulgaris*, a herb that is commonly burned in the area of the illness as part of this traditional practice. Burns resulting from moxibustion may be full or partial thickness and are usually small and circular. Herbs and complementary medical treatments may result in chemical burns mimicking those burns resulting from abuse. Garlic has been reported to cause burns in patients when crushed and applied directly to the skin (**248**)[25–28].

A variety of conditions may be mistaken for burns of the anus and genitalia. Accidental ingestion of senna may present with erythema and blister formation (**249**). This typically has an overall diamond shape with linear borders and sparing of the peri-anal area and the gluteal cleft[2]. Lichen sclerosis et atrophicus is a chronic dermatologic inflammatory condition seen most often in postmenopausal women and prepubertal girls[29,30]. It occurs 10 times more often in females than in males, suggesting that hormones may play a role; however, a specific etiology is unknown. Girls most often present with anogenital involvement. The chief complaint is often intense genital itching or burning, and pain with urination. Constipation is also a frequent presenting sign and is due to withholding secondary to the pain associated with defecation. Bleeding may be reported. Vaginal discharge can precede development of the skin lesions in some cases. The classic finding on physical examination is parchment-like atrophic plaques in a figure-of-eight distribution around the vulva and anus (**250**). The skin is extremely friable. Intraep-

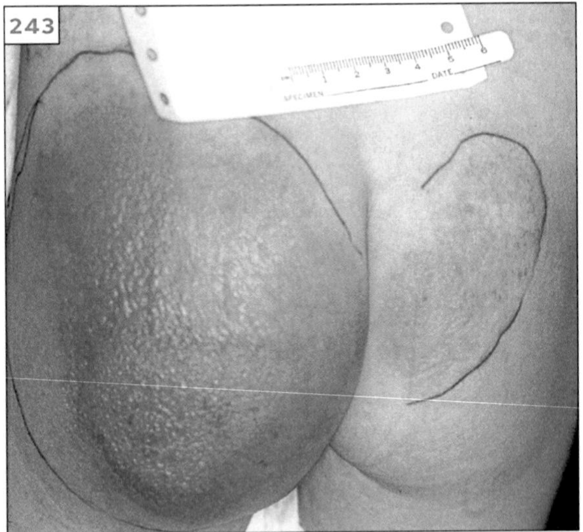

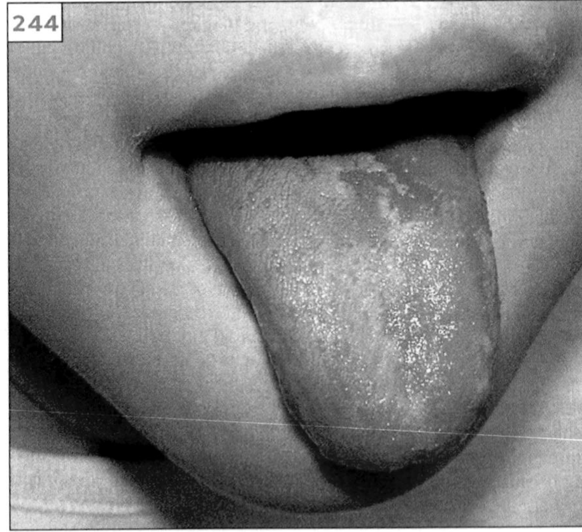

243 A child who presented with redness and painful swelling of her buttocks. An abusive burn was suspected. Further history and disclosure from the child suggested the presumptive diagnosis of a spider bite. Photograph courtesy of Mary E. Smyth.

244 A 4-year-old girl referred by protective services for suspected inflicted burns on the tongue. Notice the red plaque on the tongue with a well-demarcated, irregular, white border. The patient's mother had a similar lesion. The lesion was also migratory, with longer-term presence, and had neither eschar nor signs of tissue coagulation as is seen in burns. The diagnosis was geographic tongue. Reproduced with permission from *Consultant for Pediatricians*, photograph courtesy of Sushma Nuthakki *et al.*

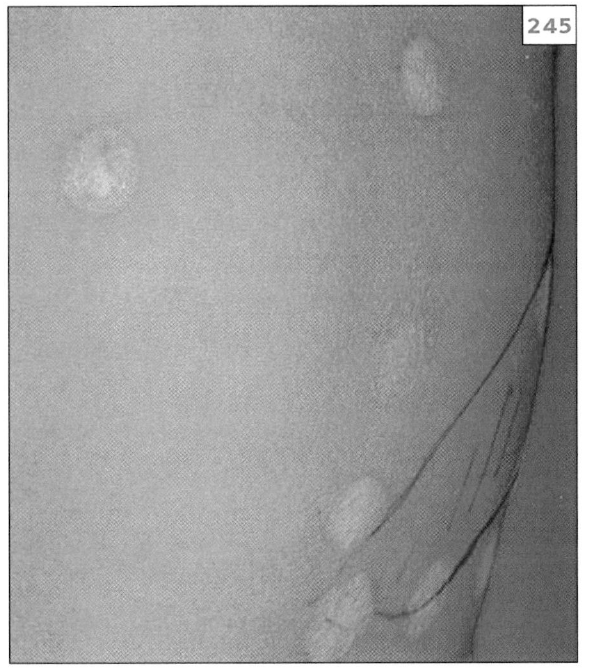

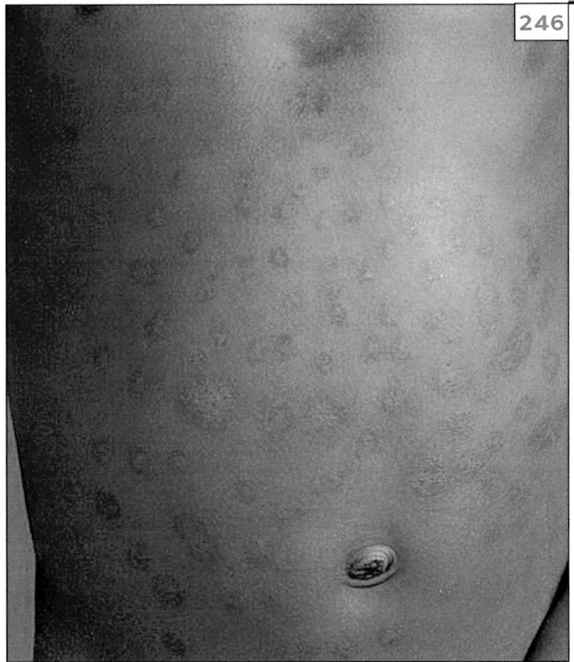

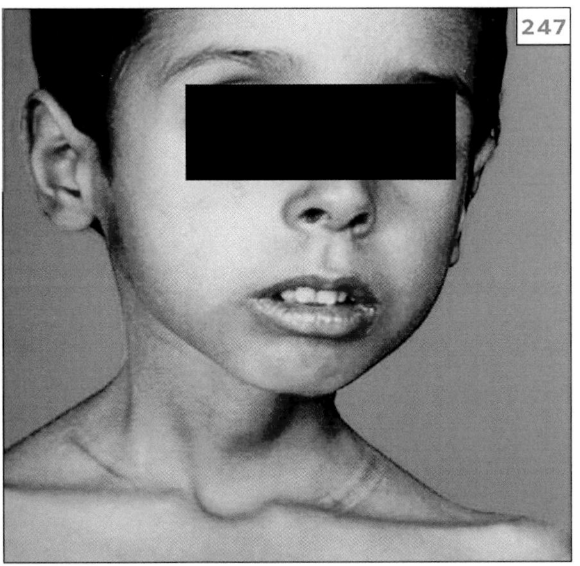

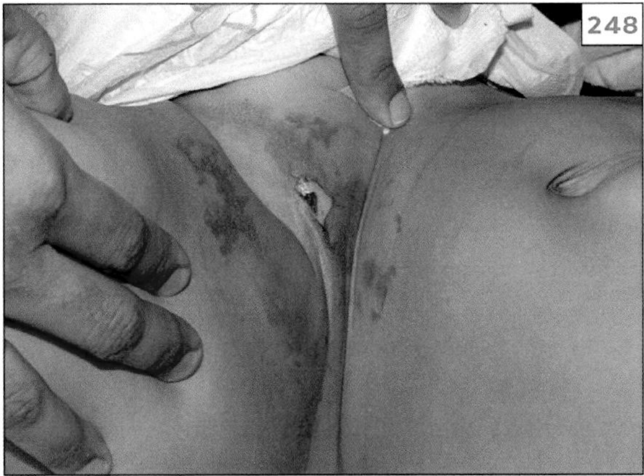

245 'Therapeutic' burns in a patient with glycogen storage disease. The diagnosis was maquas. Photograph courtesy of Hisham Nazer.

246 'Therapeutic' burns in a patient with recurrent abdominal pain. The diagnosis was maquas. Photograph courtesy of Hisham Nazer.

247 'Therapeutic' burns around the neck in a patient with celiac disease. The diagnosis was maquas. Photograph courtesy of Hisham Nazer.

248 A 16-month-old baby referred to the child protection team for suspected abuse due to a burn of unknown etiology. Further history revealed that the mother applied garlic to treat an insect bite. The diagnosis was garlic burn. Reproduced with permission from *Consultant for Pediatricians*, photograph courtesy of Dena Nazer *et al.*

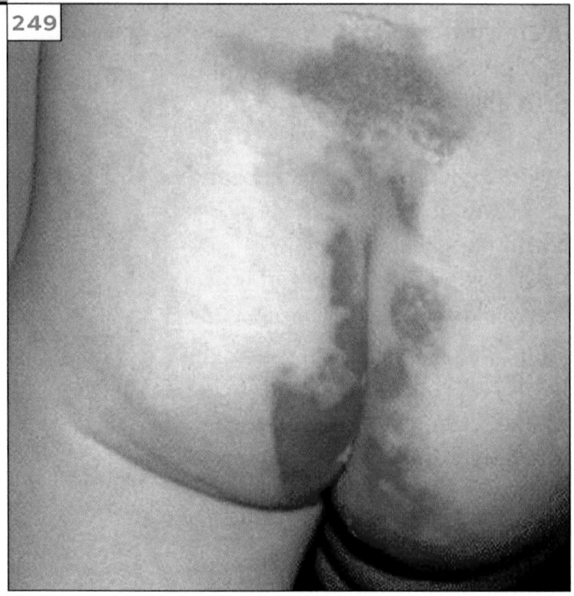

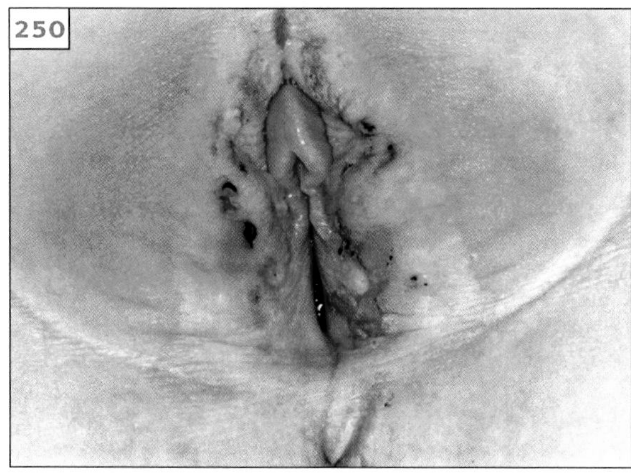

249 A 2-year-old presented with burns to her buttock and perineum. The history revealed accidental ingestion of sennosides (ExLax tablets) and resulting diarrhea. Notice that the burns extend up the back, consistent with the diarrhea. The diagnosis was senna burn secondary to accidental laxative ingestion. Reproduced with permission from *Consultant for Pediatrics*, photograph courtesy of Jaenlee F. Carver *et al.*

250 A child with a depigmented area around the labia, perineum, and anus. The diagnosis was lichen sclerosis et atrophicus. Photograph courtesy of Mary E. Smyth.

ithelial hemorrhages, purpura, and peri-anal fissures are common features. Diagnosis of lichen sclerosis is usually made on a clinical basis, but can be confirmed with a skin biopsy. In this condition, unexplained bleeding, vaginal discharge, or purpura that may look like bruises lead to a concern about sexual abuse. Group A beta-hemolytic streptococcal vulvovaginitis or peri-anal infection mostly affects girls aged 3–10 years. Symptoms include erythema, discomfort, dysuria, and vulvar discharge.[31] Diagnosis is made by culture. Often there is a history of recent streptococcal pharyngitis or asymptomatic infection may be found. Other causes of vulvovaginitis are *Staphylococcus aureus*, *Hemophilus influenzae*, *Klebsiella pneumoniae*, and *Shigella flexnerii*.

Teaching points

- There are a variety of conditions that can be mistaken for bruises or burns.
- The physician should evaluate alternative explanations when abuse is being considered, especially when there are unusual lesions inconsistent with classic abuse patterns.
- In some cases, alternative explanations can be excluded based on history, physical examination, and basic laboratory findings; however, certain conditions may require sophisticated testing and referral to a consultant for definitive diagnosis.
- Some cultural practices are associated with inflicted (but not abusive) lesions; the degree of injury, presumed intent, and the cultural acceptability of the practice need to be considered in making an abuse assessment.

Chapter 5

IMAGING CHILD ABUSE

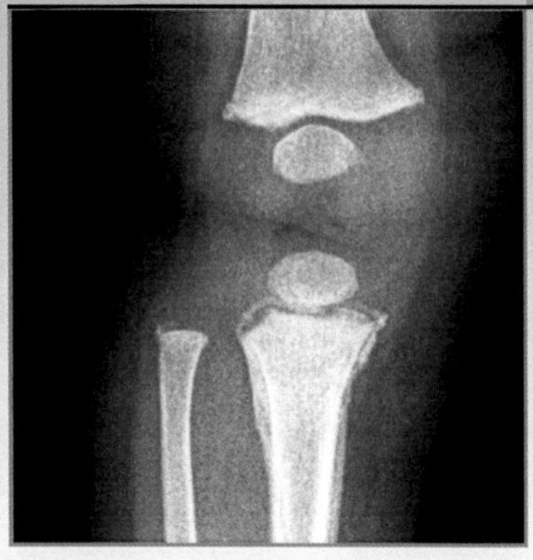

Aparna Joshi MD and
Thomas L. Slovis MD

Historically, radiology has played a significant role in the recognition of physical findings of child abuse. In his seminal article of 1946, the pediatric radiologist John Caffey became the first to note an association between long bone fractures and subdural hematomas in infants[1]. Caffey later hypothesized that these injuries were nonaccidental, inciting many investigators in radiology and pediatrics to study child abuse further. Among them was pediatric radiologist Fred Silverman, who in 1953 described three infants with fractures as a result of unrecognized trauma[2]. In 1955, pediatrician Paul Woolley and radiologist William Evans correlated the presence of multiple bony injuries in infants with social histories pointing to injury-prone environments[3]. C. Henry Kempe, Fred Silverman, and colleagues followed with their landmark paper in 1962 describing the battered child syndrome[4]. Since the 1980s, pediatric radiologist Paul Kleinman and his colleagues have contributed greatly to our understanding of the subject with radiographic and pathologic examination of skeletal specimens from fatally abused children[5].

Introduction

Diagnostic imaging continues to be a key component in the assessment of children for nonaccidental trauma (NAT). Specifically, diagnostic imaging allows detection of skeletal injury, intracranial injury, and abdominal visceral injury due to inflicted trauma. In fact, the radiologist may be the first to suspect nonaccidental trauma based on the recognition of injuries that are suggestive of physical child abuse or that are not explained by the history provided. Since almost any injury may be inflicted, it is important to take into consideration the developmental capabilities of the child, as well as the history provided for mechanism of injury when determining whether an imaging-detected abnormality may be nonaccidental. For example, although long bone fractures result quite commonly in older children from accidents, a long bone fracture in a nonambulatory, 4-month-old infant should be regarded as highly suspicious for inflicted injury (**251**). Similarly, a displaced femur fracture in a child whose caregiver explains that it was incurred by the child falling from a sofa should be viewed as suspicious for nonaccidental injury. The great force (F) needed to fracture a femur cannot be attained by such a mechanism, since force equals mass (m, child's weight) times acceleration (a, speed attained while falling)[6], $F = m \times a$.

Imaging examinations cannot be interpreted in isolation from the clinical history and physical examination, and any injury that is seen on radiographs which does not have a suitable mechanism of injury to explain its presence needs further investigation. Some injuries demonstrated on radiologic examinations have a high specificity for nonaccidental trauma. These include metaphyseal fractures, posterior rib fractures, and interhemispheric subdural hemorrhage. The following sections will address and illustrate each of these in greater depth. For more in-depth discussion on the diagnostic imaging of child abuse, the reader is referred to Kleinman's authoritative textbook on the topic and several comprehensive review articles[5–9].

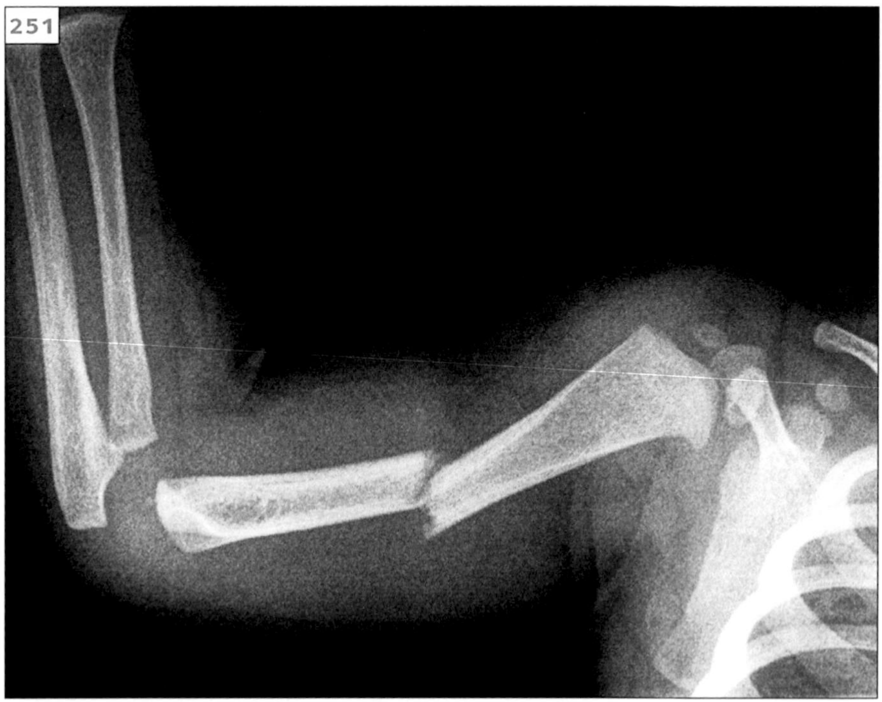

251 Long bone fracture in a young, nonambulatory infant. A lateral view of the right arm in a 3-month-old abused infant shows a mildly displaced right humeral mid-diaphyseal fracture.

Skeletal injury

Skeletal injuries are the most common noncutaneous injuries seen in NAT, as fractures are documented in up to 55% of physically abused children[10]. Fractures are much more common in younger children, with studies showing 78–94% of inflicted fractures occurring in children under 3 years of age[11,12]. Skeletal injuries in NAT are more frequently the result of indirect forces from torsion, traction, or acceleration–deceleration mechanisms, although direct blows may obviously result in injury as well. Fractures have also been described in association with sexual abuse[13].

The entire skeleton must be assessed in cases of suspected NAT to document the extent and nature of the skeletal injuries. This should initially be accomplished by means of a radiographic skeletal survey. The examination must be meticulously performed so that the radiologist can detect even the most subtle injuries. Although some investigators have shown scintigraphy to be more sensitive than radiography in detection of abnormalities[14], the technical expertise and equipment needed to perform and interpret high-quality scintigraphic examinations in small children are not as widely available as those needed for high-quality radiographic examinations and have the additional disadvantage of requiring conscious sedation (**252**). In children between 12 months and 3 years of age, either radiographic survey or scintigraphy is acceptable. The radiographic survey is used as the primary means of evaluation, supplemented with scintigraphy in more difficult cases. Beyond the age of 3 years, the added utility of a global screening of the skeleton is questionable, as the child is able to give a more complete history and demonstrate more localized findings, so at this point radiographic evaluation of the skeleton is limited to sites of clinically suspected injury.

The American College of Radiology Practice Guidelines and Technical Standards outline some recommendations on how to perform a technically satisfactory skeletal survey, including imaging

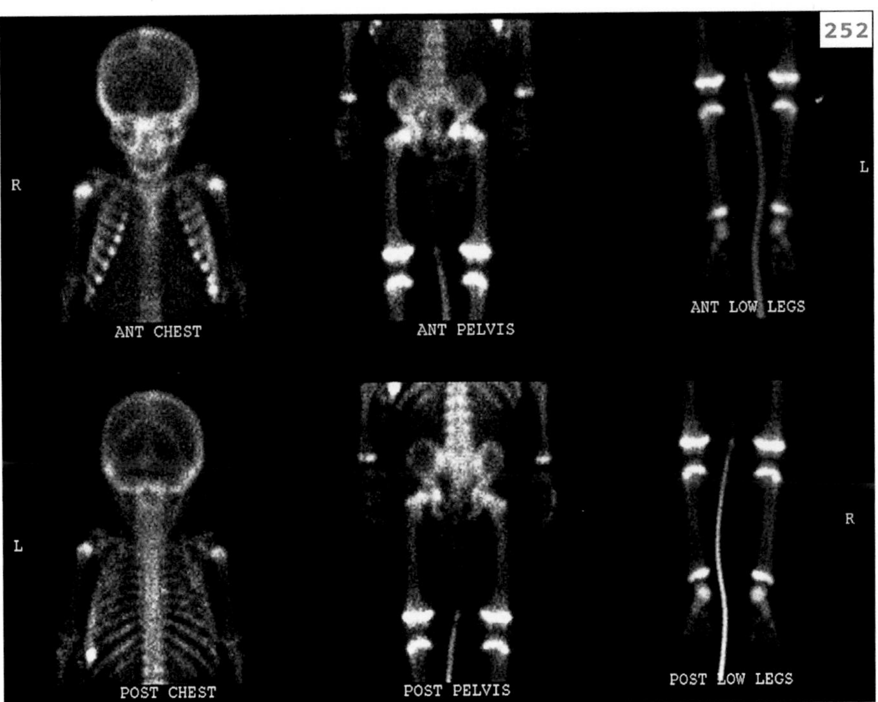

252 Skeletal scintigraphy. Planar images from a whole body bone scan in this 22-month-old abused child show increased activity in the posterolateral left 10th rib and the left superior pubis, where fractures were confirmed by plain radiography and computed tomography, respectively. Note the bands of relatively high uptake in normal metaphyses throughout the skeleton.

protocol and equipment specifications[15]. Rather than a 'babygram' image of the entire skeleton on a single radiograph, tightly collimated views of each portion of the anatomy are obtained with attention to proper positioning. At a minimum, anterior–posterior (AP) and lateral views of the axial skeleton are obtained along with AP/PA views of the appendicular skeleton (*Table 10*). At the Children's Hospital of Michigan, the imaging protocol is modified: the lateral view of the thorax is replaced with a lateral view of the thoracic spine and bilateral oblique views of the entire thorax to improve sensitivity for rib fractures, and lateral views of the humeri, forearms, femora, and lower legs are obtained in addition to the frontal views to show subtle long bone fractures that may not be visible on a single view. A high-detail imaging system should be used in infants, while in toddlers

Table 10 **Radiographic skeletal survey views[15]**

Skull: frontal and lateral
Cervical spine: anterior–posterior and lateral
Thorax: anterior–posterior and lateral (to include ribs, thoracic and upper lumbar spine)
Pelvis: anterior–posterior (to include the mid-lumbar spine)
Lumbosacral spine: lateral
Humeri: anterior–posterior
Forearms: anterior–posterior
Hands: posterior–anterior
Femurs: anterior–posterior
Lower legs: anterior–posterior
Feet: posterior–anterior/anterior–posterior

Table 11 **Specificity of radiologic findings after child abuse**

High specificity	Classic metaphyseal lesions
	Posterior rib fractures
	Scapular fractures
	Spinous process fractures
	Sternal fractures
Moderate specificity	Multiple fractures, especially bilateral
	Fractures of different ages
	Epiphyseal separations
	Vertebral body fractures and subluxations
	Digit fractures
	Complex skull fractures
Common, but low specificity	Subperiosteal new bone formation
	Clavicular fractures
	Long bone shaft fractures
	Linear skull fractures

Modified from Kleinman PK (ed.). (1998). *Diagnostic imaging of child abuse*, 2nd edn. Mosby, St Louis, p. 9.

and older children, general medium-speed systems may be needed to image larger body parts because of concerns over the dose of radiation. When a digital radiographic system is employed, it should have sufficiently high spatial resolution and good dose-efficiency characteristics. As always in pediatric imaging, technical factors should be adjusted so that the radiation dose to the patient is minimized while maintaining the necessary diagnostic image quality.

While the distribution of fracture location in abused children varies in many studies depending on the age and referral pattern of the population examined, there are some common findings. The long bones, skull, and ribs are the most common sites for inflicted fractures. The femur, tibia, and humerus are the three most commonly injured long bones in abused children. Overall, long bone diaphyseal fractures are the most common fractures seen in child physical abuse. However, in infancy, rib, skull, and metaphyseal fractures predominate. The difference in pattern of injury in infancy can be explained both on the basis of changes in applied mechanism of injury depending on the size of the child, as well as by intrinsic alterations in the skeleton and its response to traumatic forces with age. As mentioned previously, any fracture that is discrepant with the provided history must be further evaluated for potential abuse. However, some fractures are highly specific for inflicted trauma (*Table 11*). These include the classic metaphyseal lesion, rib fractures, sternal fractures, spinous process fractures, and scapular fractures. Though long bone diaphyseal fractures are the leading type of inflicted fracture, occurring four times more frequently than metaphyseal fractures[16], they are less specific for physical abuse. Other less specific injuries include subperiosteal new bone formation, linear skull fractures, and clavicle fractures[5,17].

The classic metaphyseal lesion (CML) is nearly pathognomonic for inflicted injury and is seen primarily in infants. For many years, the pathogenesis was believed to be avulsion of the metaphyseal margin by tightly adherent periosteum in this location, leading to a 'corner'- or 'bucket-handle'-shaped fragment of bone (**253–258**). However, the meticulous histologic and radiologic examination of numerous autopsy specimens by Kleinman and colleagues beginning in the mid-1980s[18,19] showed that the CML is not simply an avulsion of the metaphyseal margin, but rather a planar fracture through the weakest portion of metaphysis (**259**). Histologically, the fracture plane in the center of the bone is through the primary spongiosa near the chondro-osseous junction, while near the periphery of the bone, the fracture plane undercuts the subperiosteal new bone collar. This results in a disk-shaped fragment that is thicker peripherally than centrally. The 'corner'- or 'bucket-handle'-shaped appearance of the fragment on radiographs can be explained by radiographic projection (**259**). The lesion may also be seen on radiographs as metaphyseal irregularity (**260**) or as transmetaphyseal linear lucency. The CML is seen more frequently in the lower extremities than the upper, especially in the proximal tibia, distal tibia, and distal femur (**259**). Interestingly, metaphyseal fractures are often not accompanied by pain or bruising, so the only evidence of their existence is radiological, supporting the need for careful attention to all metaphyses on interpretation of a skeletal survey[17,20].

Subperiosteal new bone formation may be seen in the long bones of abused infants with or without associated fracture (**261**). In infants, the periosteum is not as strongly anchored to the underlying bone as it is in older children, so even indirect injury from violent shaking can cause elevation of the osteogenic layer of the periosteum from the cortical surface by hemorrhage. Subperiosteal new bone formation is a nonspecific finding that may also occur in cases of infection, metabolic bone disease, and accidental injury. Physiologic apposition of new bone is a normal phenomenon in young infants and should not be mistaken for new bone formation secondary to abuse (see below).

Rib fractures are highly specific for infant abuse in children without metabolic bone disease[21,22]. The mechanism of injury explains the locations of rib fractures posteriorly, laterally, and anteriorly (**262–274**): an assailant's tight grip around the infant's thorax results in compression and deformation of the ribs, such that the posterior rib is levered on the transverse process of the associated thoracic vertebra, the lateral rib is flexed, and the anterior rib is stressed, particularly at the costochondral junction[23]. Rib fractures related to birth trauma have been reported only rarely. Rib fractures from cardiopulmonary resuscitation are also very unusual and have not been shown to occur posteriorly[24]. Sternal fractures (**275–278**) and scapular fractures (**279, 280**) are other thoracic fractures that have a high specificity for NAT.

Long bone fractures (**251, 281**) are the most common type of fracture seen in NAT, but because of their nonspecific nature and frequent occurrence in accidental injury, it is of paramount importance to correlate the imaging findings with the child's developmental abilities and the history provided, as mentioned above. The spiral or oblique appearance of these fractures (**281**) is thought by many to imply NAT as an etiology, but they are encountered in accidental trauma as well and are not specific[25,26].

Many studies have proven the process of dating fractures to be an imprecise one, although general ranges of time since injury can be given[5,7]. Absence of any subperiosteal new bone formation indicates that a diaphyseal fracture is usually less than 7–10 days old. Any amount of subperiosteal new bone formation suggests a fracture greater than 10 days old. Periosteal new bone and callus formation are seen on radiographs between 2 and 4 weeks after the injury.

Recent experience has taught us that follow-up skeletal surveys are often useful in confirmation and clarification of skeletal injuries in NAT[27–29]. Even on technically adequate skeletal surveys, acute nondisplaced fractures are difficult to visualize, but a follow-up survey performed approximately 2 weeks after the initial examination (to allow time for the aforementioned periosteal new bone and callus to develop) can show these initially subtle fractures to better advantage. Not only do follow-up surveys show additional fractures that are not initially evident, but they have utility in confirming or refuting questionable fractures. Follow-up studies are particularly helpful for evaluating questionable rib and metaphyseal fractures.

Several other conditions have radiologic findings that may be confused with those of inflicted skeletal injury. The more commonly seen differential diagnostic entities are metabolic bone disease (especially rickets), osteomyelitis, accidental trauma, birth injury, drug-induced changes, physiologic apposition of new bone, and some normal variants. Although a discussion of the entire differential diagnosis is beyond the scope of this chapter, a couple of these deserve special mention. Physiologic apposition of new bone (**282**) is seen in young infants between the ages of 1 and 5 months along the diaphyses of the femur, tibia, and humerus; it is bilateral and symmetric in its distribution, usually under 2 mm in thickness. Rickets (**283, 284**) can cause metaphyseal irregularity, fractures, and subperiosteal new bone formation, so it may be occasionally confused with inflicted injury, especially in the healing stage, but is characterized by bony demineralization and increased distance between the metaphysis and epiphysis. Findings of rickets are most pronounced at the knees and wrists, which are places of rapid bone growth. Toddler's fracture (**285, 286**) is a nondisplaced oblique fracture of the tibia in infants who cruise or toddlers who have just learned to walk; it is caused by the child turning while the foot is planted.

Osteogenesis imperfecta (OI) is sometimes also raised as a possible explanation for fractures in abused children. OI, an uncommon disorder of type I collagen production with an incidence of 1 in 20,000 births, predisposes affected individuals to fractures with only minimal trauma. The clinically based Sillence classification of OI divides the disease into four categories: type I (**287–289**), a mild phenotype with only mild osteoporosis on radiographs, but important clinically evident features of blue sclerae and sometimes dentinogenesis imperfecta; type II, which is always prenatally lethal and manifested radiographically with severe skeletal deformities due to innumerable fractures (**290**); type III, a moderately severe phenotype which presents early in life with severe osteoporosis and many fractures (**291, 292**); and type IV, another phenotypically mild form, but with normal sclerae. Types II and III cannot be confused with NAT because of the lethality of type II and the profound osteopenia and multiple fractures of type III. Type I should be clinically evident based on abnormality of sclerae, but the more uncommon type IV may pose some difficulty in differentiation from NAT. Fortunately, the majority of patients with type IV OI will have a positive family history and most of the rest will have some other physical or radiographic manifestation, such as Wormian bones (**287–289**), dentinogenesis imperfecta, deafness, bowing deformity (**291, 292**), ligamentous laxity, or short stature[30,31]. It has been hypothesized that a sporadic case of type IV OI without any of these other manifestations might be encountered only once every 100–300 years in a population of 500,000[32].

Radiologists experienced with OI emphasize that all types exhibit radiographically discernible generalized osteopenia, and that fracture patterns highly specific for NAT, such as the CML and scapular or sternal fractures, are not seen with OI. When evaluating skeletal survey radiographs obtained for abuse, it is important to always look for manifestations of OI, such as generalized osteopenia (**287–289**), Wormian bones, and dentinogenesis imperfecta. If bony mineralization is normal, OI can be excluded, but if bone density is decreased or equivocal, further clinical evaluation and, if necessary, biochemical analysis of collagen from dermal fibroclast culture or genetic testing may be warranted[30].

In 1993, Paterson and colleagues proposed the idea that there is a temporary variant form of osteogenesis imperfecta, termed 'temporary brittle bone disease,' postulating that copper deficiency might be the underlying cause of this entity[33]. Since then, the existence of temporary brittle bone disease has been hotly debated and Paterson's scientific methodology has been widely criticized[31,34-36]. Currently, temporary brittle bone disease is considered a hypothetical, if not fictitious, entity without an accepted scientific basis (see Chapter 4, Cutaneous conditions mimicking child abuse, for additional discussion).

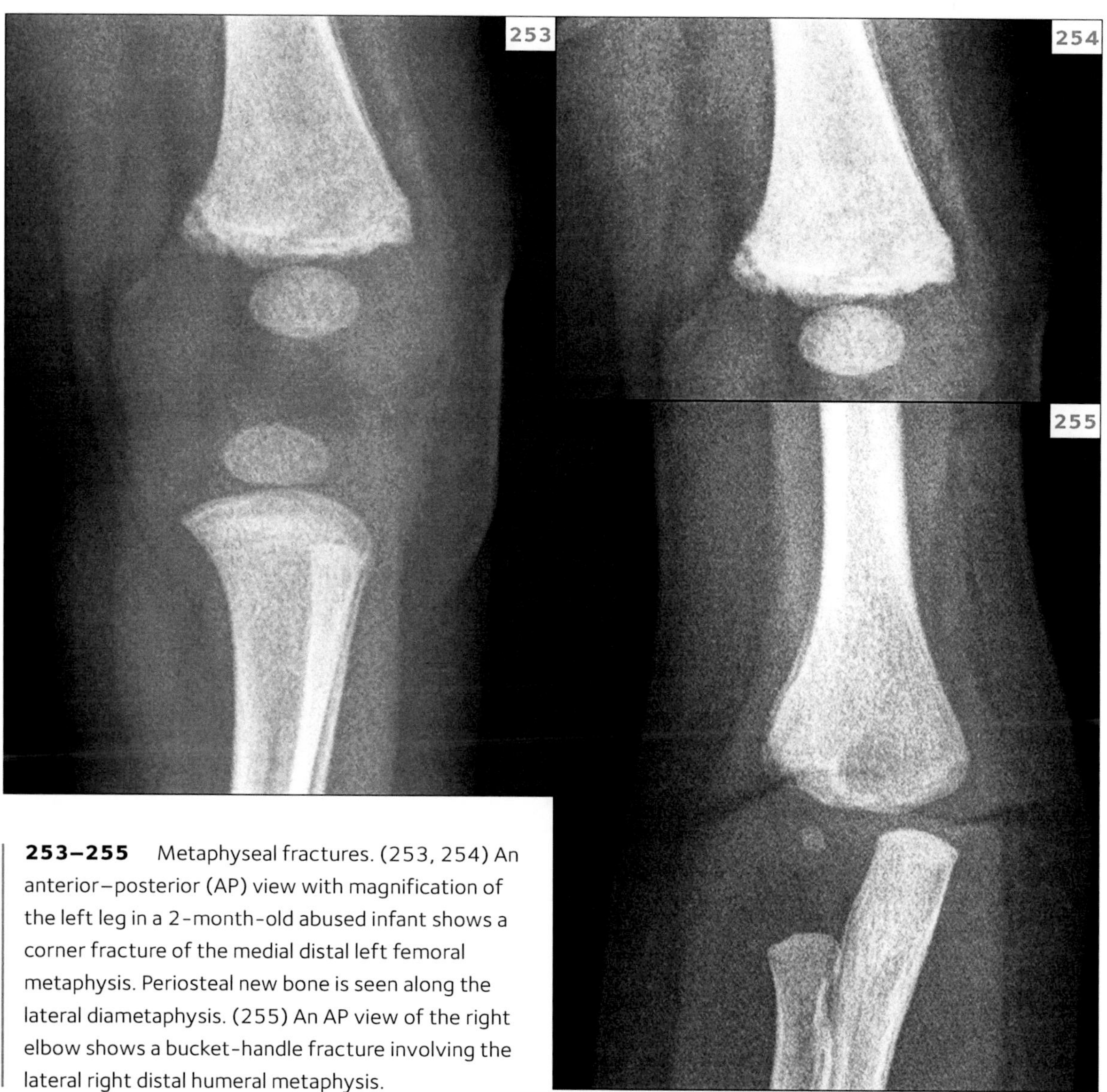

253–255 Metaphyseal fractures. (253, 254) An anterior–posterior (AP) view with magnification of the left leg in a 2-month-old abused infant shows a corner fracture of the medial distal left femoral metaphysis. Periosteal new bone is seen along the lateral diametaphysis. (255) An AP view of the right elbow shows a bucket-handle fracture involving the lateral right distal humeral metaphysis.

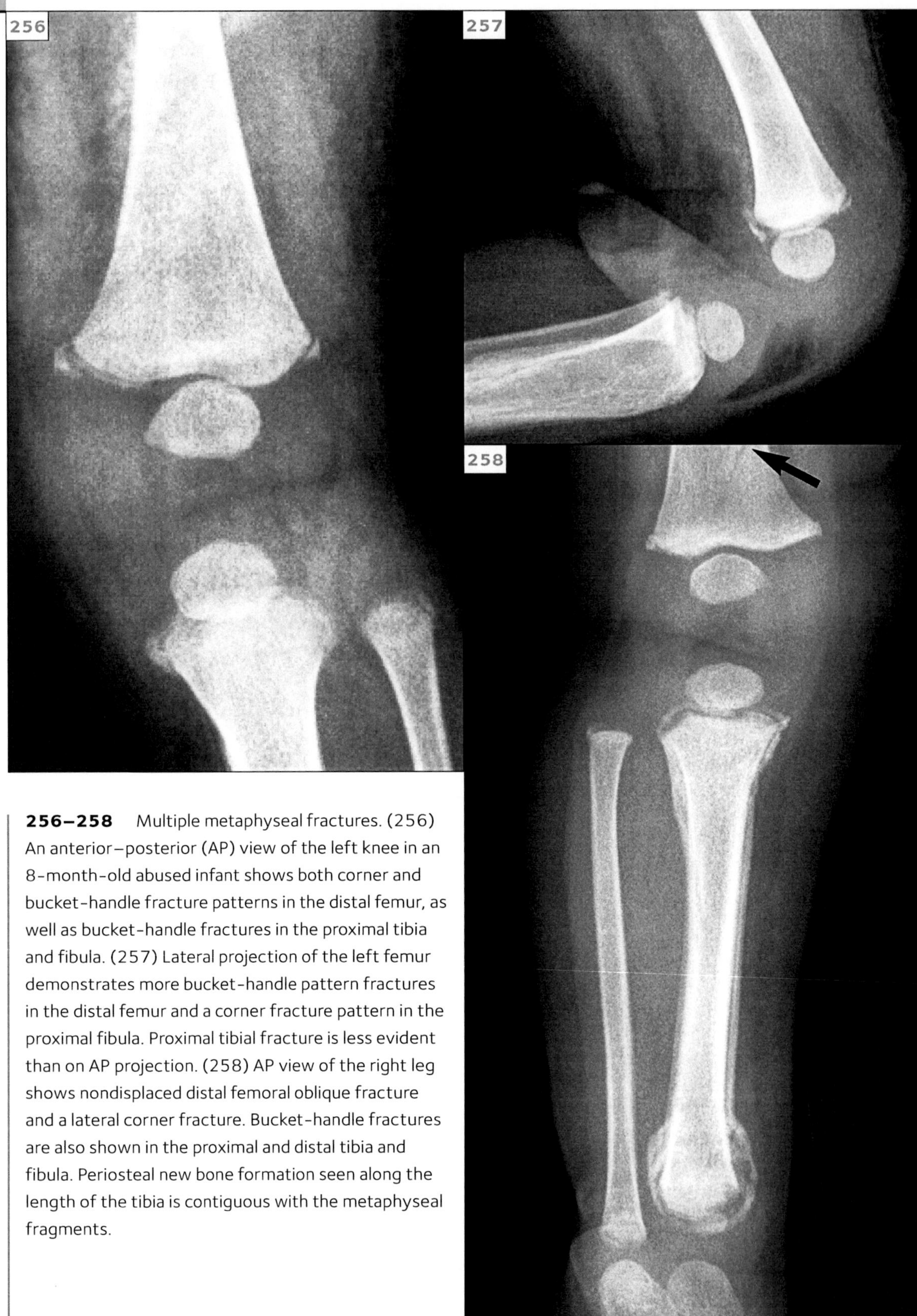

256–258 Multiple metaphyseal fractures. (256) An anterior–posterior (AP) view of the left knee in an 8-month-old abused infant shows both corner and bucket-handle fracture patterns in the distal femur, as well as bucket-handle fractures in the proximal tibia and fibula. (257) Lateral projection of the left femur demonstrates more bucket-handle pattern fractures in the distal femur and a corner fracture pattern in the proximal fibula. Proximal tibial fracture is less evident than on AP projection. (258) AP view of the right leg shows nondisplaced distal femoral oblique fracture and a lateral corner fracture. Bucket-handle fractures are also shown in the proximal and distal tibia and fibula. Periosteal new bone formation seen along the length of the tibia is contiguous with the metaphyseal fragments.

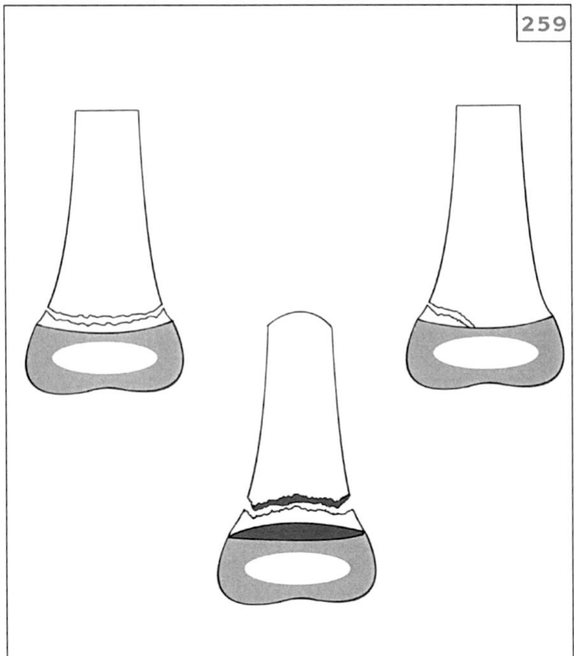

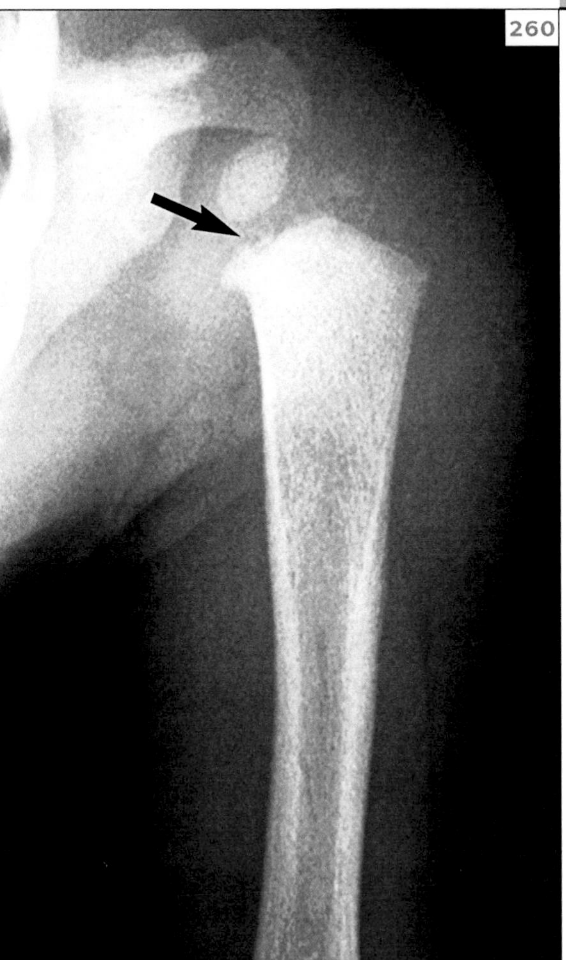

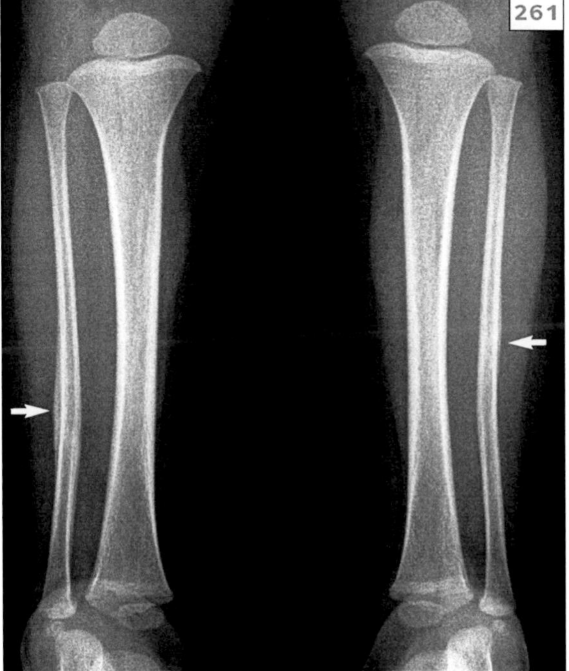

259 A schematic representation of the metaphyseal fracture and its appearance in various projections. Reproduced with permission from Slovis TL, Haller JO, Joshi A (2004). *Pediatric Imaging*, 3rd edn. Springer, Heidelberg.

260 Metaphyseal fracture. Anterior–posterior view of the left humerus in an abused 9-month-old infant who would not move her left arm shows slight metaphyseal irregularity and a more subtle bucket-handle pattern fracture of the proximal humeral metaphysis.

261 Periosteal new bone formation. An anterior–posterior view of both legs in an abused 2-year-old shows mild periosteal new bone formation along both fibular diaphyses. There is mild medial bowing of both fibulae and slight endosteal sclerosis suggesting healing nondisplaced fractures.

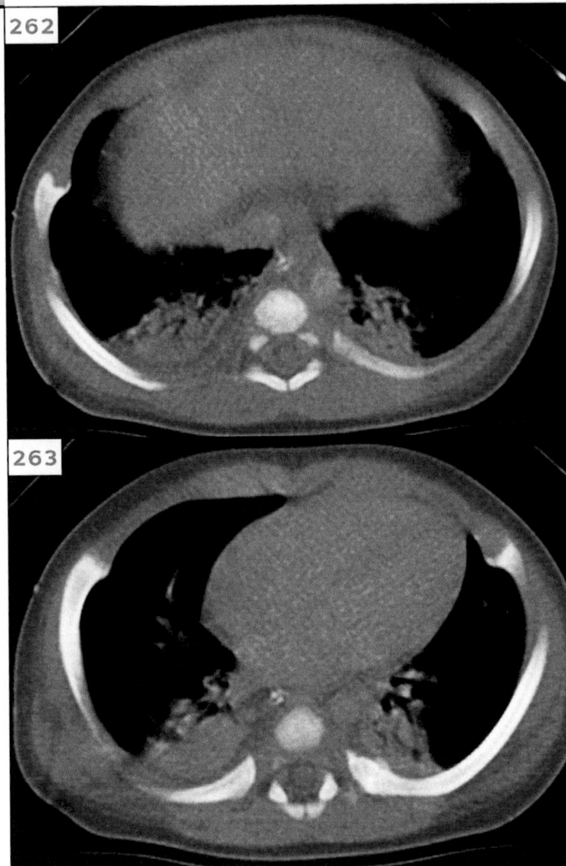

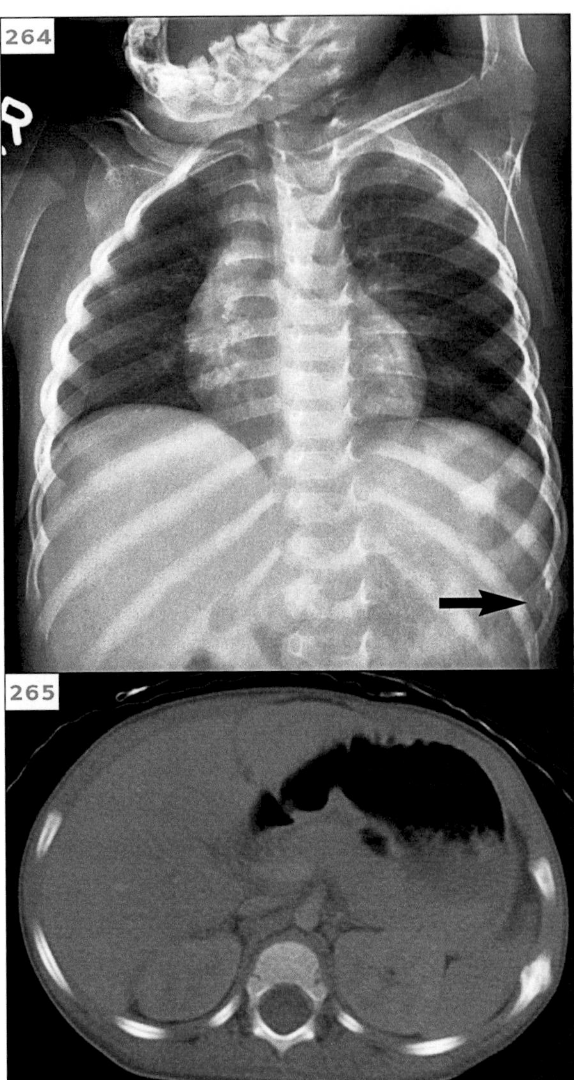

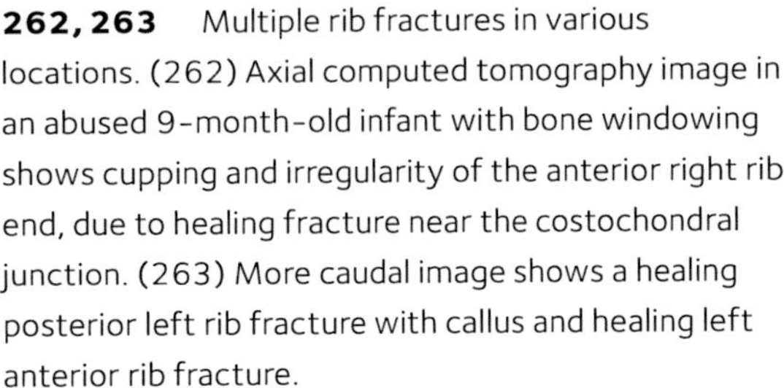

262, 263 Multiple rib fractures in various locations. (262) Axial computed tomography image in an abused 9-month-old infant with bone windowing shows cupping and irregularity of the anterior right rib end, due to healing fracture near the costochondral junction. (263) More caudal image shows a healing posterior left rib fracture with callus and healing left anterior rib fracture.

265, 265 Healing rib fracture. A 22-month-old with healing left posterolateral rib fracture with callus (264) on rib radiographs and (265) on computed tomography.

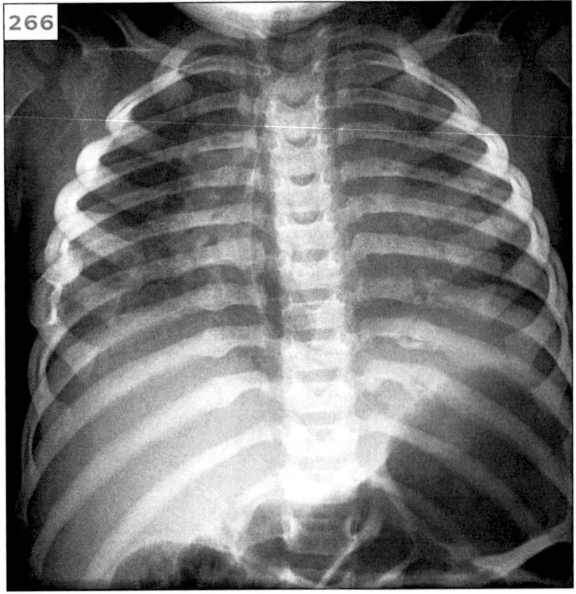

266 Multifocal healing rib fractures. An anterior–posterior radiograph of the chest in this 12-month-old fatally abused child demonstrates multiple healing rib fractures, posteriorly and laterally.

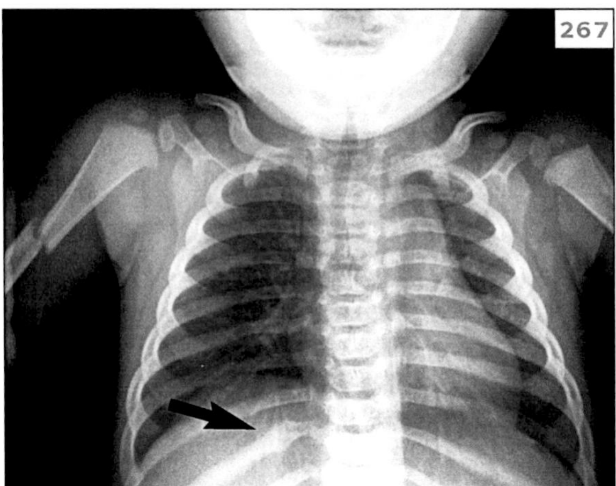

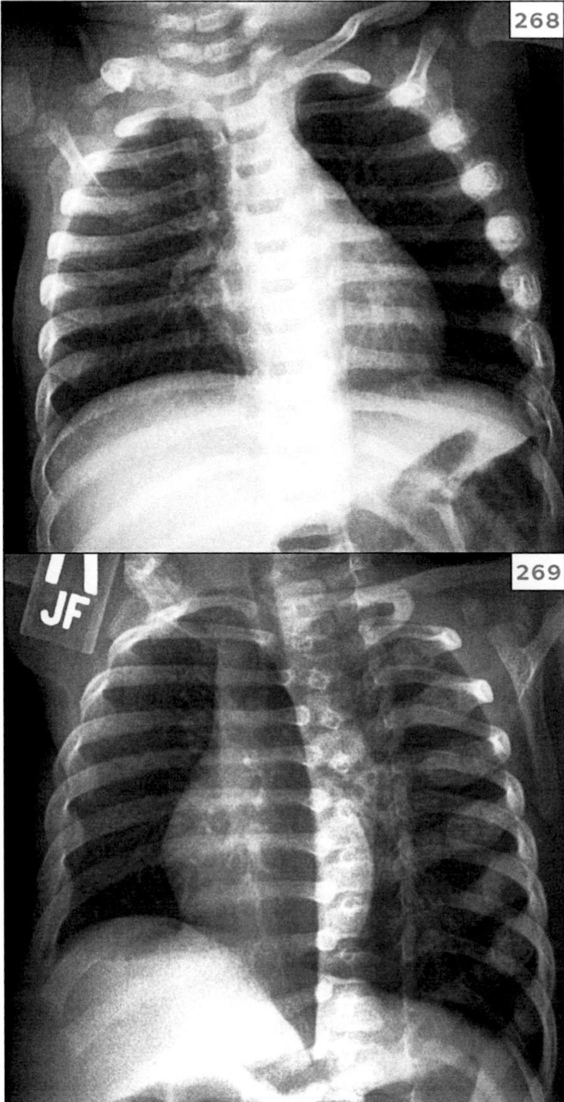

267 Healed rib fracture. An anterior–posterior radiograph of the chest in a 3-month-old abused infant demonstrates a healed rib posterior 10th rib fracture and a transverse humeral shaft fracture.

268, 269 Healing rib fractures. (268) Anterior–posterior and (269) right posterior oblique views of the thorax in this 4-month-old abused infant show multiple healing left lateral rib fractures (ribs 2–8) with callus, better seen on the oblique view, as well as a right clavicle fracture with abundant callus.

270 Healing rib fractures. Anterior–posterior views of the thorax in a 2-month-old abused infant show healing fractures of the right 4th to 7th ribs with callus formation.

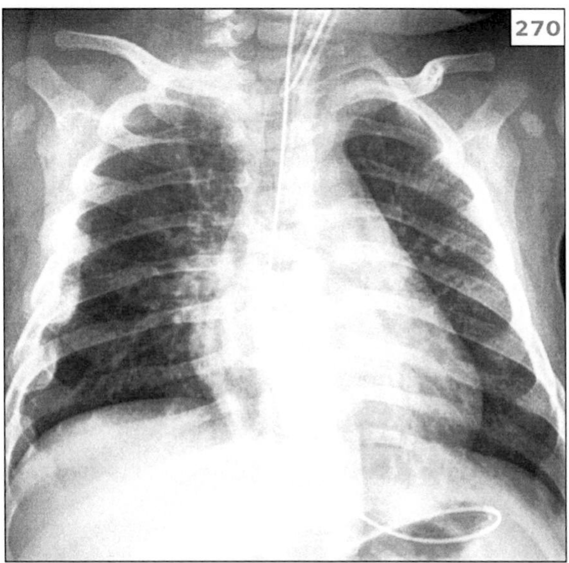

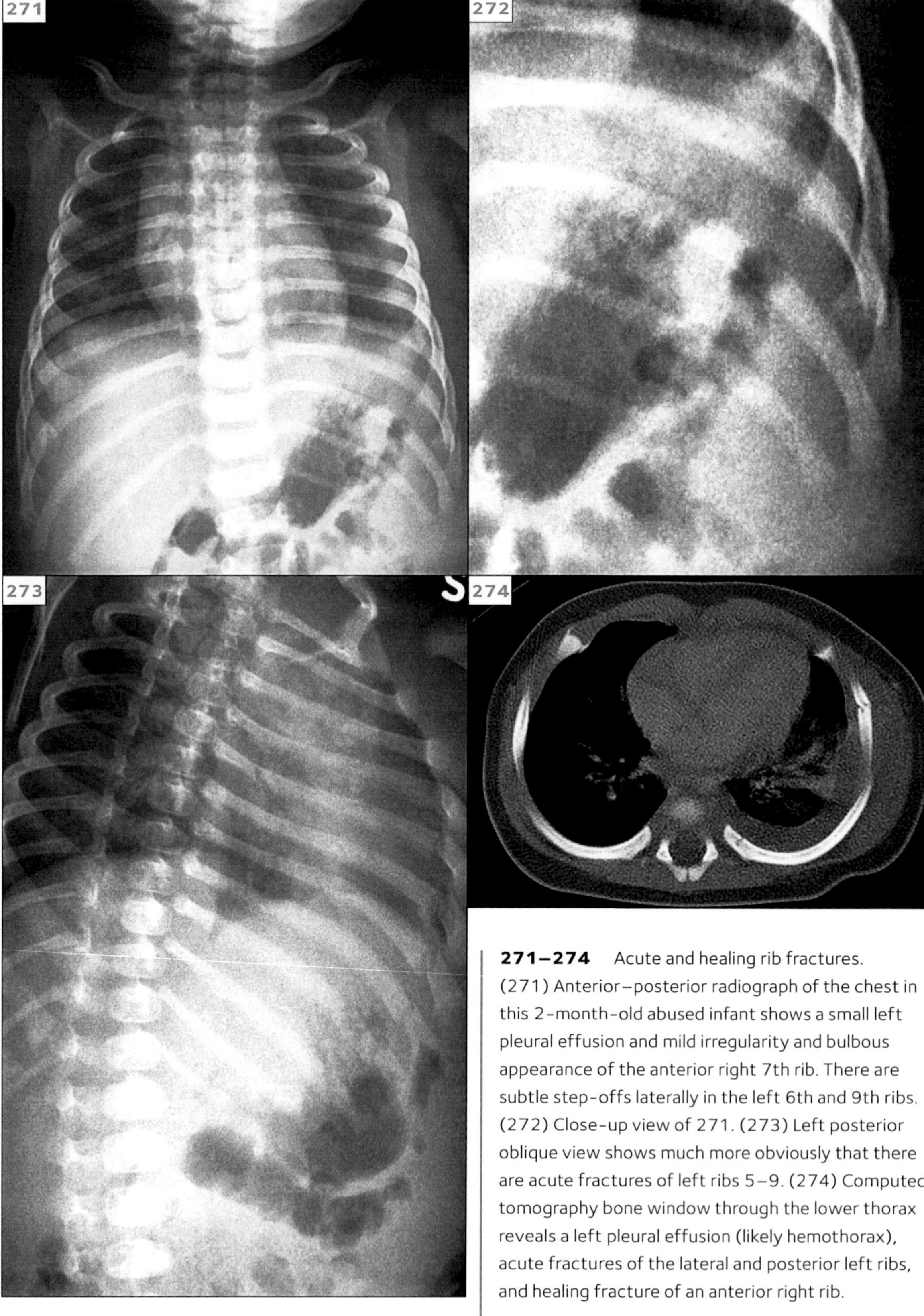

271–274 Acute and healing rib fractures. (271) Anterior–posterior radiograph of the chest in this 2-month-old abused infant shows a small left pleural effusion and mild irregularity and bulbous appearance of the anterior right 7th rib. There are subtle step-offs laterally in the left 6th and 9th ribs. (272) Close-up view of 271. (273) Left posterior oblique view shows much more obviously that there are acute fractures of left ribs 5–9. (274) Computed tomography bone window through the lower thorax reveals a left pleural effusion (likely hemothorax), acute fractures of the lateral and posterior left ribs, and healing fracture of an anterior right rib.

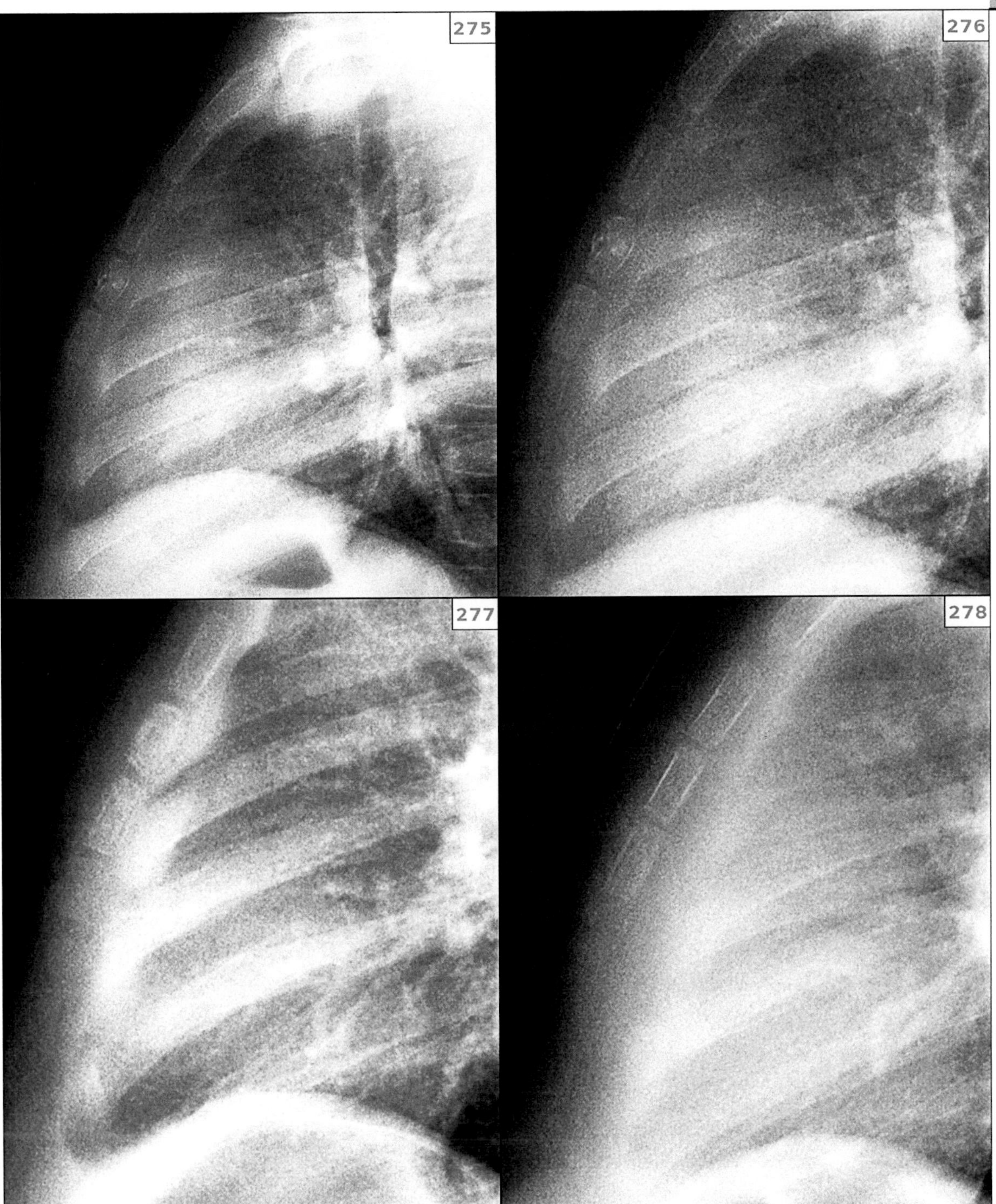

275–278 Sternal fracture with healing. (275, 276) Lateral chest radiograph with magnified view in this 2.5-year-old child shows a fracture of the second sternal segment. (277) Follow-up 1 month later shows healing with sclerosis in the involved segment. (278) Follow-up 4 months after the initial film shows complete healing.

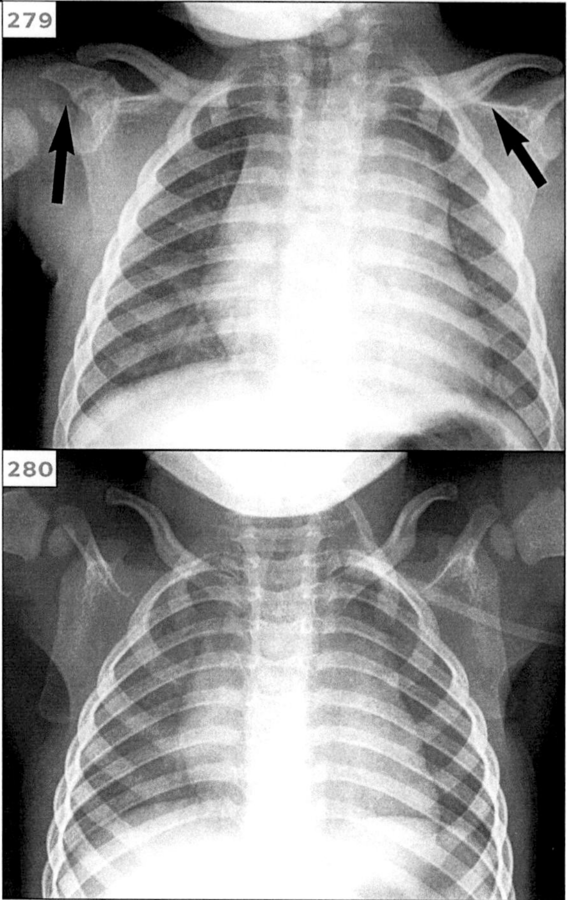

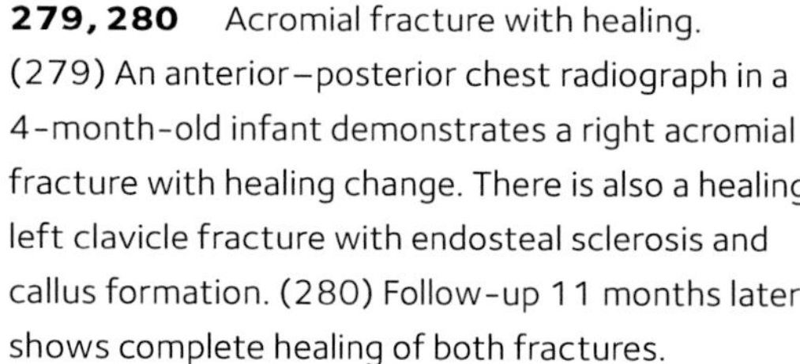

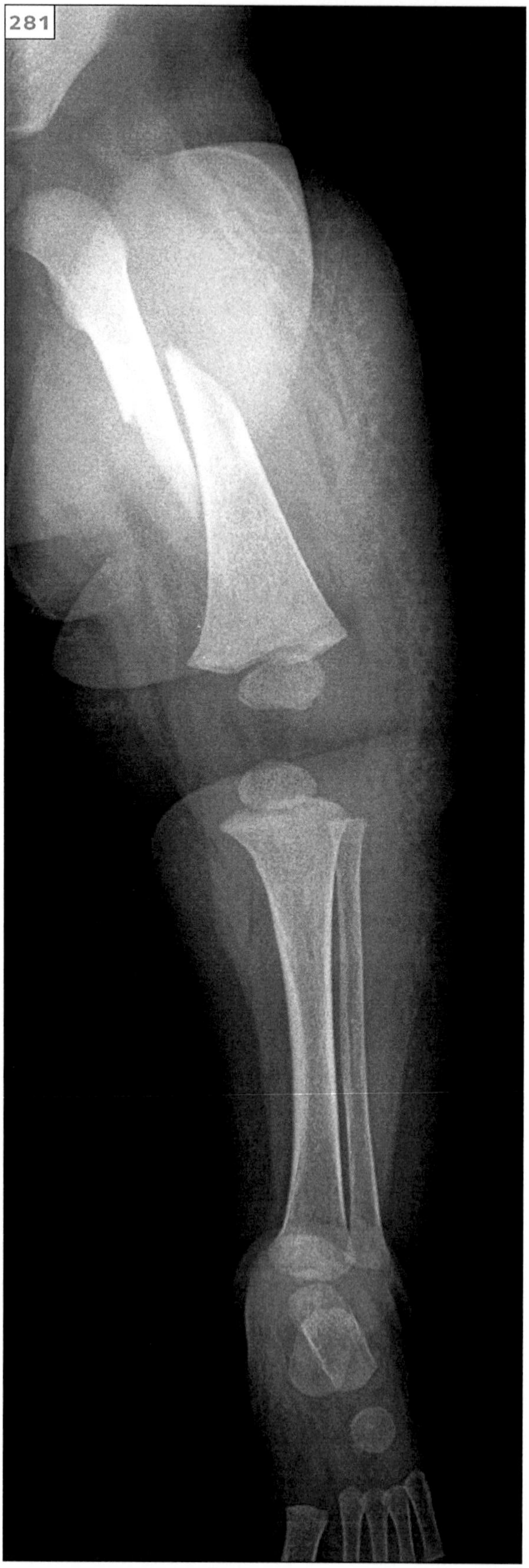

279, 280 Acromial fracture with healing. (279) An anterior–posterior chest radiograph in a 4-month-old infant demonstrates a right acromial fracture with healing change. There is also a healing left clavicle fracture with endosteal sclerosis and callus formation. (280) Follow-up 11 months later shows complete healing of both fractures.

281 Spiral femoral shaft fracture. An anterior–posterior radiograph of the left leg in a 6-month-old shows a mid-diaphyseal fracture of the left femur with lateral displacement of the distal fragment by more than one full shaft's width. Note also adjacent soft tissue edema.

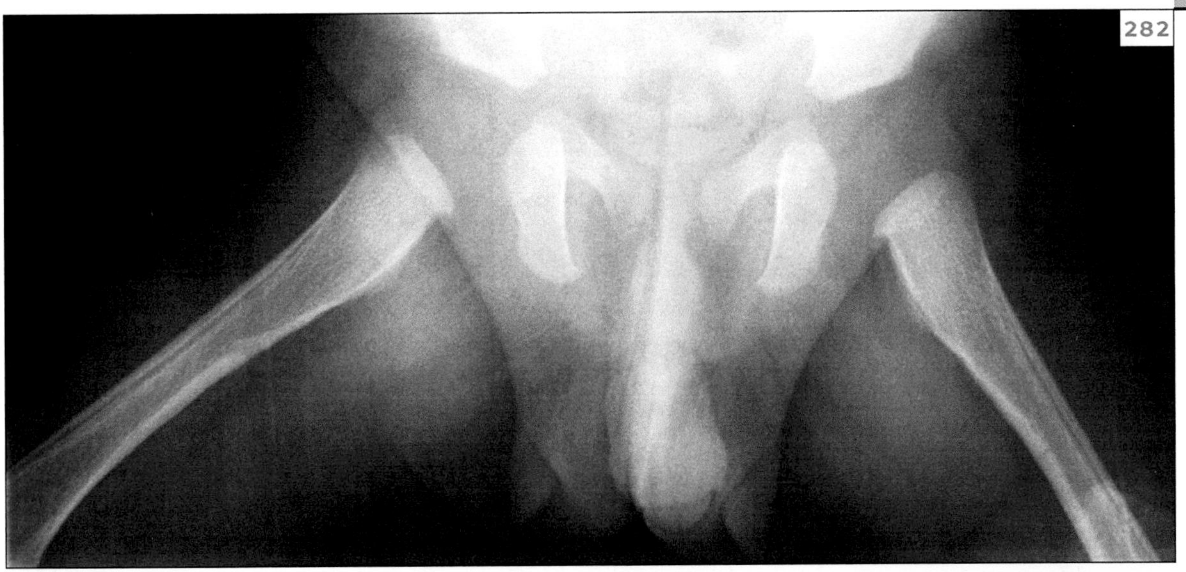

283

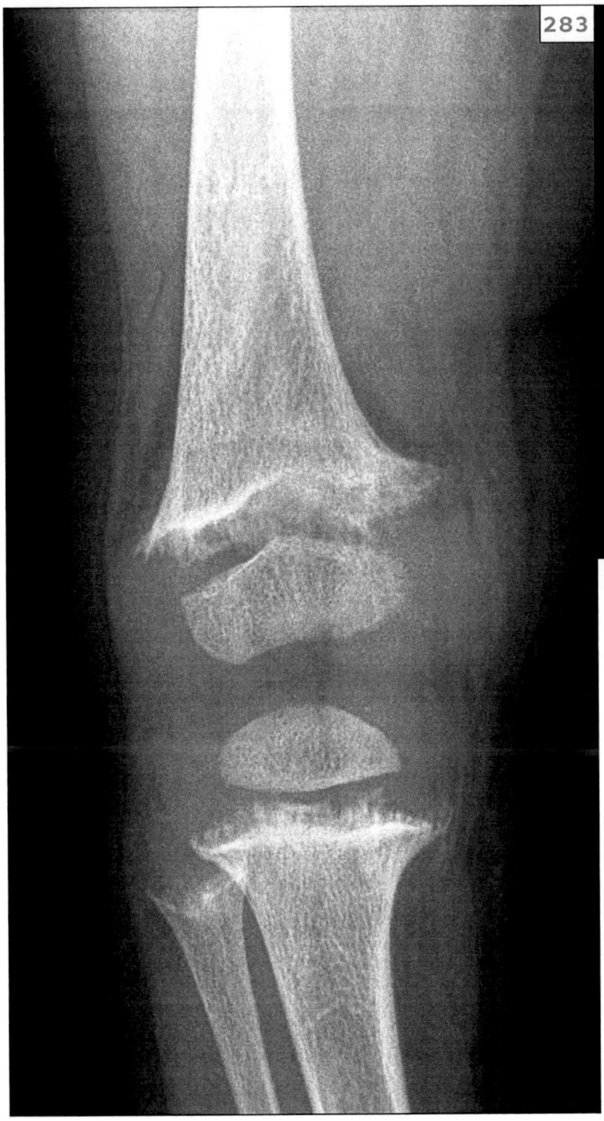

284

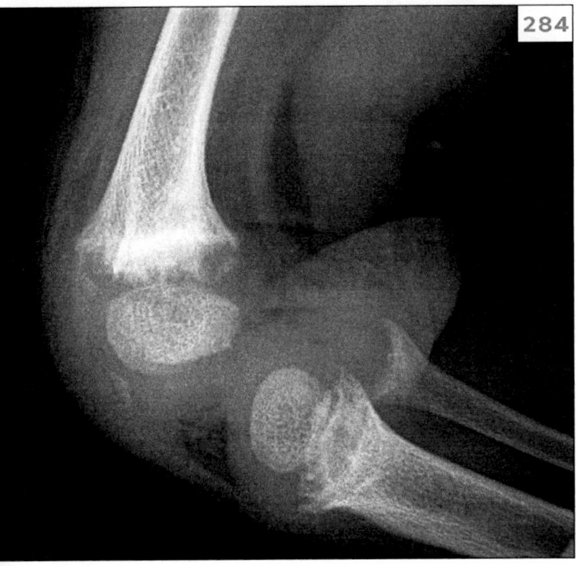

282 Anterior–posterior radiograph of the pelvis and femora in a 5-month-old child shows normal physiologic apposition of new bone along the femoral diaphyses.

283, 284 Healing rickets. (283) Anterior–posterior and (284) lateral knee radiographs in a 22-month-old with rickets shows metaphyseal widening, cupping, and fraying, and increased space between the metaphysis and epiphysis in the distal femur and the proximal tibia and fibula. Linear sclerosis at the metaphysis indicates healing has begun.

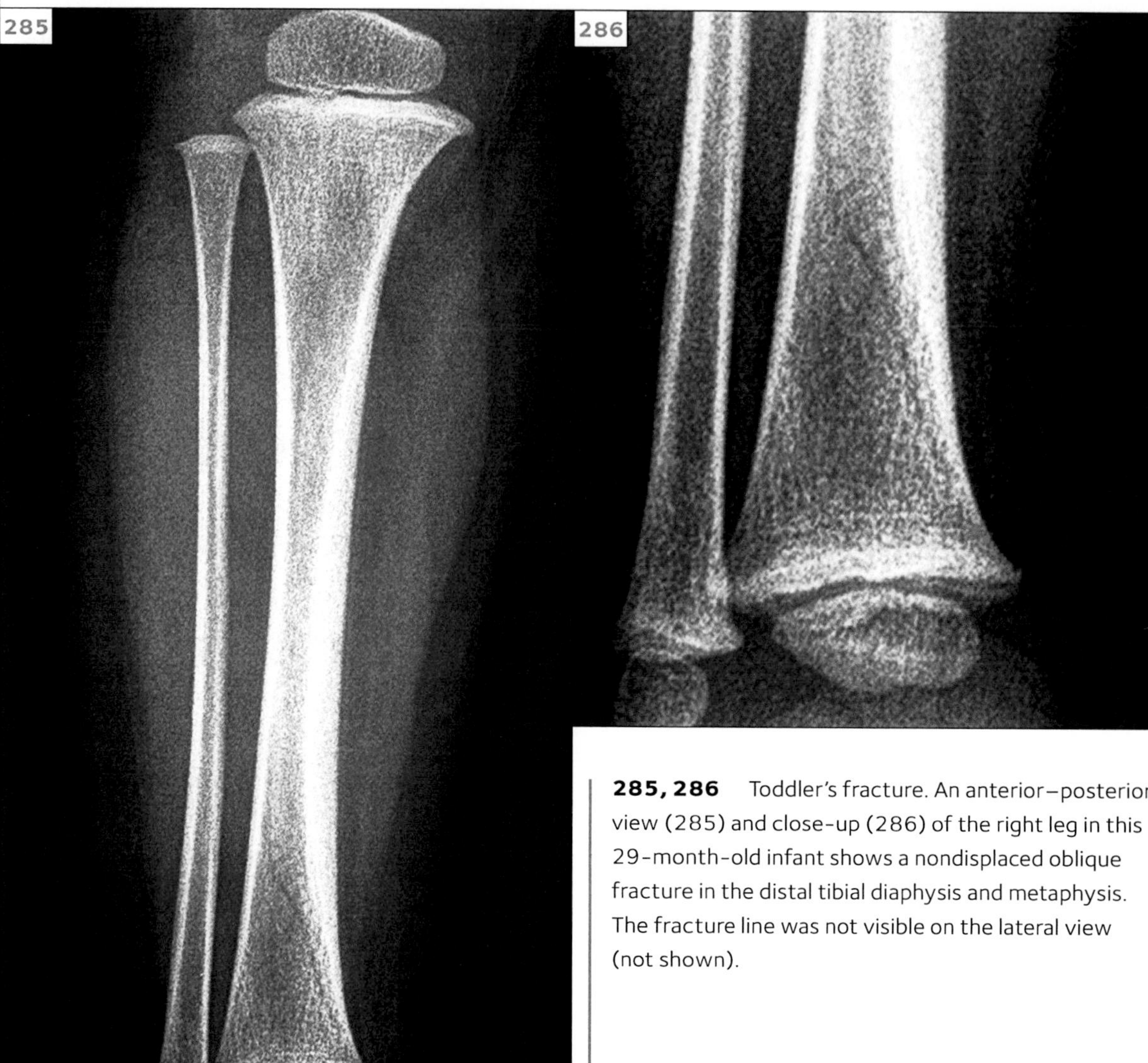

285, 286 Toddler's fracture. An anterior–posterior view (285) and close-up (286) of the right leg in this 29-month-old infant shows a nondisplaced oblique fracture in the distal tibial diaphysis and metaphysis. The fracture line was not visible on the lateral view (not shown).

287

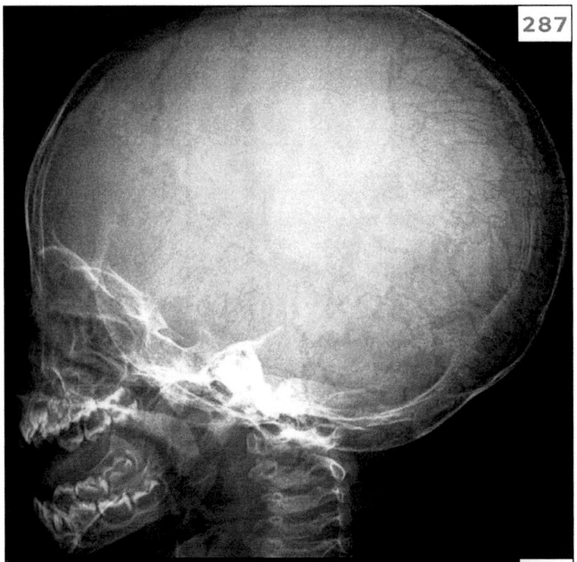

288

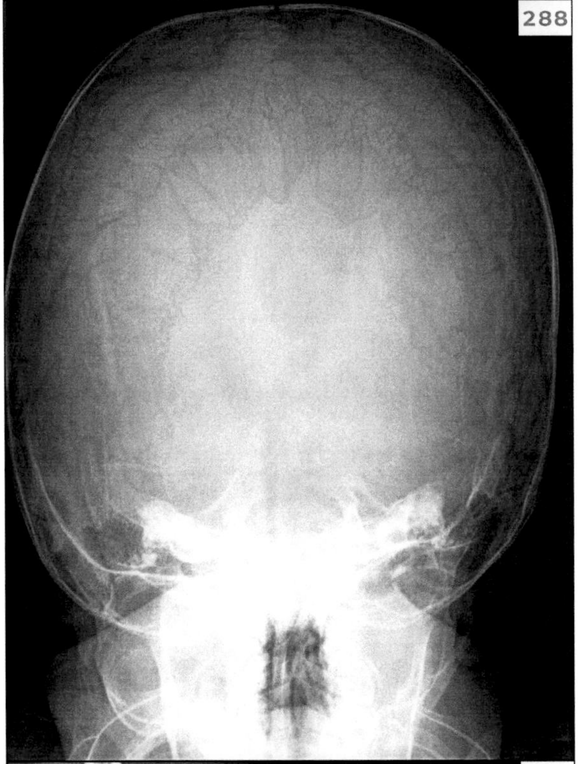

289

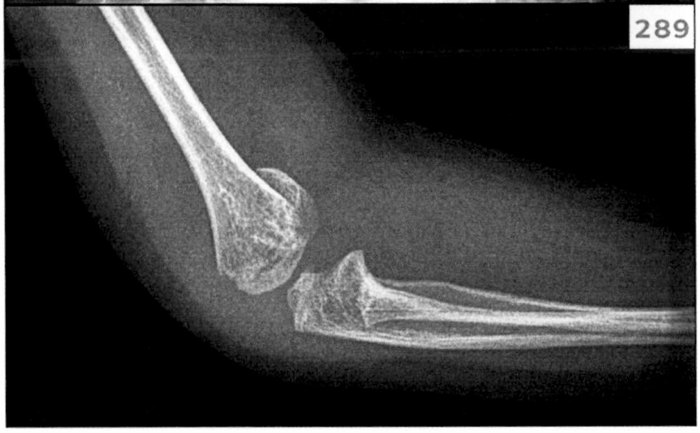

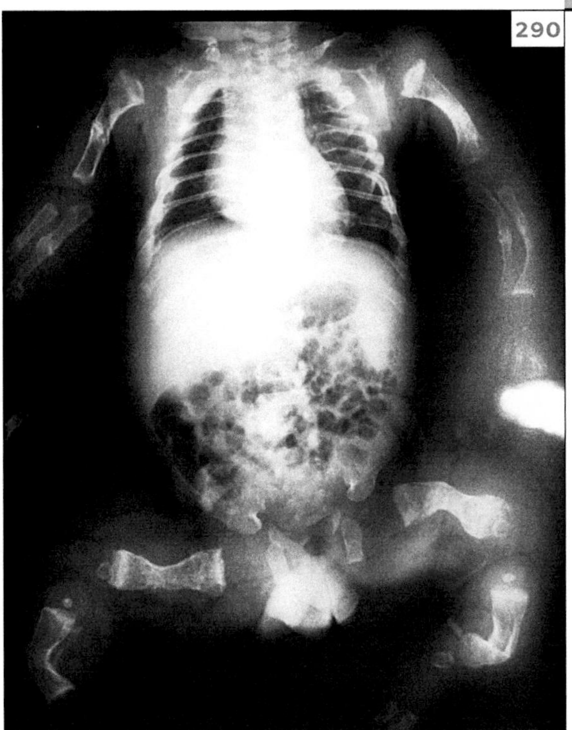

287–289 Type I osteogenesis imperfecta. (287) Lateral and (288) Towne views of the skull at 11 months of age show numerous Wormian bones. (289) Lateral view of the elbow at 19 months of age shows a fracture of the humeral condyle incurred after minimal trauma. Note the generalized bony demineralization.

290 Type II osteogenesis imperfecta. This newborn's long bones are bowed, deformed, and shortened from multiple *in utero* fractures.

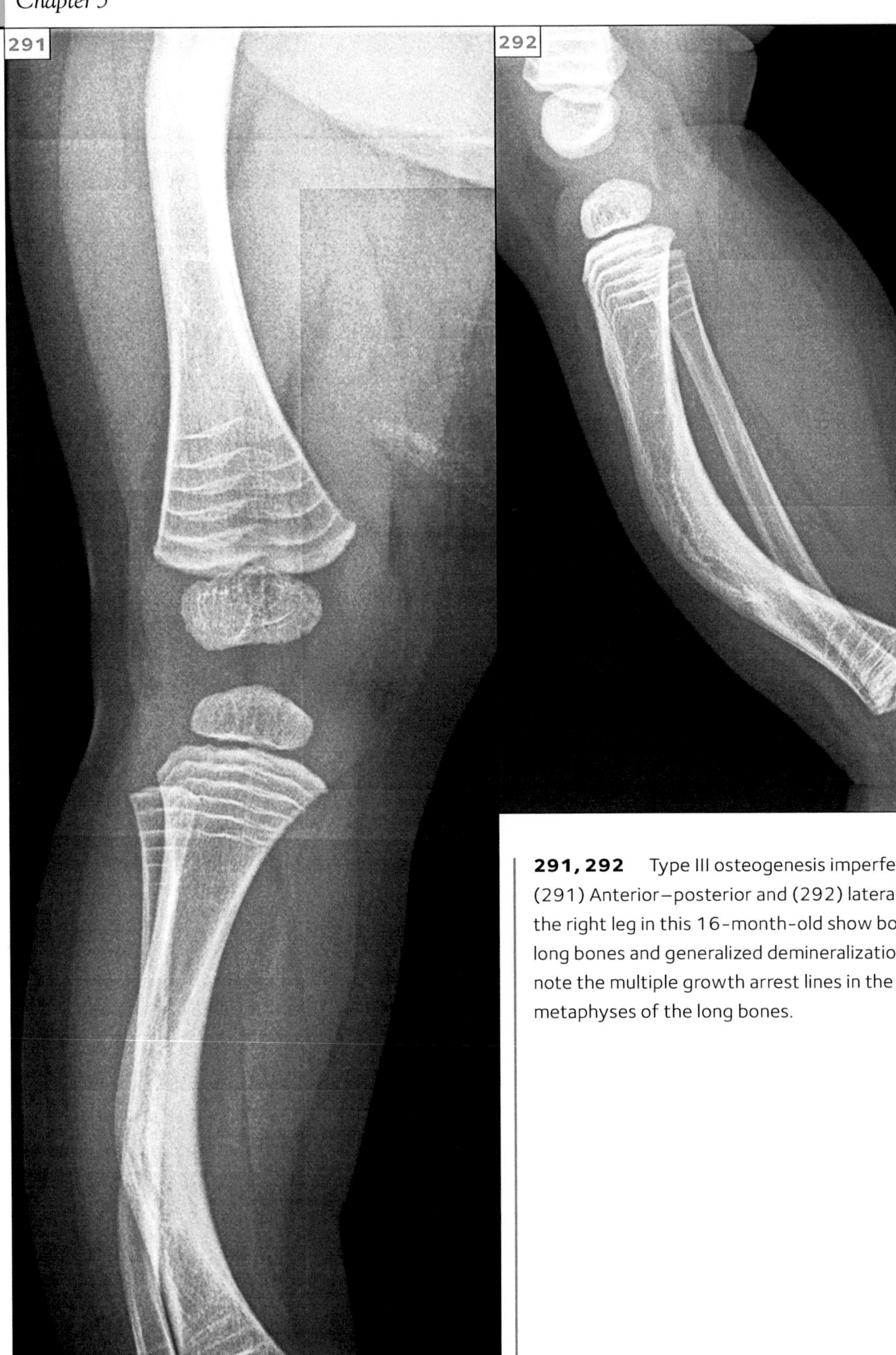

291, 292 Type III osteogenesis imperfecta. (291) Anterior–posterior and (292) lateral views of the right leg in this 16-month-old show bowing of the long bones and generalized demineralization. Also note the multiple growth arrest lines in the metaphyses of the long bones.

Head injury

Head injury from nonaccidental trauma has serious implications, as it may result in mental retardation or death. Inflicted head injury is seen in 7–12% of abused children and is responsible for most child abuse fatalities in infants and young children[5,7]. As with skeletal injury, most of these inflicted injuries occur in infants and toddlers because of the mechanism of abuse in infants and because of the susceptibility of the immature infant brain to acceleration–deceleration forces. Since the infant has a relatively large head compared to the neck and body and has incompletely myelinated brain tissue, acceleration–deceleration forces more readily lead to shear-strain deformation at many tissue interfaces in the brain and can result in disruption of axonal integrity and of cortical veins. Whether shaking alone accounts for these forces or whether additional impact is required has long been a topic of debate[37–40]. Certainly additional impact may provide further large deceleration forces on the brain, as well as direct force to the skull, leading to fractures. Apnea resulting from the primary injury may lead to secondary injuries such as cerebral edema, swelling, hypoxia–ischemia, and herniation.

Skull fractures are found in approximately 10% of abused children[41]. No pattern or appearance of a skull fracture is highly specific for NAT. Simple skull fractures, i.e. linear fractures which do not cross calvarial sutures and have less than 3 mm separation between fragments, are frequently seen in both accidental and nonaccidental trauma (**293**). Diastatic, depressed, or complex (comminuted) fractures may also be seen in accidental injury, although if these are seen in combination with a reported history of only minor trauma, they should be viewed as suspicious for abuse[42,43] (**294–298**). As with accidental trauma, there is poor correlation between the presence of a skull fracture and intracranial injury. The likelihood of a child incurring a skull facture by falling from a short height, such as a bed, has been shown to be quite low[44]. The likelihood of death from such a short fall is estimated to be less than one in a million[45]. Because axial plane computed tomography (CT) images are not as sensitive for the detection of skull fractures as plain radiographs, it is particularly important to include skull radiographs as part of the routine skeletal survey. Sutural diastasis alone on plain films may be seen with chronic subdural hematomas (**299**).

Subdural hematoma (SDH) is the most common intracranial imaging abnormality in NAT. There are other potential causes of SDH besides NAT, including accidental injury, birth-related trauma, metabolic and coagulation disorders, but most of these can be excluded by history and routine testing[46]. SDH in NAT typically results from shear-strain forces leading to disruption of cortical veins, often those draining into the superior sagittal sinus because of the great force produced along the falx cerebri. Hence, early or small SDH due to inflicted injury is typically seen in the interhemispheric fissure, a pattern first described by pediatric neuroradiologist Robert Zimmerman and colleagues[47]. This lesion is one that is strongly associated with abuse when seen in infancy, though it may also be seen with major accidental injury (**300–312**)[48]. SDH is also frequently seen along the cerebral convexities; in cases of NAT, convexity collections are commonly bilateral and may be remote from a fracture caused by the associated impact, as opposed to accidental epidural or subdural hematoma, which is commonly unilateral and situated just deep to a skull fracture.

On CT, acute interhemispheric SDH appears as a high-attenuation stripe in the interhemispheric fissure. Acute convexity SDH appears as a high-attenuation crescentic collection over the cerebral hemisphere. On conventional 'brain window' settings, acute convexity blood may be dense enough to be indistinguishable from the adjacent inner table of the skull, so it is important to view images on wider 'subdural window' settings to improve lesion conspicuity. Small acute convexity SDH near the vertex of the skull may not be evident on CT because of this hyperdensity.

Dating of intracranial hemorrhage by CT is not as straightforward as once thought[40]. Initial studies on evolution of blood products by CT involved blood in various intracranial locations in the adult head, which does not translate neatly to evaluation of subdural hemorrhage in a young child's head. On CT, hyperacute blood may mix imperceptibly with cerebrospinal fluid, but within hours, the acute phase of white blood within the subdural space is seen. Generally, subdural blood becomes less dense as it ages. On CT, parenchymal blood becomes imperceptible by 10 days after bleeding, and extra-axial hemorrhage probably begins to evolve away from the acute pure 'white state' even earlier. Mixed-density subdural collections may be seen as soon as 24–48 hours after the injury[40,49,50]. There is a general pattern of evolution of SDH on magnetic resonance imaging that is better for dating SDH than is CT[51]. Acute SDH (1–3 days old) is iso- to hypointense on T1-weighted images and hypointense on T2-weighted images. Early subacute SDH (3–7 days old) is hyperintense on T1-weighted images and still hypointense on T2-weighted images, but late SDH (8–14 days) is hyperintense on both T1- and T2-weighted sequences. As the SDH becomes more chronic, it becomes iso- to hypointense on T1-weighted images and hypointense on T2-weighted images.

Extra-axial hemorrhage from NAT is less frequently seen in the subarachnoid space. Subarachnoid hemorrhage results from disruption of cortical vessels by shear-strain forces. Epidural hematomas are much less common as a major component in NAT. Brain parenchymal injuries include contusion (**313**), axonal shearing injury, and hypoxic injury. In severe hypoxic injury, the cerebrum is more profoundly affected than is the cerebellum; this injury results in swelling and decreased attenuation, and so the cerebrum has lower attenuation than the basal ganglia and cerebellum, which is termed the 'reversal sign' (**314, 315**)[52].

When faced with choosing from the various imaging modalities available to evaluate intracranial injury, there are several considerations. CT is the best imaging modality to use in the acute setting in a symptomatic or neurologically impaired patient, because the short scan time ensures that a sick patient will not be away from an emergency department or critical care unit for long. It readily identifies acute hemorrhage. In the subacute setting, magnetic resonance imaging (MRI) is the more sensitive test and is frequently helpful in evaluation of head injury in NAT[53]. MRI is more sensitive than CT in detecting small subdural hematomas because of its multiplanar imaging capability. Furthermore, various MRI sequences can be employed to highlight different aspects of parenchymal injury. Early on, diffusion-weighted MRI is more sensitive than CT to the presence and extent of cytotoxic edema from injury or ischemia. Fluid attenuating inversion recovery (FLAIR) sequences in MRI are helpful in demonstrating axonal shearing injury or subdural hemorrhage. With MRI, blood and blood products are detectable for longer periods of time, and MRI allows for more accurate dating of injury. T2* gradient sequences are most sensitive for detection of chronic blood products on MRI. Ultrasound is a secondary modality in the evaluation of patients with inflicted head injury. It can be useful in differentiating diffuse enlargement of the subarachnoid space from low-attenuation subdural hematoma (**309–311**). It is best reserved for follow-up of findings seen on CT or MRI and has limited usefulness.

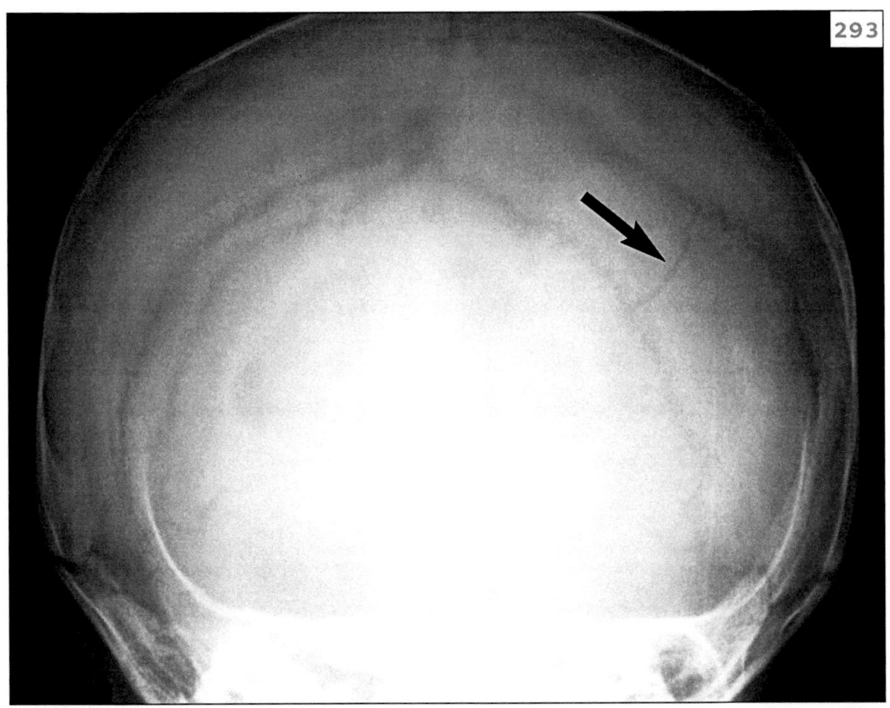

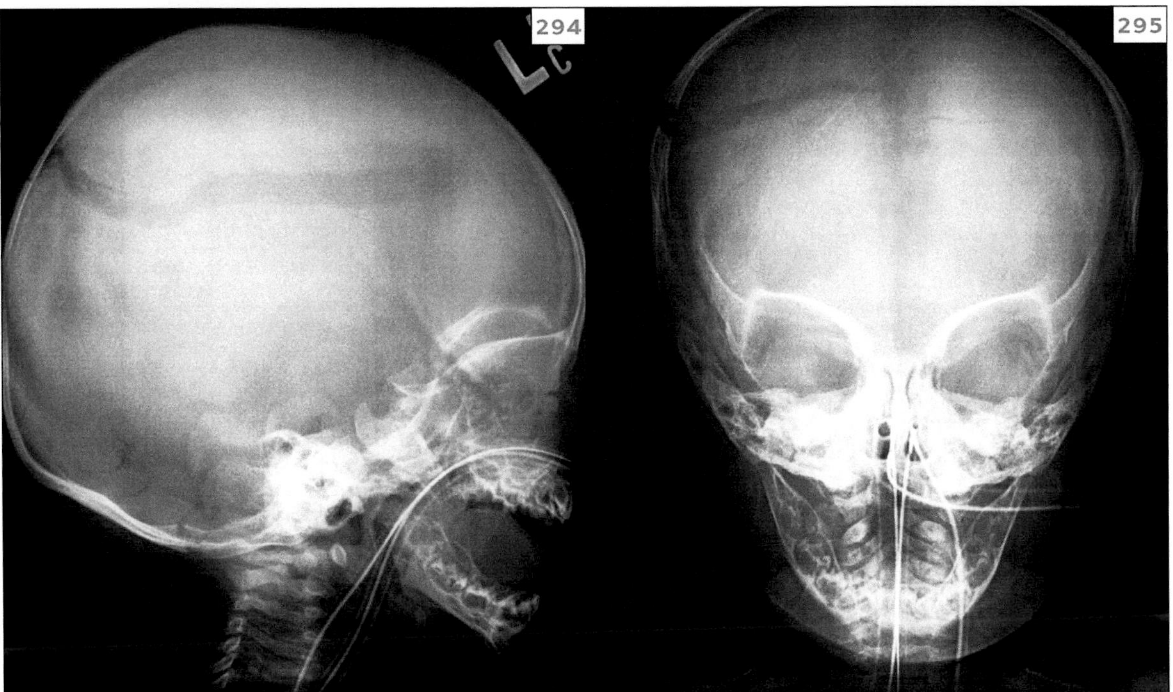

293 A Towne view of the skull in an abused 3-month-old infant demonstrates a simple linear left parietal skull fracture.

294, 295 Diastatic skull fracture. (294) Lateral and (295) frontal radiographs of the skull show a diastatic right parietal fracture in an abused 2-month-old infant. 295 reproduced with permission from Slovis TL, Haller JO, Joshi A (2004). *Pediatric Imaging*, 3rd edn. Springer, Heidelberg.

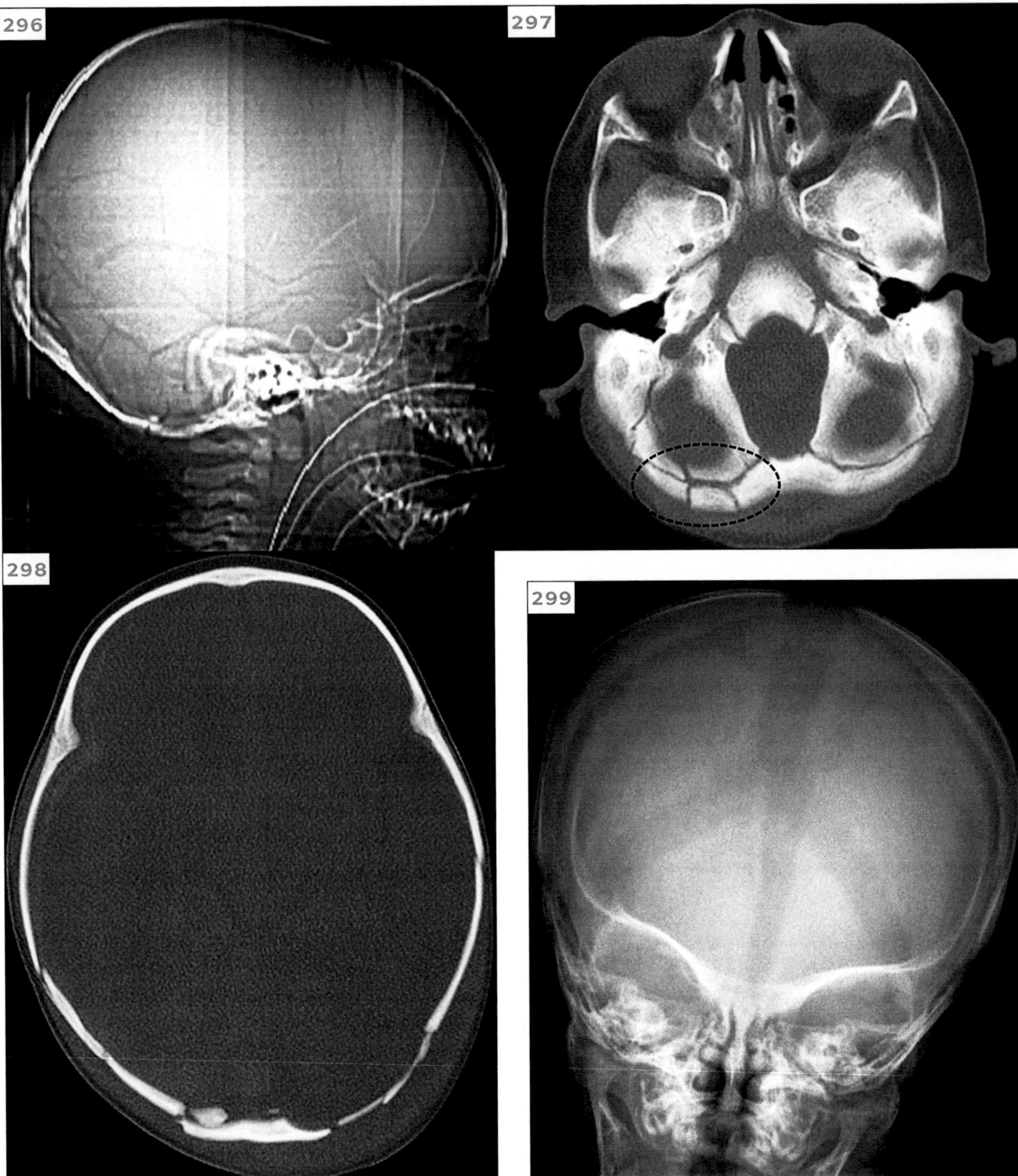

296–298 Complex skull fracture. (296) Lateral computed tomography (CT) scout view from the head of an abused 7-month-old infant shows multiple fracture lines in the occipital and parietal bones. (297) Bone window image from the CT shows multiple fracture lines and diastasis of the right occipital suture. (298) More cephalad image from the CT with bone windowing shows multiple fractures with depressed fragments and associated scalp swelling.

299 Sutural diastasis. A frontal view of the skull shows the calvarial sutures to be widened in this 4-month-old with chronic subdural hematomas.

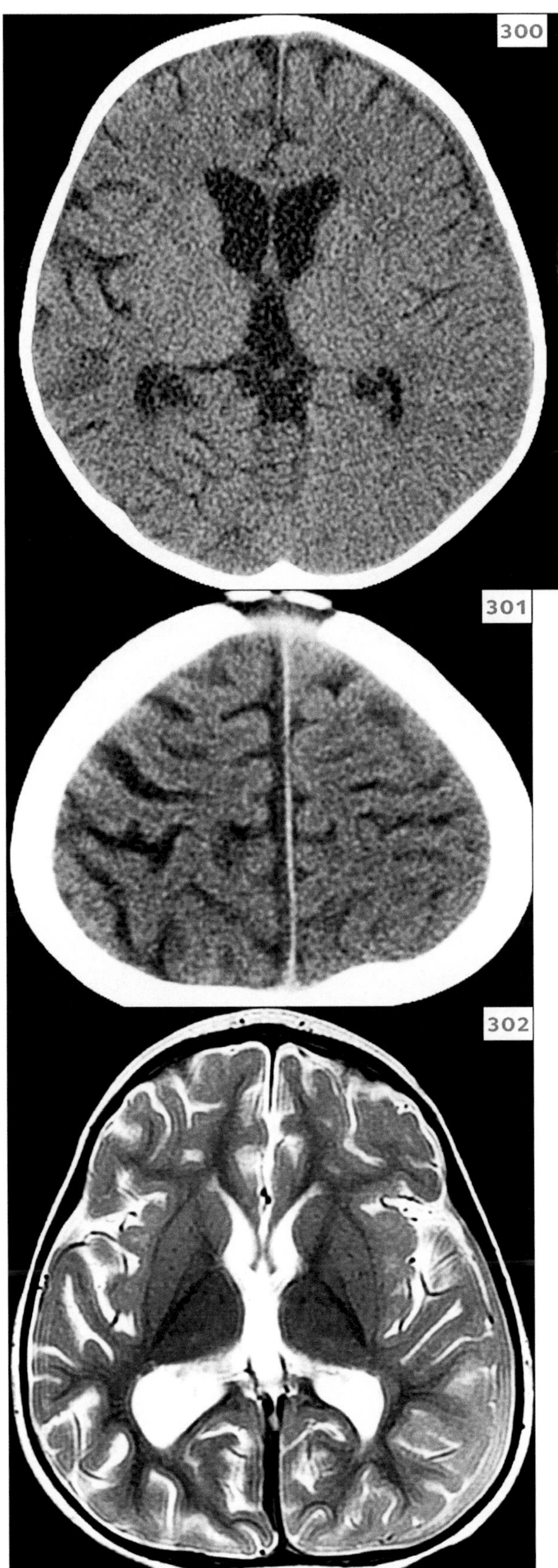

300–303 Subdural hematomas of different ages. (300) Noncontrast axial computed tomography (CT) image of the head in a 2-year-old shows an isodense subdural hematoma over the left convexity, with sulcal effacement on the left, and mild dilatation of the lateral and third ventricles. (301) A more cephalad image from the same CT examination reveals a right parafalcine low attenuation collection near the vertex. (302) Axial fast spin echo (FSE) T2 and (303) coronal FSE T2 magnetic resonance images confirm the presence of the iso- to mildly hyperintense left convexity subdural hematoma and hypointense right posterior parafalcine hematoma.

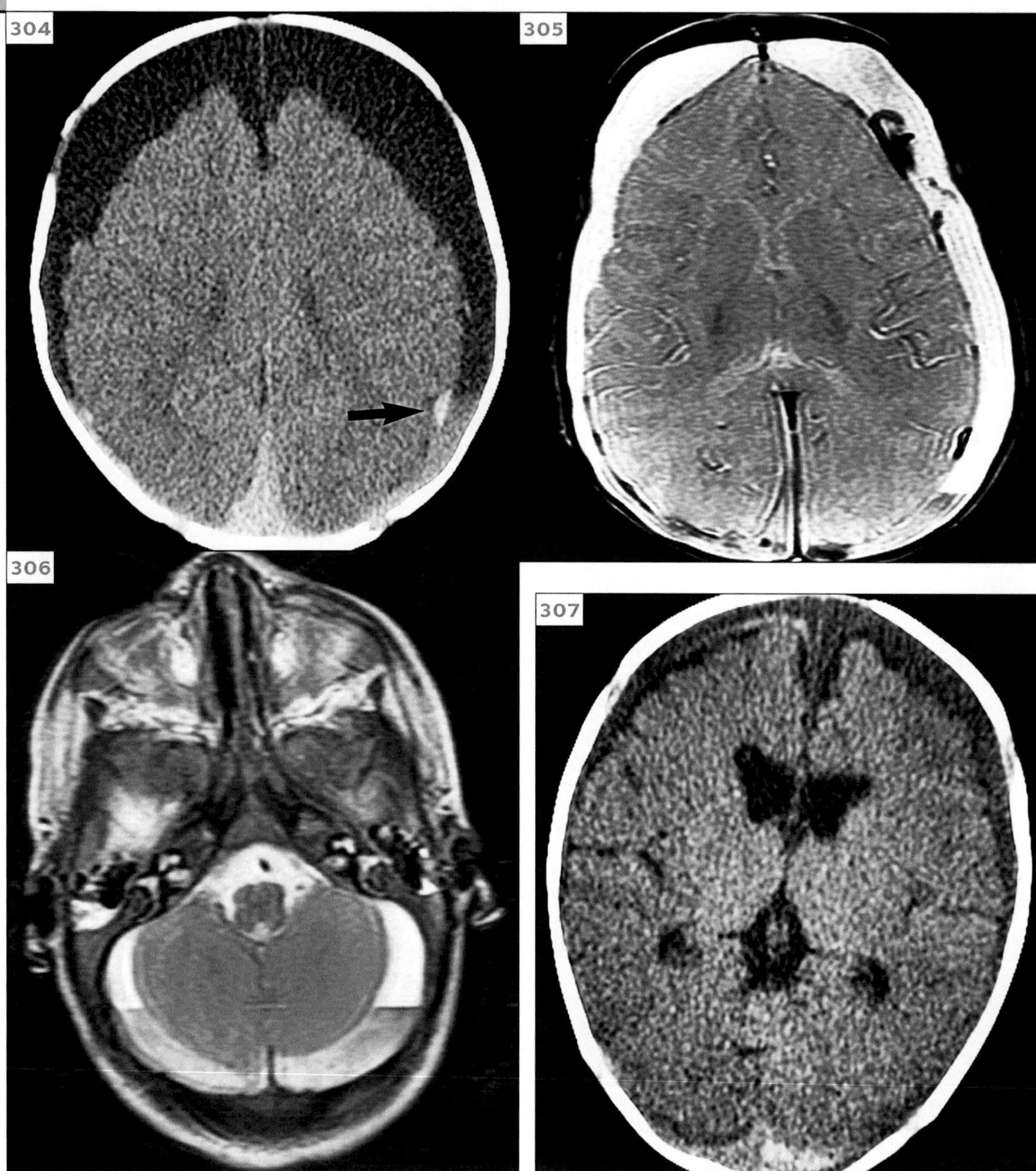

304–306 Bilateral subdural hematomas with blood of varying ages in an abused 2-month-old. (304) Axial computed tomographic image at the level of the frontal horns shows large bilateral subdural collections with a fluid-blood level, a small acute hemorrhage near the left parietal convexity and more acute blood in the interhemispheric extra-axial space posteriorly. (305) T2* gradient echo sequence shows large bilateral subdural hematomas with a fluid-blood level. Over the frontal and parietal convexities, there are hypointense areas consistent with superficial siderosis. (306) Axial T2 fast spin echo (FSE) magnetic resonance (MR) image shows subdural hematoma in the posterior fossa with fluid-blood levels.

307 Subdural hematomas. Axial noncontrast computed tomographic image of the head in this 4-month-old with chronic subdural hematomas shows more acute blood products posteriorly, as well as a membrane anteriorly in the right frontal extra-axial space. The lateral ventricles are mildly enlarged.

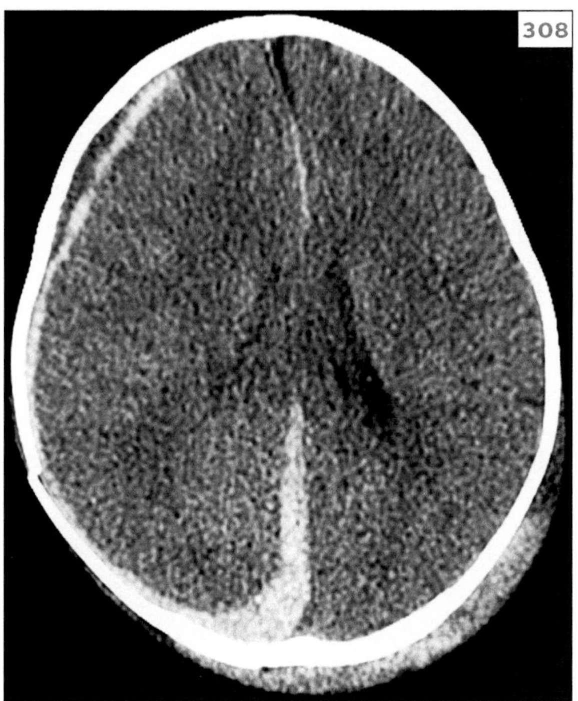

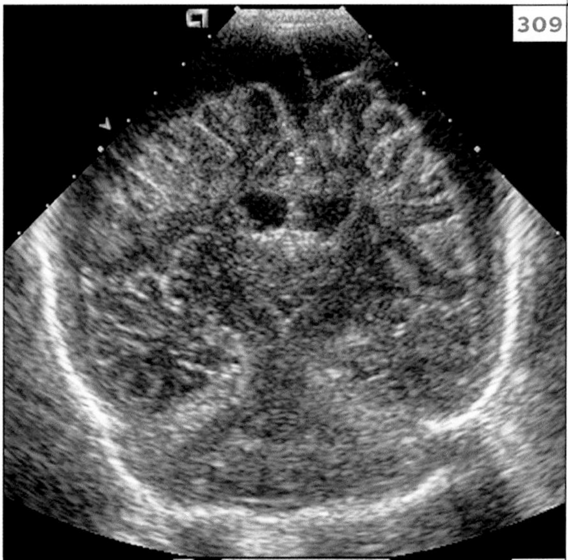

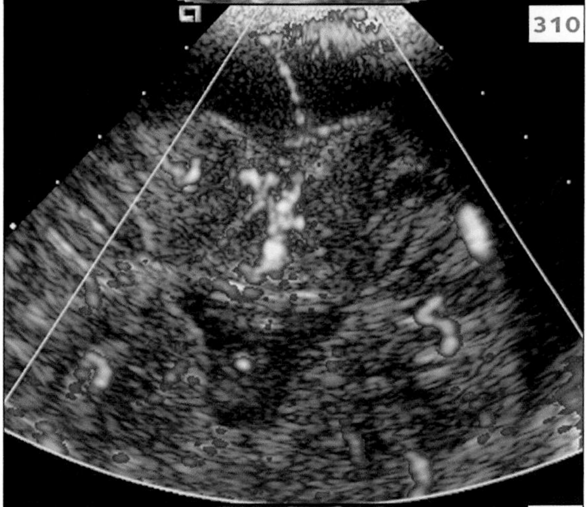

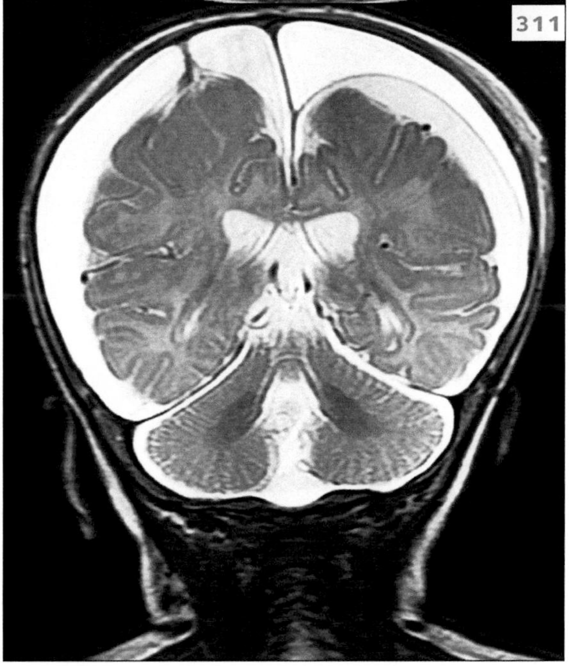

308 Subdural hematoma. Axial noncontrast computed tomographic image of the head in a 7-month-old shows an acute right subdural hematoma in the right parafalcine area, as well as over the right cerebral convexity and lower attenuation fluid (either chronic or hyperacute blood) in the right extra-axial space. There is also mild right-to-left midline shift with effacement of right-sided sulci, scalp hematoma, and a depressed skull fracture on this image.

309–311 Subdural hematoma diagnosed on ultrasound in a 4-month-old with macrocephaly. (309) Coronal transfontanelle ultrasound image demonstrates large extra-axial fluid collections bilaterally, compressing cerebral gyri and extending into the interhemispheric fissure. (310) Color Doppler ultrasound with a high-frequency linear transducer shows no bridging vessels. In contrast, bilateral large subarachnoid spaces would show multiple bridging vessels within the fluid spaces and enlarged sulci. (311) Coronal fast spin echo (FSE) T2-weighted magnetic resonance image confirms the presence of large bilateral subdural hematomas.

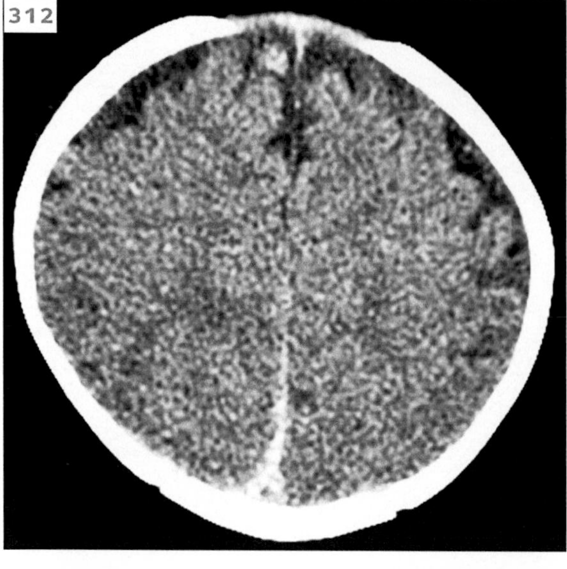

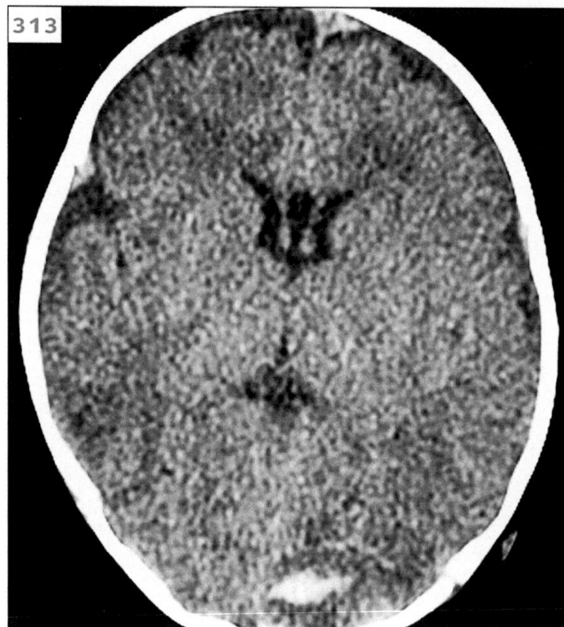

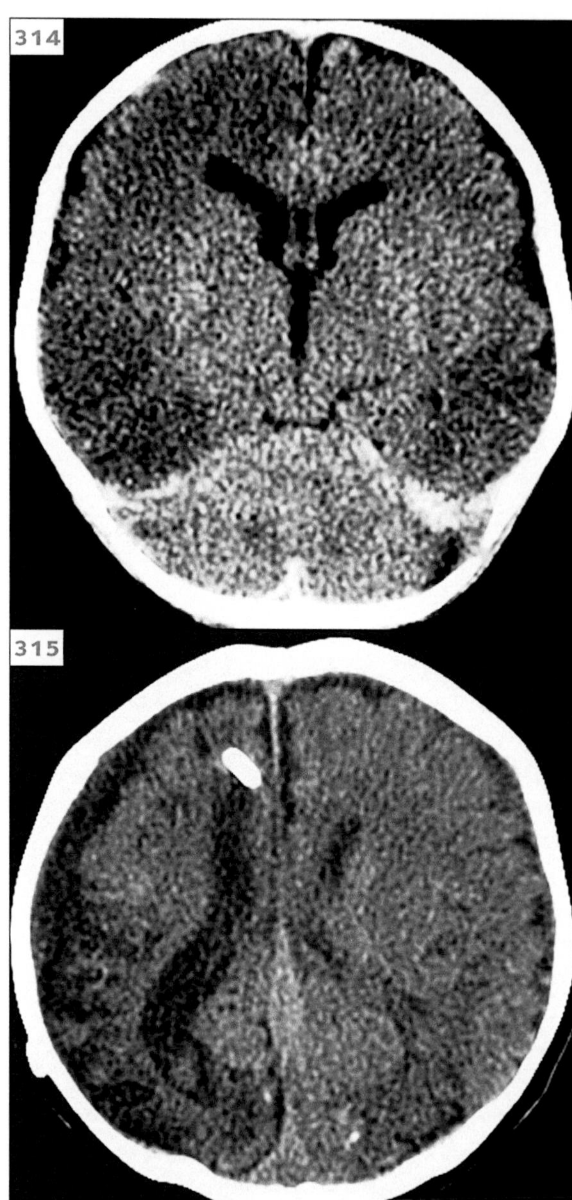

312 More subtle subdural hemorrhage. Axial noncontrast computed tomographic image of the head in a 2.5-month-old abused infant shows a thin collection of hyperdense (acute) interhemispheric blood posteriorly and small focus anteriorly. Subdural blood products were confirmed by magnetic resonance imaging.

313 Hemorrhagic contusion. Axial noncontrast computed tomographic image of the head in a 1-month-old abused infant shows hypoattenuation and loss of gray–white matter differentiation in the left occipital lobe consistent with contusion, within which there is a central hyperdense hemorrhagic focus within the lesion.

314, 315 Hypoxic injury with diffuse edema. (314) Axial noncontrast computed tomographic image of the head in a 2-month-old with seizures reveals cerebral hypoattenuation, more in the right cerebral hemisphere, and loss of gray–white matter differentiation. Normal attenuation of cerebellum and basal ganglia is maintained (reversal sign). There is a small amount of acute blood along the tentorium. (315) Follow-up computed tomography 4 months later shows encephalomalacia, worse again in the right cerebral hemisphere, a ventriculostomy catheter and dystrophic calcification in the occipital lobes.

Visceral injury

No good data exist on the overall incidence of visceral injury in physically abused children, but the literature suggests that with increasing age after infancy, nonaccidental abdominal trauma becomes a more frequent cause of death than nonaccidental head injury. These injuries may result from direct blows to the abdomen from the perpetrator's fist or foot or from deceleration injury after being thrown. Delay in seeking medical treatment and the incomplete history provided at the time of presentation contribute to the high mortality of up to 50% from such injuries. By the time the diagnosis is made, patients may be hypovolemic from hemorrhage or in septic shock from peritonitis. The most commonly injured abdominal viscera from nonaccidental trauma are the gastrointestinal tract, liver, pancreas, and adrenal gland[54–56]. The surgical issues associated with these injuries are discussed in Chapter 9, Abusive abdominal trauma.

As in accidental trauma, contrast-enhanced CT scan is the most sensitive examination for detecting abdominal visceral injury, although ultrasound is a reasonable modality with which to begin the imaging work-up in cases where signs and symptoms are vague and the child is not acutely ill. Plain radiography is of limited utility in evaluating the abdominal viscera except to display pneumoperitoneum in cases where intestinal perforation is suspected. Upper gastrointestinal examinations are especially helpful in evaluation for intramural intestinal hematoma. The abdominal visceral injuries seen on imaging examinations in cases of abuse are in most cases indistinguishable from accidental injuries, and noting any discrepancy between the provided history and the severity of injury, as seen on imaging examinations, is very important.

Intestinal injuries in nonaccidental trauma include perforations and intramural hematomas. Perforations occur most commonly in the jejunum and duodenum, and manifest on radiographic examinations as small amounts of free air with possible ascites or hemoperitoneum. Intramural hematoma, described in many cases of child abuse, commonly affects the lateral wall of the descending duodenum and may be visible on ultrasound, CT, or as a 'coiled spring' on upper gastrointestinal examination (**316**).

The liver is more commonly injured in abdominal NAT than initially recognized and is seen in nearly 50% children with inflicted abdominal trauma[55,56]. Most commonly, hepatic injuries occur in the midline, in the left lobe and caudate lobe, because of midline blows compressing the organ against the spine. Ultrasound, CT, and MRI may show parenchymal disruption with parenchymal hematoma or biloma (**317–322**). Hemoperitoneum may also be seen.

Approximately one-third of pancreatitis in children is due to trauma, including inflicted injury, and about 60% of pancreatic pseudocysts are due to trauma[57,58]. On plain radiographs, some more subtle signs of pancreatitis can be seen, including sentinel loops (focal dilatation of small bowel loops due to adjacent inflammation) and the colon cut-off sign. Ultrasound may demonstrate an enlarged gland with decreased echogenicity, possibly with adjacent fluid collections. On CT examination, the pancreas appears enlarged and of heterogeneously low density, with adjacent fat stranding and peripancreatic fluid. Lytic osseous changes from fat embolism in pancreatitis have been described in the small bones of the extremities and long bone metaphyses[59].

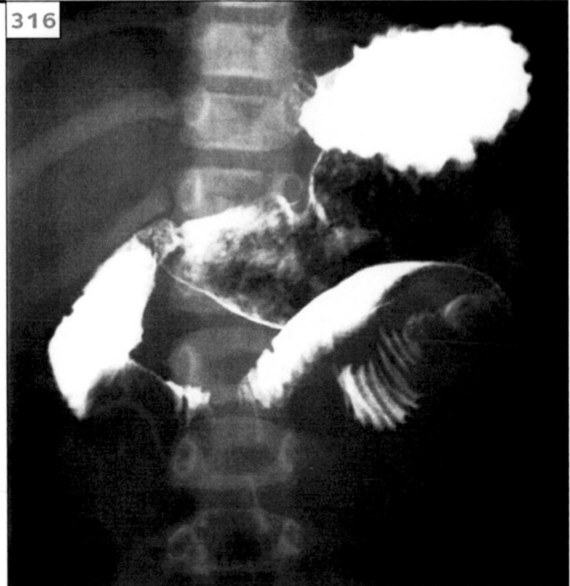

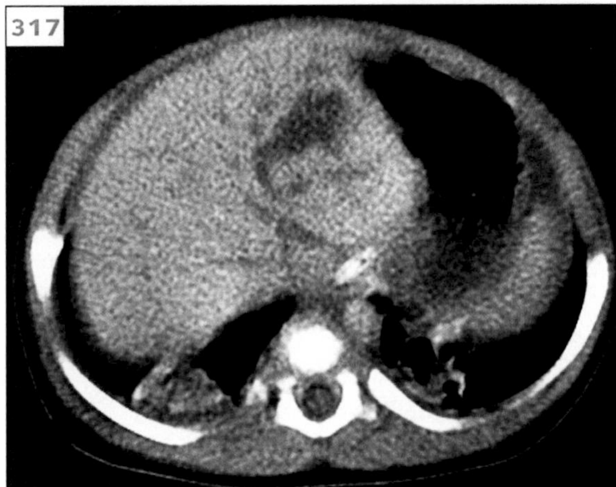

316 Duodenal hematoma. Anterior–posterior view from an upper gastrointestinal series in an 8-year-old shows an intramural filling defect in the transverse portion of the duodenum just right of the spine. Reproduced with permission from Slovis TL, Haller JO, Joshi A (2004). *Pediatric Imaging*, 3rd edn. Springer, Heidelberg.

317 Hepatic injury. Axial contrast-enhanced computed tomography scan of the abdomen in a 2-month-old male with abdominal distention shows a laceration in the medial segment of the left hepatic lobe.

Injuries to the adrenal glands are usually not isolated, but rather are seen in tandem with injuries to the above viscera[54]. Adrenal injury is more commonly seen on the right, perhaps because of drainage of the right adrenal vein directly into the inferior vena cava, making it more susceptible to changes in pressure. Ultrasound shows an enlarged and hypoechoic gland. CT and MRI demonstrate variable abnormality centrally in the gland, depending on the age of injury (**322, 323**).

Visceral injury to the kidneys, spleen, and intrathoracic viscera are less frequently seen in child physical abuse. Renal injuries, seen in 10–30% of cases of abdominal injury from abuse, may include renal contusion, renal fracture (with resultant peri-nephric hematoma or urinoma) (**324**) or renal pedicle vascular injury resulting in decreased perfusion[54,55]. The incidence of splenic injury is low in inflicted injury compared to accidental injury[54,55,60]. Also, despite the high frequency of rib fractures, injury to the intrathoracic viscera is fairly unusual, although hemothorax or pneumothorax may result (**271–274**)[61].

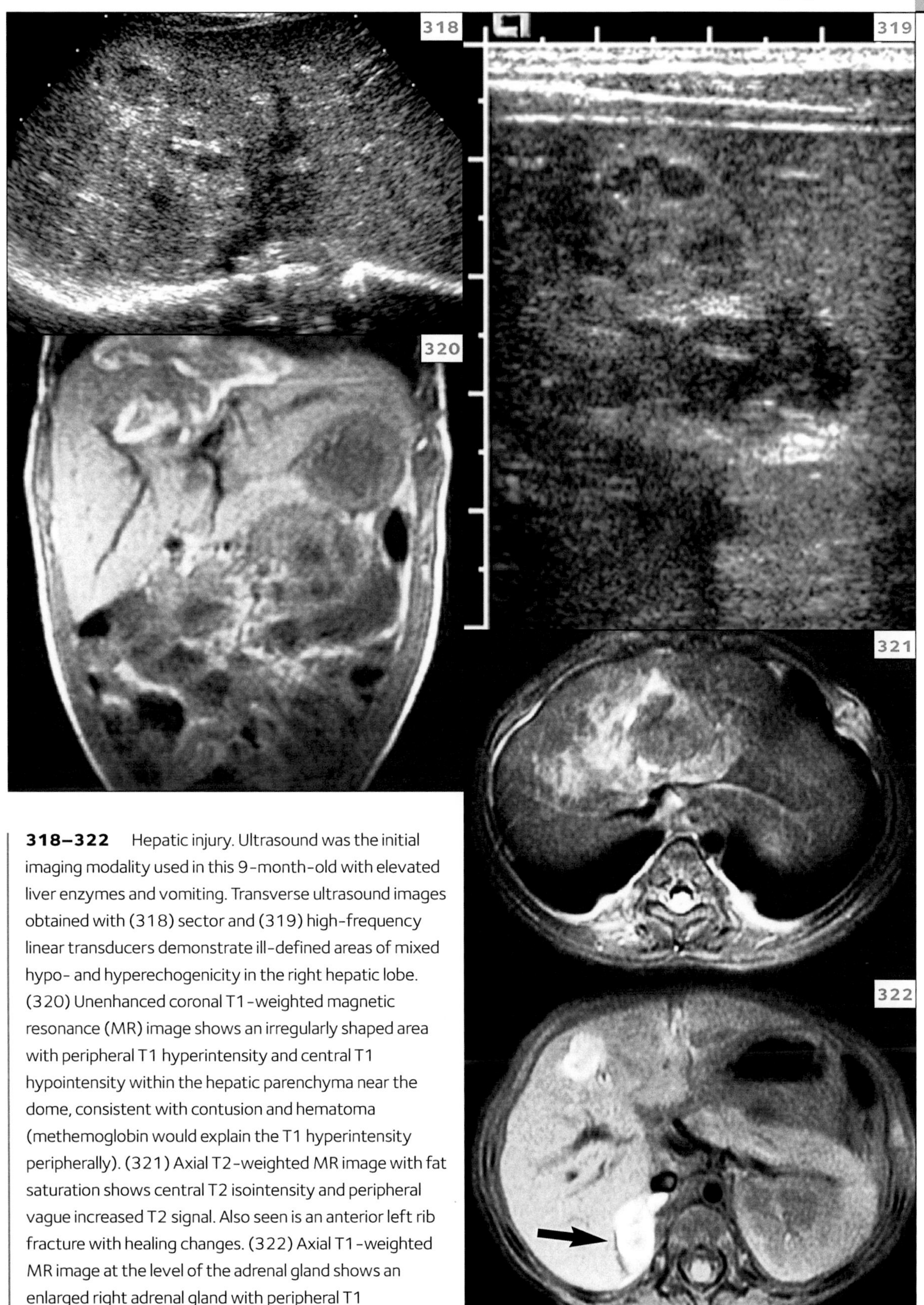

318–322 Hepatic injury. Ultrasound was the initial imaging modality used in this 9-month-old with elevated liver enzymes and vomiting. Transverse ultrasound images obtained with (318) sector and (319) high-frequency linear transducers demonstrate ill-defined areas of mixed hypo- and hyperechogenicity in the right hepatic lobe. (320) Unenhanced coronal T1-weighted magnetic resonance (MR) image shows an irregularly shaped area with peripheral T1 hyperintensity and central T1 hypointensity within the hepatic parenchyma near the dome, consistent with contusion and hematoma (methemoglobin would explain the T1 hyperintensity peripherally). (321) Axial T2-weighted MR image with fat saturation shows central T2 isointensity and peripheral vague increased T2 signal. Also seen is an anterior left rib fracture with healing changes. (322) Axial T1-weighted MR image at the level of the adrenal gland shows an enlarged right adrenal gland with peripheral T1 hyperintensity consistent with adrenal hemorrhage.

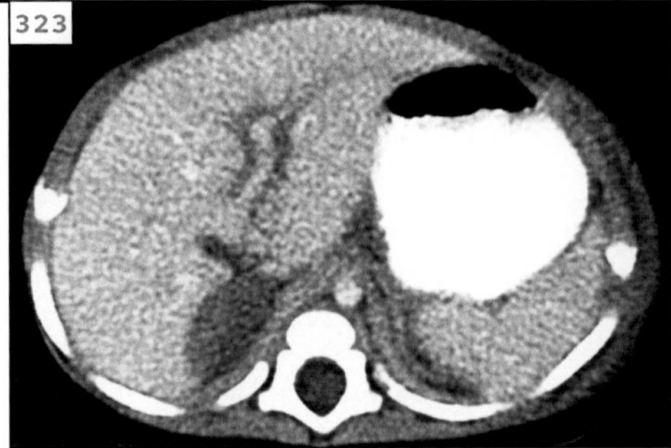

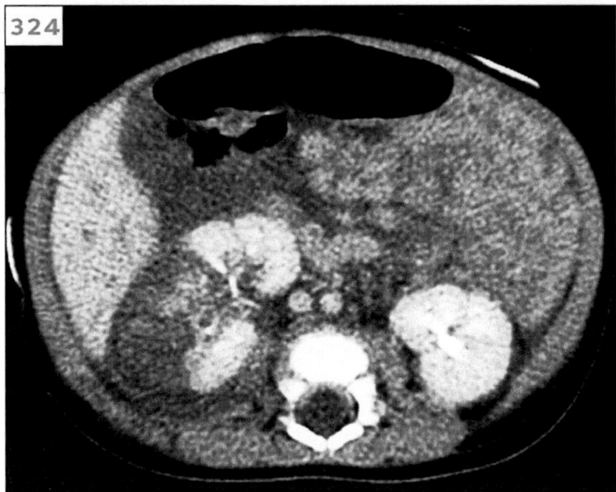

323 Hepatic injury. Axial contrast-enhanced computed tomography scan of the abdomen in a 2-month-old female with bruising demonstrates a liver laceration in the right lobe and an adjacent adrenal hematoma.

324 Renal injury. Axial contrast-enhanced computed tomography scan of the abdomen in a 2-month-old male with abdominal distention shows a right renal laceration with an area of nonenhancement interposed between two enhancing portions of the kidney, consistent with a devascularized segment and intraparenchymal hematoma.

Teaching points

- Physicians should consider the possibility of skeletal trauma in all children with suspected abuse.
- There are specific guidelines to help the physician obtain the optimal number and type of imaging studies when abuse is suspected.
- While most bone injuries in abused children are nonspecific and similar to those with accidental trauma, there are a number of specific fractures that need to be identified.
- Head injuries pose special concerns for imaging, and the physician needs to know what type of imaging is indicated and when to best document the findings while meeting the needs of the child and clinical team.
- Imaging abdominal trauma follows guidelines for accidental injuries, and it is inconsistency of the history given and the severity and nature of the internal injuries that are more predictive of the mechanism rather than the injury itself.

Chapter 6

OCULAR TRAUMA

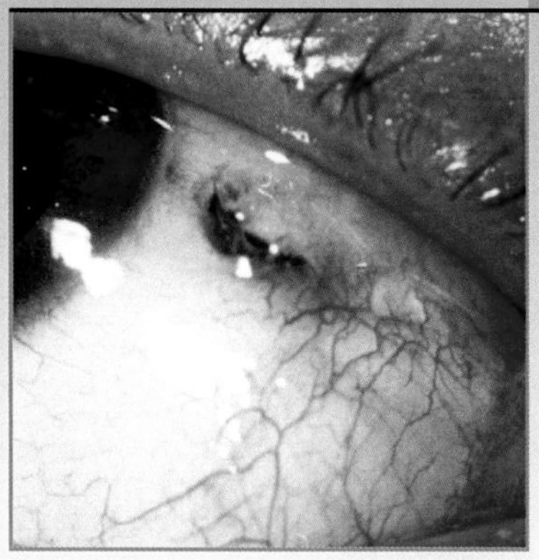

John D. Roarty MD, MPH

In 2001, there were 1,990,872 eye injuries in the United States, as reported by the National Hospital Ambulatory Medical Care Survey[1]. Up to 35% of all eye injuries are in the pediatric age group. In 2005, there were 7,523 pediatric eye injuries requiring hospitalization in the United States[2]. MacEwen *et al.*[3] reported that among their 415 Scottish residents admitted with ocular injury, 22% were under 15 years old, at an annual rate of 8.85 per 100,000 population. Of these, 70% were male, one-sixth were under 4 years old, with a slight preponderance of the right eye (52%), occurring at home (73%), and with blunt trauma causing the majority (65%) of injuries. Similar findings were noted in Helsinki, where roughly one-third of eye injury patients were children, 80% of these were boys, and most (92%) occurred at home[4].

Introduction

Assaults or child abuse account for only a small proportion (1%) of eye injuries[4,5]. Most eye injuries are not intentionally inflicted, but occur during activities which, while not maltreatment in themselves, may involve some degree of improper supervision or ineffective or improperly used protective gear. Sports injuries are common, especially with baseball, basketball, tennis, and hockey[6]. Of severe sports-related eye injuries, 5% occurred with safety or prescription eyewear[7]. Fireworks, bungee cords, fishhooks, needles, knives, pencils (**325**), and pens have all been reported. Motor vehicle airbag accidents damage the cornea with significant endothelial cell loss[8]. Firearm-related eye injuries have decreased over the last 10 years, but pediatric homicide has increased[9].

Recurrent conjunctivitis as a manifestation of Munchausen syndrome by proxy has been reported[9]. Nonaccidental pediatric injuries can be associated with eye trauma in 40% of cases[10]. While the characteristic lesion of abusive head trauma has been noted to be the retinal hemorrhage, progressively more serious injuries have been identified, and ocular findings other than retinal hemorrhages must be considered[11]. In a study of 23 children dying from nonaccidental trauma over 4 years, Green *et al.*[12] noted that retinal hemorrhage and detachment are more common at the periphery and optic disk than at the equator, that optic injury is strongly correlated with the degree of central nervous system injury, and that vitreous traction is likely the cause of intra-ocular pathology. Sexually transmitted disease, external ocular trauma, orbital injury and cranial nerve palsies[13] may be manifestations of nonaccidental trauma.

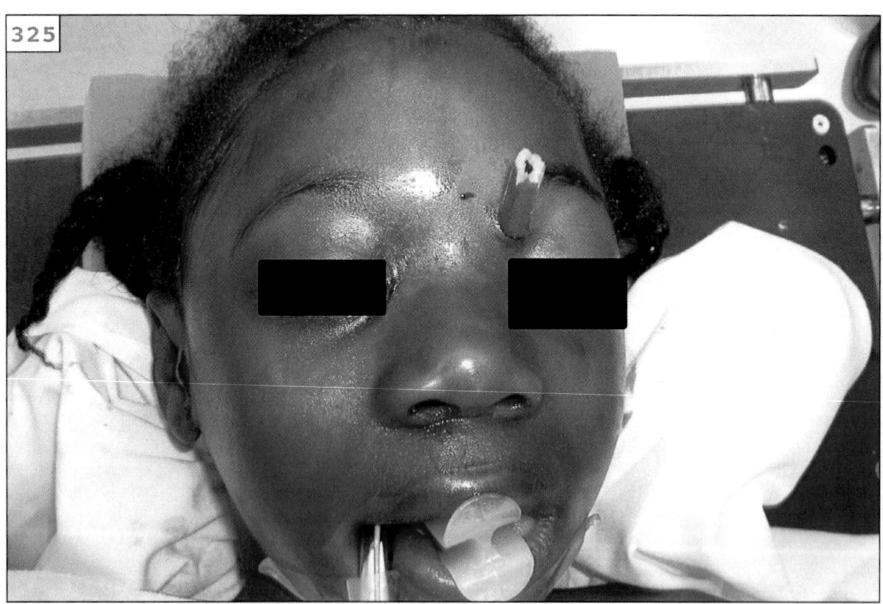

325 Patient who has suffered orbital penetration after a fall on a pencil. There is no globe injury.

Examination

A thorough history of the injury, with past medical history, including birth history, is necessary. Inconsistencies in the history aid in diagnosis. A basic eye examination is needed on the initial evaluation of the pediatric patient with ocular trauma. An external peri-orbital examination, a motility examination, and an assessment for an afferent pupillary defect can often be assessed with the help of the parent. A formal visual acuity determination is important; its form depends upon the child's age. A formal vision test at near or distance can be obtained with Snellen letters, a matching test (HOTV), the 'E' game, or Allen figures. If the largest letter cannot be seen, any characterization by 'fix and follow', count fingers, hand motion, or light perception is still valuable.

An external examination of the head, lids, and adnexa will detect lid trauma, peri-ocular bruising, a mass, or palpable orbital rim defects. Evaluation of the anterior segment for conjunctival injury, corneal injury, hyphema, or cataract is best undertaken with the slit lamp, if available. However, a penlight examination is still useful. Fluorescein staining with use of a cobalt blue light on the cornea can identify a corneal abrasion, a foreign body, or infection. Fluorescein can also highlight leakage of the aqueous fluid from a corneal laceration. A Wood's lamp offers more magnification and an ultraviolet light source. In the primary care setting, the direct ophthalmoscope can view the optic nerve and macular area well. The retina and optic nerve are examined most thoroughly with pupillary dilation and indirect ophthalmoscopy.

An intra-ocular pressure is useful in the diagnosis of a rupture of the globe. Normal intra-ocular pressure ranges from 10 to 21 mmHg. With a rupture of the globe, the intra-ocular pressure is often less than 8 mmHg. Prior to pressure measurement, proparacaine is instilled in the eye. Goldmann applanation tonometry on the slit lamp is safe with a cooperative child. The intra-ocular pressure is measured as a reflection of the tear film surface tension. Indentation tonometry with the Shiotz tonometer, Tono-Pen tonometry, or palpation applies pressure to the surface of the cornea. With a rupture of the globe, excessive indentation could result in an expulsive choroidal hemorrhage. The Shiotz tonometer weighs 16.5 g (**326**).

If the child is too young or uncooperative, sedation is required. With some injuries, the eyelids are too swollen to open easily. Lid retractors, a lid speculum, or bent paper clips can hold the lids back. If the examination is difficult and there is a concern for a ruptured globe, it is best to shield the eye and refer to an ophthalmologist without an examination.

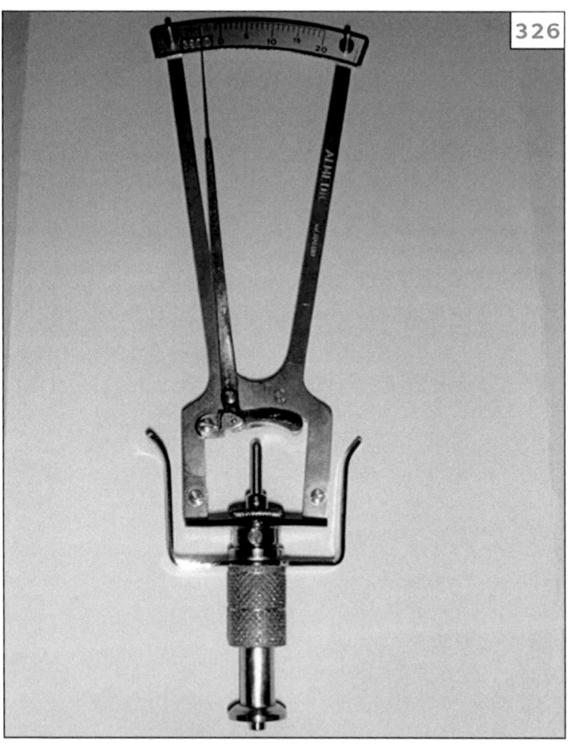

326 The Schiotz tonometer which is used to measure intra-ocular pressure.

Orbital trauma

Penetrating orbital trauma may be subtle or remote (**327**). A left eye ptosis is related to a remote bullet entry site as seen in this teenaged child. The entry site is temporal. Removal of the bullet resulted in complete lid function in this case (**328**). Imaging followed by careful intra-operative exploration may be needed to determine the extent of the injury to the orbit or globe.

Peri-orbital ecchymosis, unilateral or bilateral, may indicate trauma. However, it may be associated with a coagulopathy, or neuroblastoma with periosteal infiltration as in this patient (**329**). Blunt trauma may result in a fracture of the floor of the orbit. This may lead to entrapment of the inferior rectus muscle in the fracture. This results in an elevation deficit (**330**). Computed tomography will demonstrate the fracture and entrapped muscle. Sudden forced elevation of the eye may lead to a vasovagal or an emetic response with an entrapped inferior rectus.

A lid laceration may occur with a sharp instrument or a tear injury as in this dog bite (**331**). A lid margin laceration requires careful anatomic closure to maintain the functional status. Notching and contracture occurs when the margin structures are not opposed (**332**). A laceration of the upper or lower canaliculus of the tear duct drainage system will hinder drainage and cause overflow epiphora. Careful exploration of lacerations in the medial canthal area are mandatory. A margin laceration in the medial canthal area can be hidden as seen here (**333, 334**). Temporal displacement of the puncta may be a clue that there is a lid margin laceration (**335, 336**). Repair of the canaliculus is accomplished with a silicon stent across the laceration to ensure patency. A lid laceration may also localize a corneal or scleral injury.

Intentional thermal injuries to the lids may be extensive but are usually associated with limited ocular injury at the time of exposure because of the protective Bell's response (**337**). Acute corneal opacification from a chemical exposure indicates more severe damage (**338**). Chemical exposure has a prolonged contact time and can lead to corneal melting and long-term scarring.

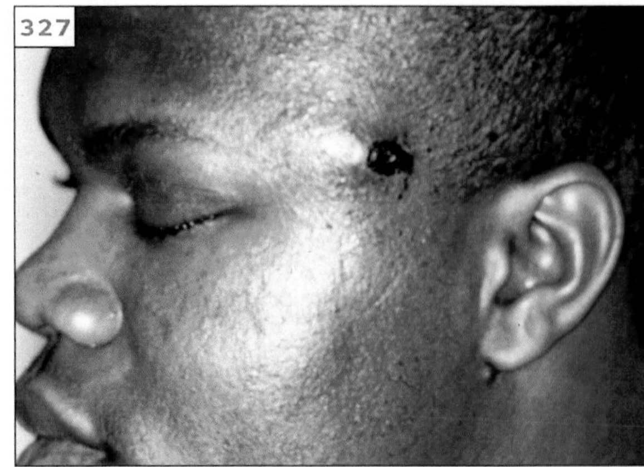

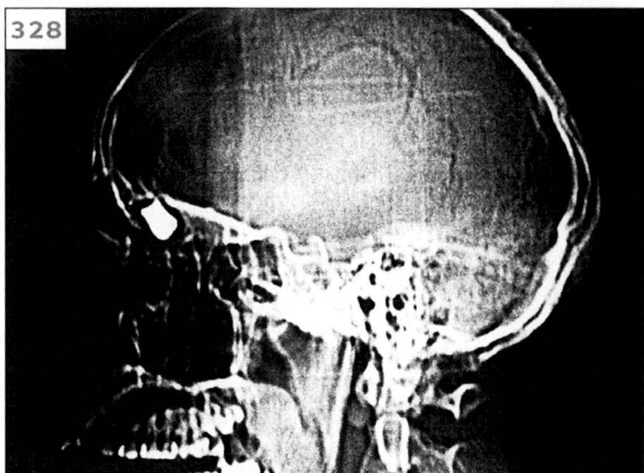

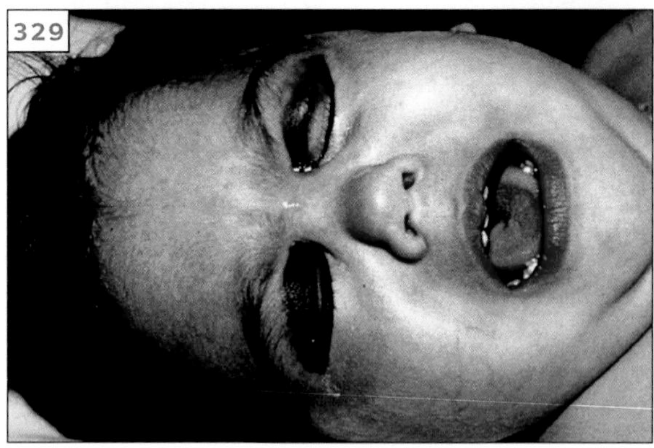

327 This figure shows a teenaged patient with a lateral bullet entry.

328 A plain radiographic view of a bullet in the orbit.

329 A patient who presented with bilateral peri-orbital ecchymosis secondary to neuroblastoma.

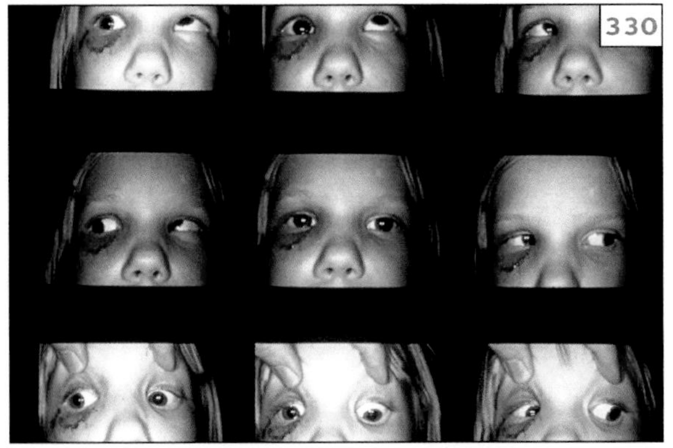

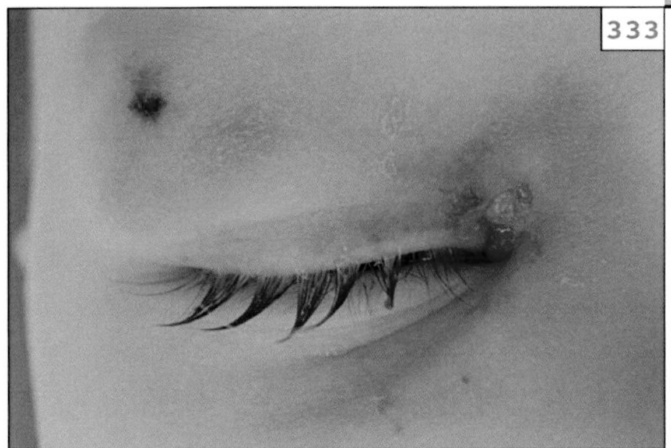

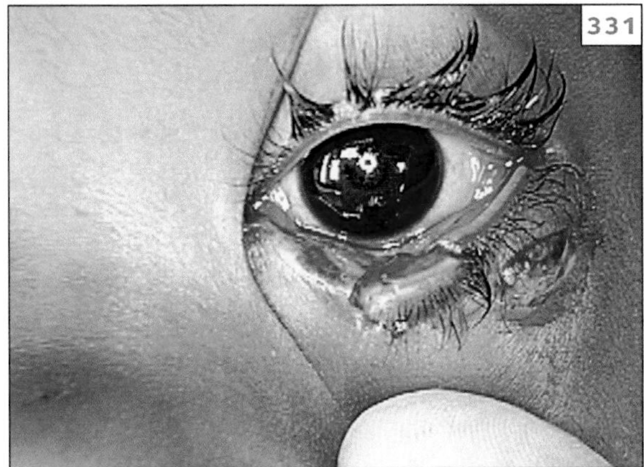

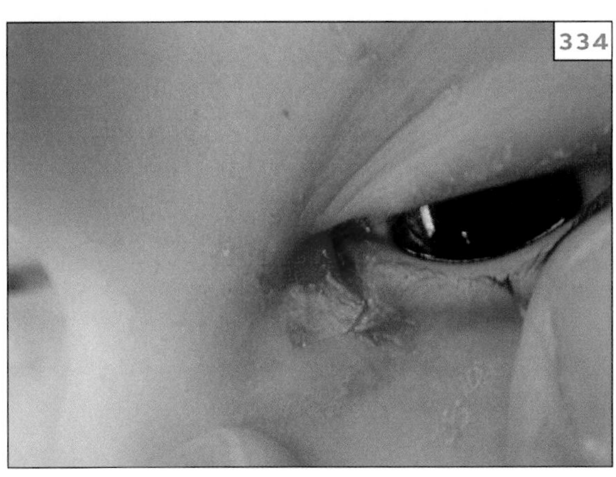

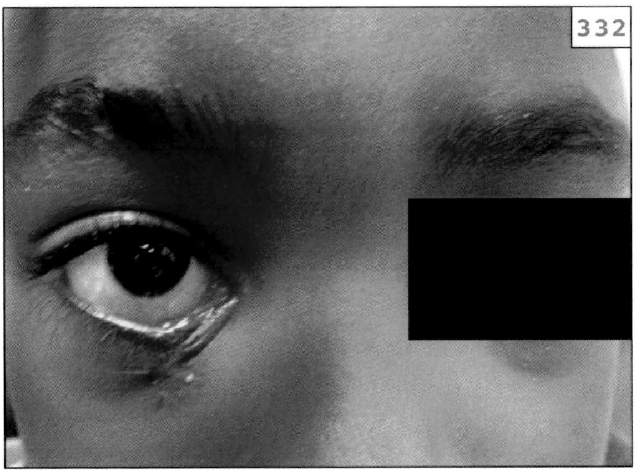

330 A female patient with limited upgaze right eye secondary to orbital floor fracture with entrapment.

331 This illustrates lid lacerations resulting from a dog bite.

332 Lid margin with contracture due to poor closure.

333 Lid margin medial canthal laceration.

334 Lid margin medial canthal laceration with lateral traction.

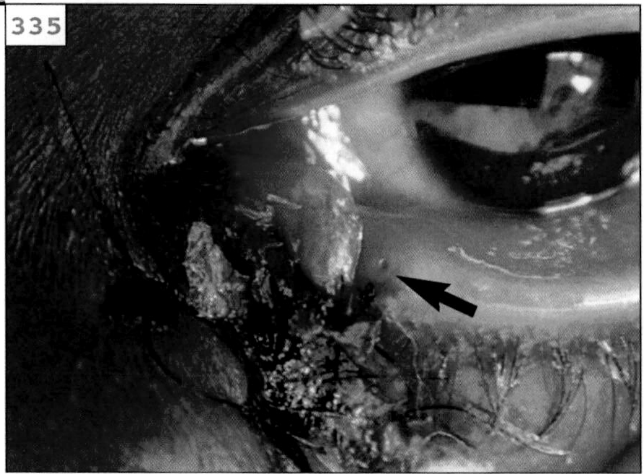

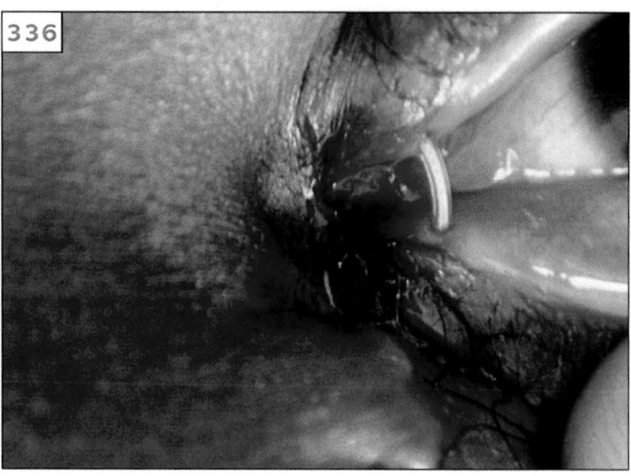

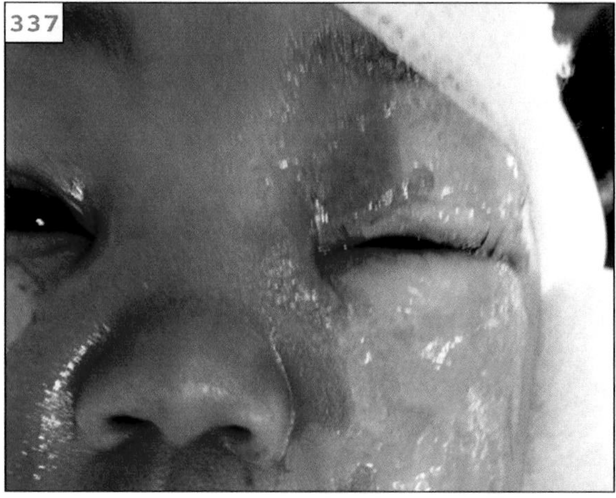

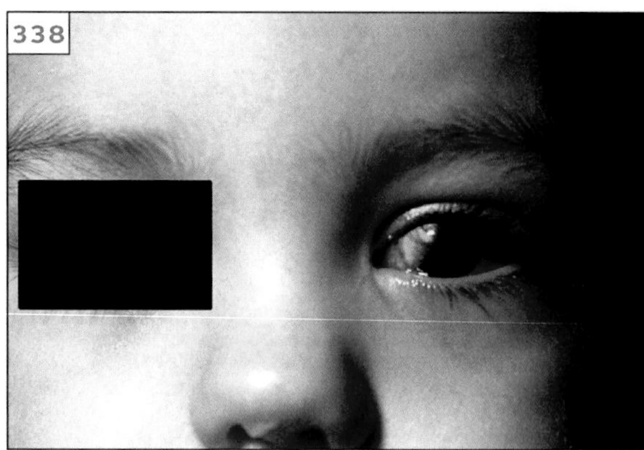

335 Pre-operative, canalicular laceration with temporal displacement of puncta.

336 This figure shows the normal postoperative position after canalicular laceration repair.

337 A deep thermal facial burn is illustrated.

338 Alkaline eye injury resulting in corneal edema.

Anterior segment

Subconjunctival hemorrhage is common and usually benign (**339**). The conjunctiva tends to be flat. However, conjunctival lacerations can be masked by subconjunctival hemorrhage. Many conjunctival lacerations do not need suturing. If there is prolapse of Tenon's capsule, the subconjuctival tissue, closure is warranted.

Open globe injuries in the pediatric age group are due to penetrating injury (79%), blunt trauma (13%), or perforating injury (8%)[10]. Blunt external trauma may result in a rupture of the globe without obvious corneal or scleral perforating injury. Signs of a possible rupture may include conjunctival chemosis (edema) with or without subconjunctival hemorrhage (**340**), an irregular pupil (**341**), and low intra-ocular pressure. Intra-ocular pressure is often less than 4 mmHg, with normal being 10–21 mmHg. The most common locations for a rupture from blunt trauma are at the limbus (**342**) and behind the intra-ocular muscles. Pigmented uveal tissue can be seen in the wound. The thickness of the sclera is 1 mm at the optic nerve. The thinnest area of sclera is behind the extraocular rectus muscles, 0.5 mm thick.

Penetrating scleral or corneal lacerations may be subtle (**343**) or obvious with uveal tissue in the wound (**344**). Iris, lens, or uveal tissue may become incarcerated in the wound. Extensive lacerations and the attendant hypotony lead to expulsive choroidal bleeding (**345**) as seen in this teenager hit with a glass bottle. These eyes will lose all sight and result in enucleation. Corneal or scleral lacerations require suturing (**346**). Vascularization of the wound may occur if the sutures are not removed within 8–12 weeks (**347**). A central location of the corneal laceration and associated ocular damage determine the visual prognosis. Posterior lacerations of the sclera often contain uveal tissue. The risk of a retinal detachment is greater with posterior penetration.

Hyphema is a collection of blood in the anterior chamber from a tear in the iris stroma or root (**348**). Blunt trauma is the primary cause. It may be microscopic and only seen with a slit lamp examination. In the anterior chamber, red blood cells may occlude the trabecular meshwork and result in a significant intra-ocular pressure elevation. Significant ocular hypertension can result in a retinal vascular event or ischemic optic nerve damage. This risk is enhanced in patients with sickle cell disease. Management is generally outpatient with topical glaucoma medications, oral acetazolamide, or intravenous mannitol. The use of an antifibrinolytic agent, such as aminocaproic acid, in the treatment of pediatric hyphema is controversial[13,14]. An iris injury may disinsert the root of the iris and result in irregular pupil (**349**). Other anterior segment injuries are cataract and subluxation of the lens (**350**). Vitreous red blood cells or vitreous pigment at the slit lamp indicate a possible retinal tear or penetration of the globe (**351**).

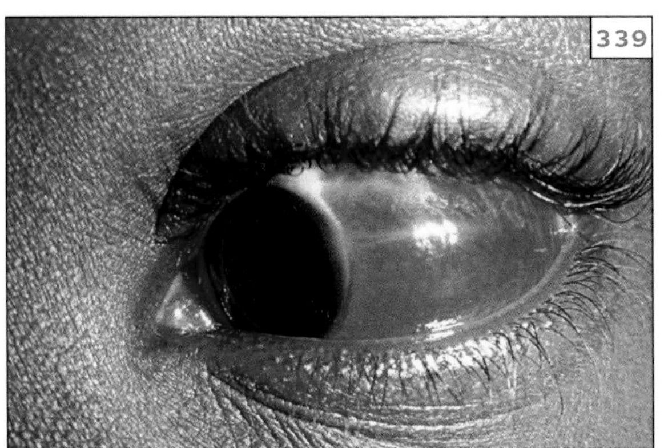

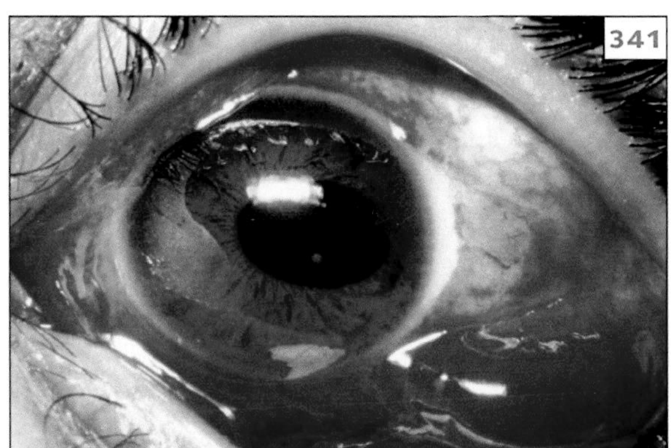

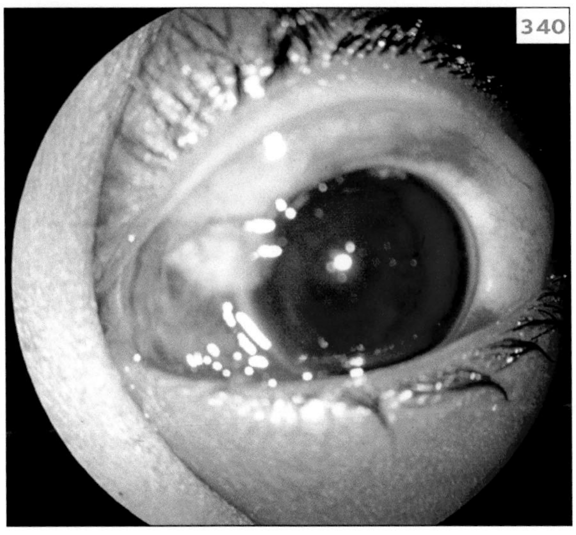

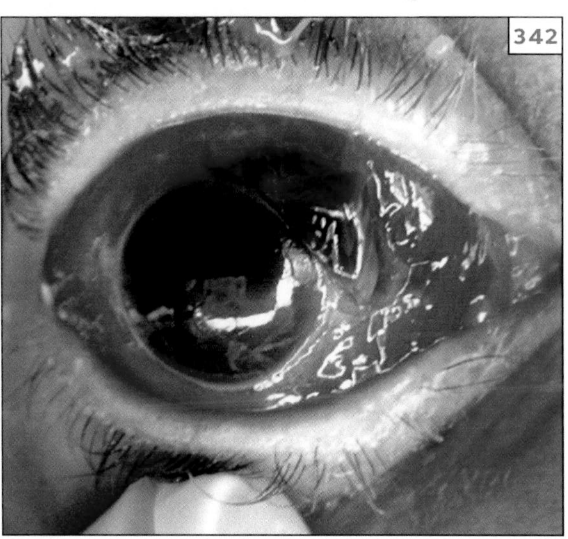

339 This figure shows subconjunctival hemorrhage.

340 Conjunctival edema (chemosis) is shown with ruptured globe.

341 This figure shows an irregular pupil with ruptured globe.

342 This figure illustrates uveal prolapse at the limbus with ruptured globe.

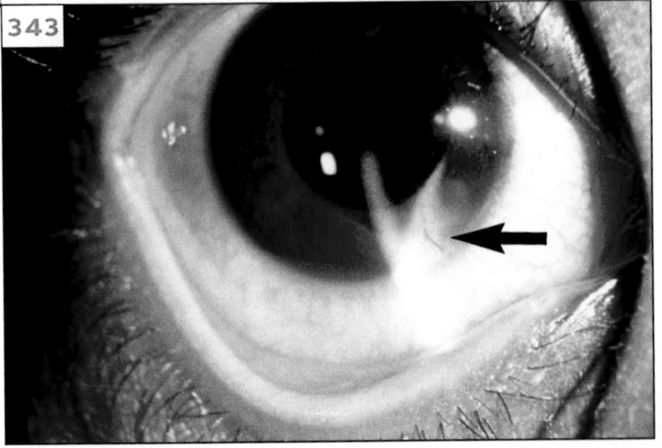
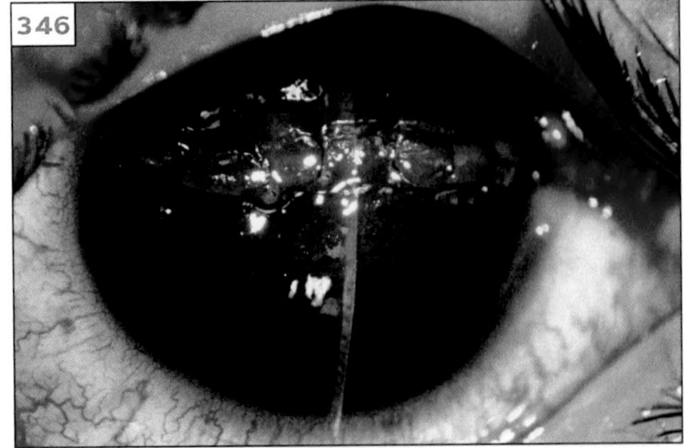
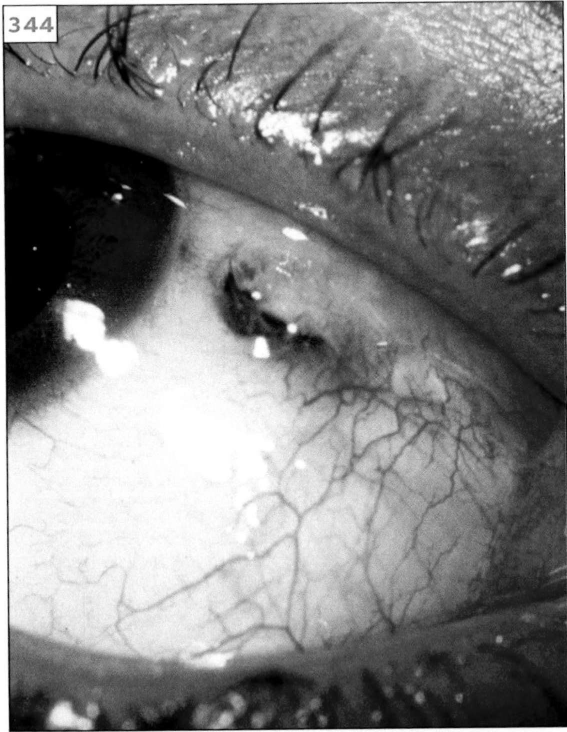
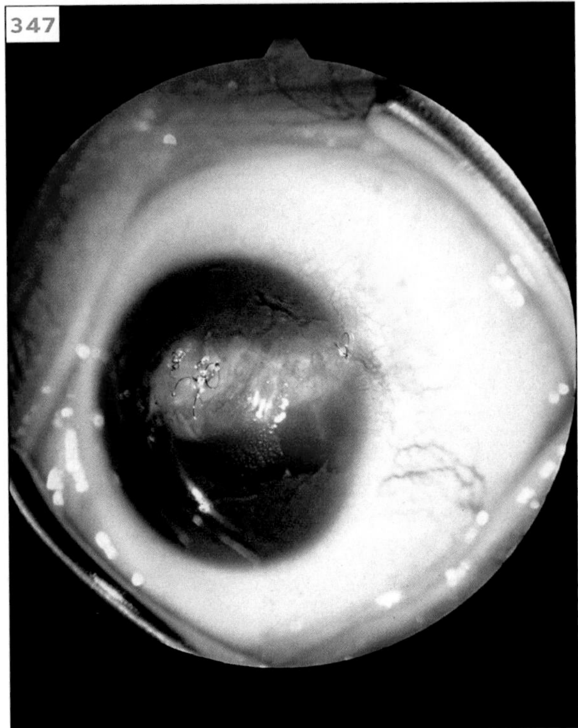
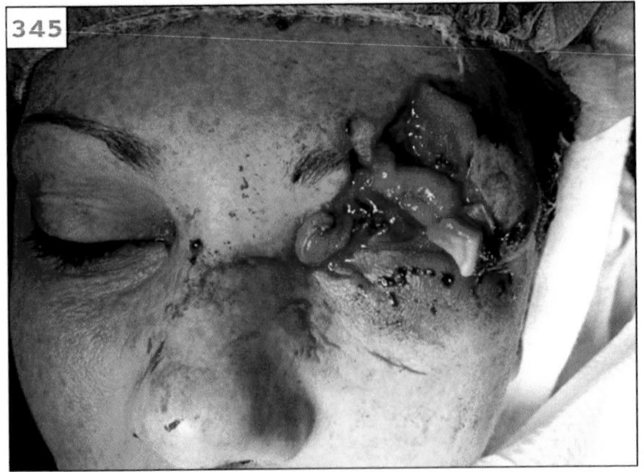

343 Subtle corneal laceration with incarcerated iris tissue.

344 Scleral laceration with uveal prolapse.

345 Extensive lid and corneal–scleral laceration with expulsive choroidal bleeding.

346 This figure shows a sutured corneal laceration.

347 Sutured corneal laceration with wound vascularization.

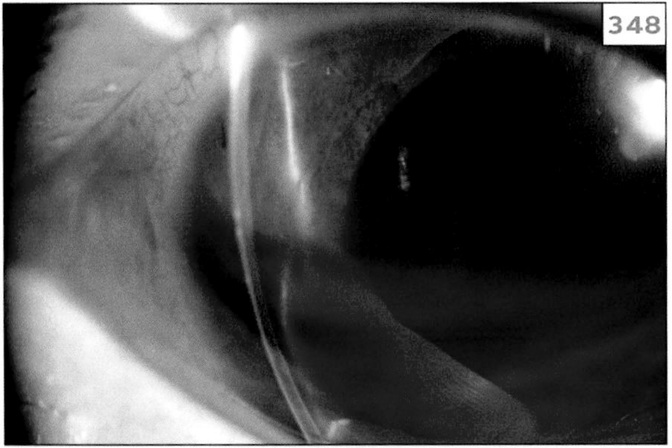

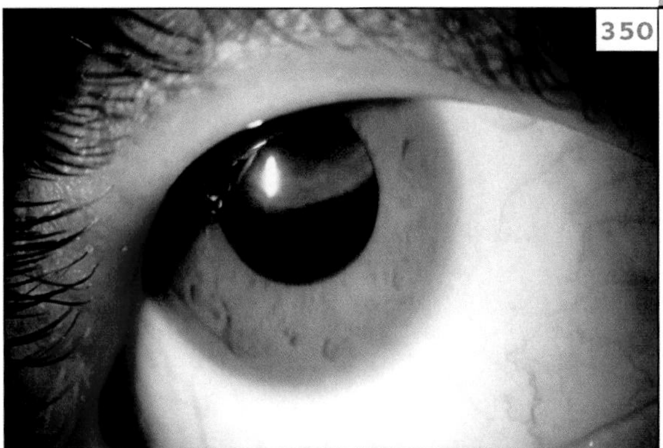

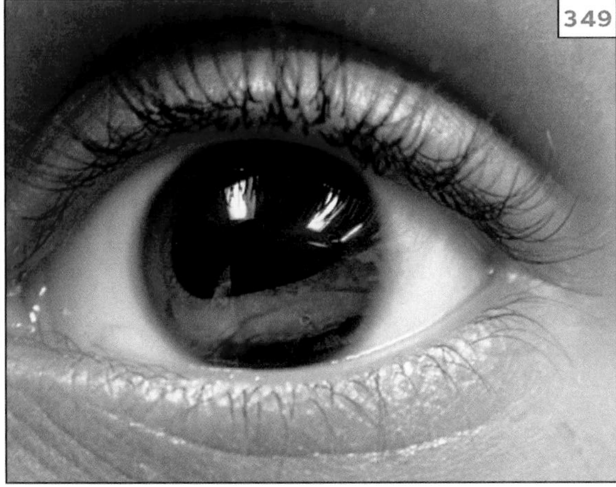

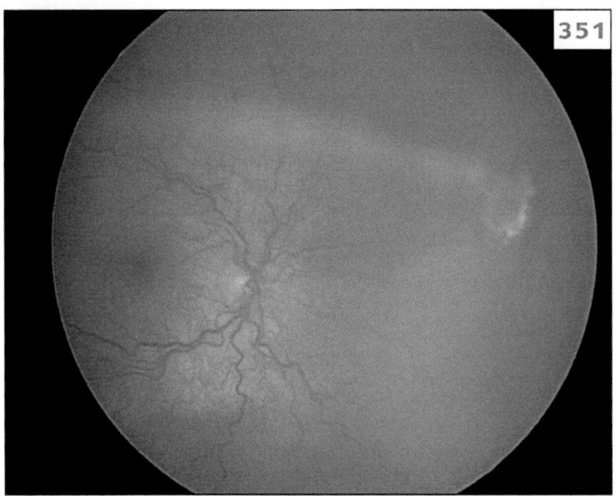

348 This figure shows an example of hyphema.

349 Iris root tear with blunt trauma.

350 Subluxed lens with blunt trauma.

351 Nasal posterior exit wound from metallic foreign body.

Fundus

Nonaccidental, repetitive, violent, acceleration–deceleration head injury (shaken baby syndrome) may cause retinal hemorrhaging, retinal folds, and cranial nerve palsies. Retinal hemorrhage occurs in 60–72% of nonaccidental head trauma and in 0–20% of accidental head trauma[15,16]. While children under 3 years of age are most susceptible, retinal hemorrhage and cerebral edema were reported in an 8-year-old boy from repetitive shaking[17]. In a large study, a severe shaking injury and retinal hemorrhaging was associated with subdural bleeding (93%), cerebral edema (44%), subarachnoid bleeding (16%), and parenchymal bleeding (8%)[18]. Intra-ocular hemorrhage may be vitreous, pre-retinal, intraretinal, or subretinal. Retinal hemorrhages are multilayer with nonaccidental acceleration–deceleration head injuries.

Accidental head injury with severe brain injury is rarely associated with retinal hemorrhaging. If at all present, retinal hemorrhages are limited to the posterior pole and are few in number[19–21]. A coagulopathy or chronic disease (hypertension or diabetes) may also cause multilayer hemorrhaging. History, age, and laboratory evaluation would eliminate these possibilities. A few scattered retinal hemorrhages may result from forceful vomiting[22], cardiopulmonary resuscitation[23], febrile seizures[24], and birth-related trauma. Both vaginal deliveries and cesarean sections have been associated with a few scattered retinal hemorrhages[25,26]. Overall, however, retinal hemorrhages are rarely, if at all, caused by these events. A number of studies have examined the occurrence of retinal hemorrhage after seizures, and none was found except in a premature infant with other risk factors. Also, significant retinal hemorrhages have not been found after pediatric cardiopulmonary resuscitation or severe coughing.

After abuse, the most common location of hemorrhages is around the optic nerve. Hemorrhages may be few (**352**) or too numerous to count into the periphery (**353**). Retinal involvement is usually bilateral, but can be unilateral. Asymmetric distribution of hemorrhage is common. Nerve fiber layer hemorrhage ('flame-shaped') is the most common (**354**). These hemorrhages are streaky, following the anatomy of the nerve fibers. Preretinal blood obscures the retinal vessels on the retinal surface. It may appear as a droplet on the retinal surface (**355**). Deeper intraretinal bleeding takes on the characteristic of 'dot and blot' hemorrhages under the normal retinal vessels (**356**). Hemorrhages may develop pale centers with accumulation of white blood cells (**357**). A subretinal hemorrhage is between the retina and choroid or within the choroid. This can elevate the retina significantly, casting a deep red color (**358**).

Retinal folds may indicate an acceleration–deceleration head injury[27]. Perimacular folds have been reported with documented accidental trauma[28,29]. Perimacular folds along the arcades (**359, 360**), macular holes, and peripheral retinoschisis cavities can be seen[30,31]. Residual retinal hyper- or hypopigmentation may result (**361**). Rapid acceleration–deceleration tractional force on the retina occurs from the tight adherence of the vitreous gel of the eye to the retina in the pediatric patient. Retinal folds are associated with severe neurologic trauma[32]. Blunt trauma may cause retinal commotio (edema) with whitening of the retina (**362**), retinal tear or detachment. Severe increased intracranial pressure will cause optic nerve edema. An acceleration–deceleration injury alone may result in severe hemorrhaging, but no optic nerve edema[33].

Motility

A motility examination should include an assessment of the primary position, left, right, up, and down as a minimum. The position of the corneal light reflex can help determine the position of the eye. An orbital floor fracture with a restrictive strabismus has previously been described. However, serious neurologic trauma may present with a fourth or sixth nerve palsy.

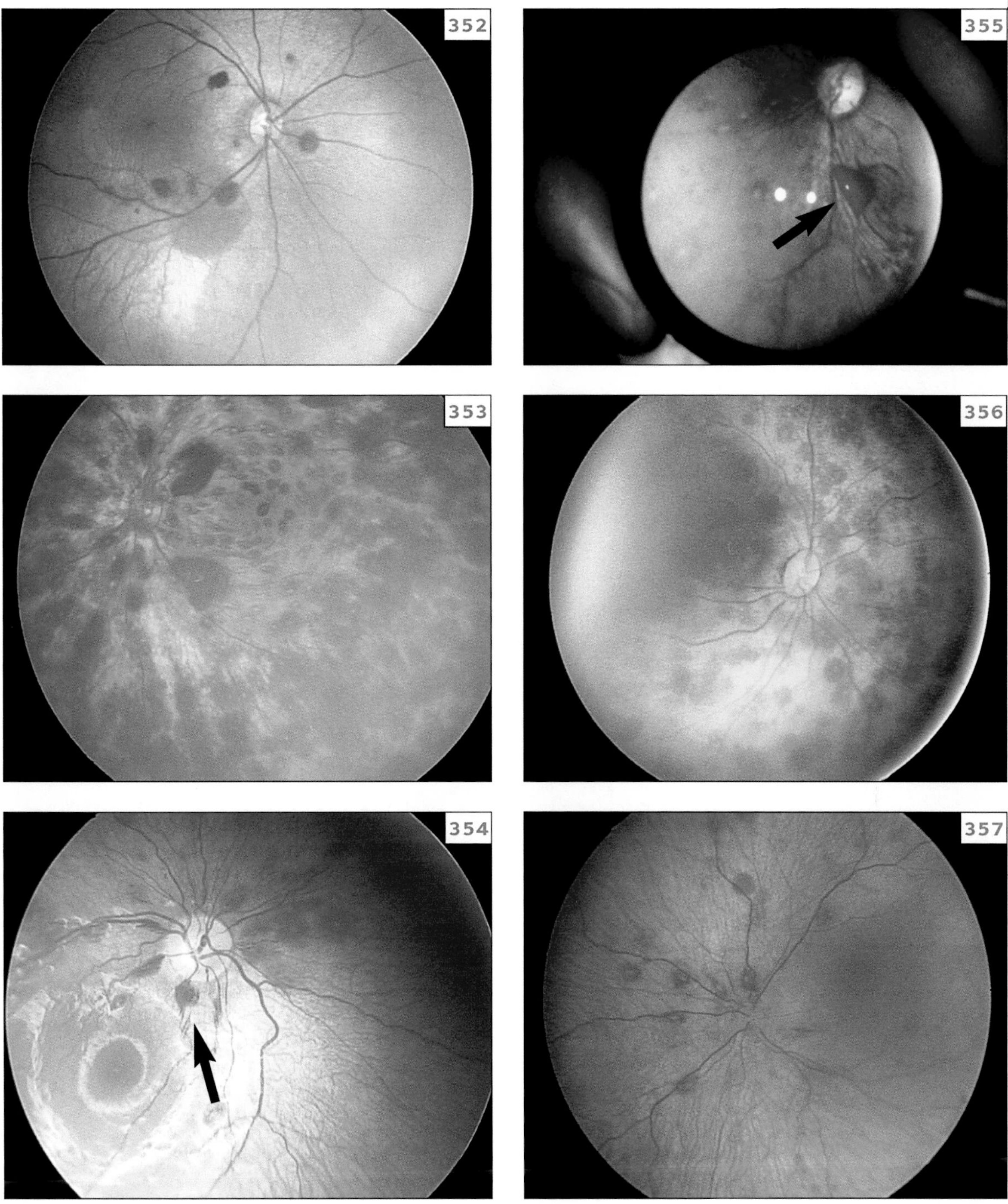

352 Mild retinal hemorrhage associated with repetitive neurologic trauma.

353 Severe retinal hemorrhage associated with repetitive neurologic trauma.

354 Nerve fiber layer ('flame-shaped') hemorrhages.

355 Preretinal hemorrhage on retina obscuring blood vessel.

356 Intraretinal (rounded, 'dot and blot') hemorrhages.

357 Retinal hemorrhage with white center (similar to 'Roth spots').

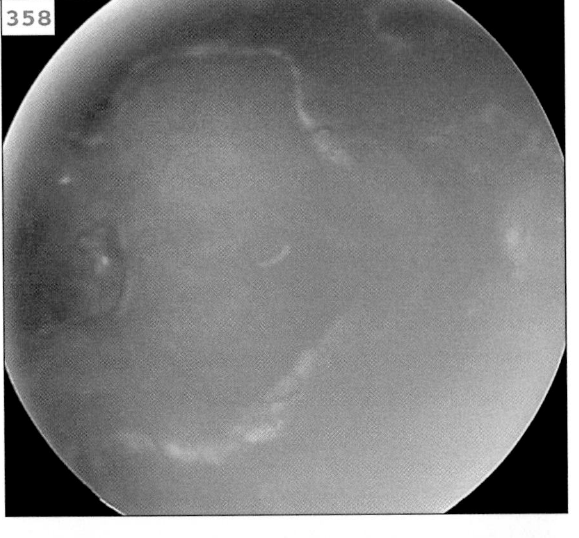

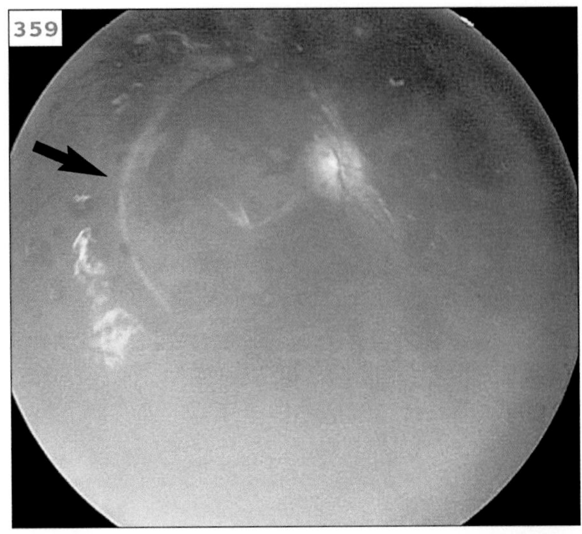

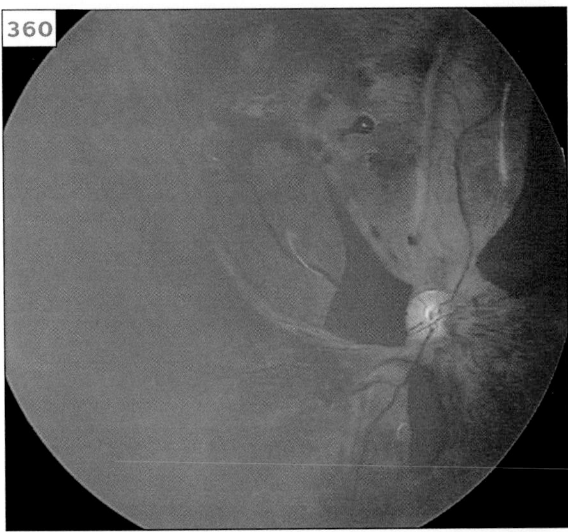

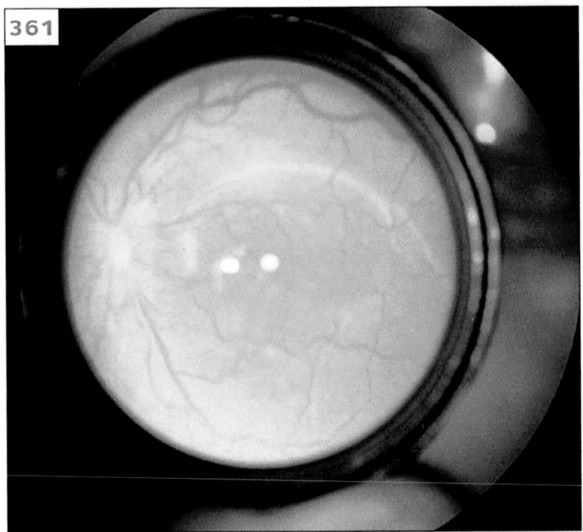

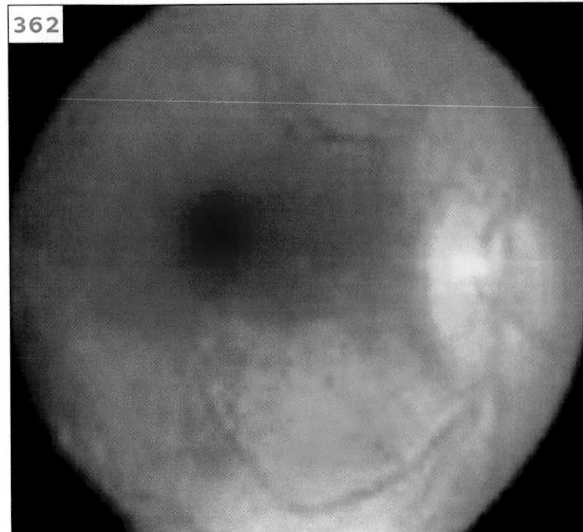

358 Subretinal choroidal bleeding (note peripheral elevation).

359 Arcuate retinal fold (white fold following the vessel arcades).

360 Linear retinal fold (tracking the vessel).

361 This figure shows a depigmented healed retinal fold.

362 Commotio (swelling) of retina (whitish area outside the fovea).

Treatment

A suspected rupture of the globe should be shielded and referred to an ophthalmologist. With blunt trauma or a shaking injury, retinal hemorrhaging requires confirmation by an ophthalmologist. Retinal hemorrhages will fade within 4 weeks in general to as late as 4 months[33]. A thorough retinal examination for retinal hemorrhages or retinal folds with a detailed retinal drawing or a photograph should be done for legal documentation. Long-term visual prognosis is dependent on the presence of a macular lesion or an occipital intracranial injury[34].

Teaching points

- There are almost 2 million eye injuries annually in the United States and approximately one-third of them involve children.
- The majority of pediatric eye injuries are considered to be accidental, but many involve improper supervision and some are the direct result of child abuse.
- Peri-orbital bruising, hyphema, and retinal injury have been seen with direct blows and acceleration–deceleration injuries. Thorough examination and documentation requires an ophthalmologist and specialized imaging equipment.
- Retinal hemorrhages, especially when extensive and extending to the anterior retina, and involving multiple layers, have not been shown to be caused by innocent or trivial forces.

Chapter 7

OTOLARYNGOLOGIC MANIFESTATIONS OF ABUSE AND NEGLECT

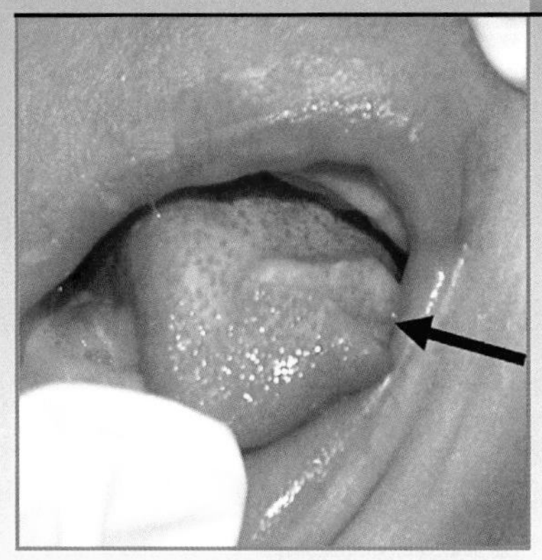

Russell A. Faust PhD, MD and Philip V. Scribano DO, MSCE

Studies indicate that orofacial injuries are manifest in 50–75% cases of child maltreatment – more than any other anatomic region.[1–3] It is essential that physicians and child advocates recognize these signs when present. In order to detect these signs, the examining physician must be familiar with them, with their mechanisms, and whether there might be less ominous explanations for these signs[4].

Introduction

Fitting a detailed examination for abuse within the otolaryngologic examination efficiently and with subtlety can be challenging[5]. It is important not to miss features of maltreatment in the following areas: head and scalp, ear, face, nose, and oropharynx. Thus, a systematic approach, which consistently includes a complete examination as a matter of routine regardless of the level of suspicion for abuse, will maximize the success in identifying the child at risk, rather than performing the evaluation only if known risk factors exist. This provides for the most thorough and efficient examination technique.

Table 12 **Ear findings in abuse**
Auricular hematoma
Ecchymoses of the auricle
Laceration of the auditory meatus
Tympanic membrane perforation
Ossicular discontinuity
Total hearing loss associated with vertigo
Facial nerve paresis
Cerebral spinal fluid otorrhea
Persistent otitis media with effusion

Head and scalp

During the examination directed by the presenting complaint, the physician should be systematically screening for findings that are suspicious for maltreatment. There may be few or no external signs, even though serious internal injury is present[6]. See Chapter 2, Bruises, for a discussion of external findings of the head and scalp[7–10].

Ear

Suspicious lesions of the ear include those listed in *Table 12*. Lacerations of the external auditory meatus, hematomas, or ecchymoses of the auricle (resulting from a pinch or slap) should be noted. Tympanic membrane perforation or ossicular discontinuity should be documented; this combination of findings is especially suspect as resulting from a forcible slap to the external ear with an open hand. Chronic, recurring trauma can result in deformed auricles and sensorineural hearing loss, documented by audiometry. The combination of unilateral ear bruising, radiological evidence of ipsilateral subdural hematoma with severe edema, and hemorrhagic retinopathy ('tin ear syndrome') is considered pathognomonic of physical abuse (**363**).[11]

Particular attention should be paid to any injury associated with total hearing or balance loss, facial nerve paralysis, or cerebrospinal fluid (CSF) otorrhea or rhinorrhea. Accidental injuries of the auricle are uncommon. Injuries of the external auditory meatus and the area behind the ear are rare and should be considered intentional. It can be challenging to distinguish a tympanic membrane perforation resulting from infection and rupture from the perforation caused by trauma; the presence of hemotympanum in the absence of purulence should be viewed with suspicion. If the child's history is known to the examining physician, a lack of infectious history and the existence of other suspicious findings or behaviors can guide the diagnosis of abuse as a possible cause.

The finding of facial nerve paresis combined with any other evidence of trauma is a red flag for significant injury, and computed tomography (CT) scan evaluation of the temporal bone seeking a fracture should be performed. Cerebrospinal fluid otorrhea – even as a solitary finding – is cause for suspicion, since it rarely is a spontaneous occurrence, and can reflect a blow of significant force, resulting in either temporal bone fracture or rupture of the membranous inner ear.

Many traumatic tympanic membrane perforations will heal spontaneously without surgical intervention. Standard treatment includes a period of topical otic drops to that ear to help irrigate dried blood, prevent infection, and keep the tympanic membrane moist to foster healing. Ossicular discontinuity with resulting conductive hearing loss may require surgical intervention for ossicular chain reconstruction. Recurrent auricular hematomas are common in wrestlers, but unusual in other sports and extremely rare from other accidental trauma. Hematomas of the pinna are properly managed by surgical incision and drainage, followed by placement of a bolster for several days to prevent recurrence.[12]

Within the head and neck region, factitious illness (also referred to as pediatric condition falsification or Munchausen by proxy) most commonly involves the ear. This syndrome should be suspected whenever persistent or recurrent unexplained illness affects a child, and when unusual signs or symptoms occur only in the presence of one caregiver (see Chapter 13, Munchausen syndrome by proxy). In the field of otolaryngology, chronic otitis, persistent tympanic membrane perforations, persistent cerebrospinal fluid otorrhea, and sinusitis have been reported as manifestations of this syndrome. Since otitis media, tympanic membrane perforations, and sinusitis are relatively common in the pediatric population, the diagnosis of factitious illness can be difficult to make[13,14]. Other examples include reports of apnea, nystagmus, and headache.

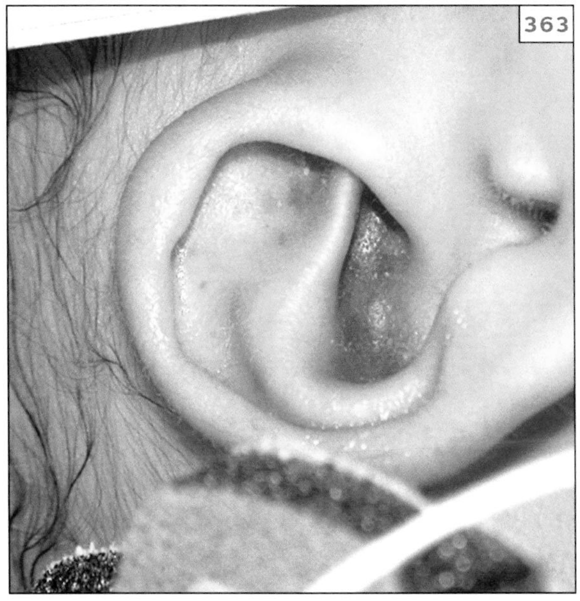

363 A 2-month-old seen in the intensive care unit with acute subdural hemorrhages, bilateral diffuse, multilayered retinal hemorrhages, and ecchymoses of the auricle (so-called 'tin ear')[11].

Face

The child's face is the area of the body most often injured in physical abuse, and should be carefully examined for the signs listed in *Table 13* (see Chapter 2, Bruises, for additional information on bruising). The most common sign of open-hand blows to the face is multiple parallel marks representing the fingers (**364**). Whether or not facial fracture is the reason for referral or chief complaint, or is incidentally found during the examination, facial fracture in a child should always be suspect for abuse unless the circumstances of the trauma are consistent. As with all evidence of previous fractures, multiple healed fractures are highly suggestive for abuse, as are facial fractures in infants (**365**)[15,16]. Facial asymmetry may reflect previous trauma with fractures or soft tissue injury. Asymmetry associated with the diagnosis of hemifacial microsomia (Goldenhar syndrome) should not be confused with such signs of trauma. Acute fractures associated with asymmetry reflect displacement and will require reduction and, probably, surgical fixation. Ecchymoses of the cheek are suspicious, since this soft tissue does not overlie any bony prominence and thus requires a significant impact for bruising to occur. Risk of accidental injury to the face is similar to that for the head and scalp, with unstable toddlers at greatest risk.

Table 13 **Abusive injuries of the face**
Asymmetry
Bruises
Scars
Lacerations
Burn marks
Periorbital ecchymoses
Scleral hemorrhage
Focal neurological findings, e.g. deviated gaze or unequal pupils
Facial fracture, including evidence of past fractures
Bruising of the buccal area of the cheek

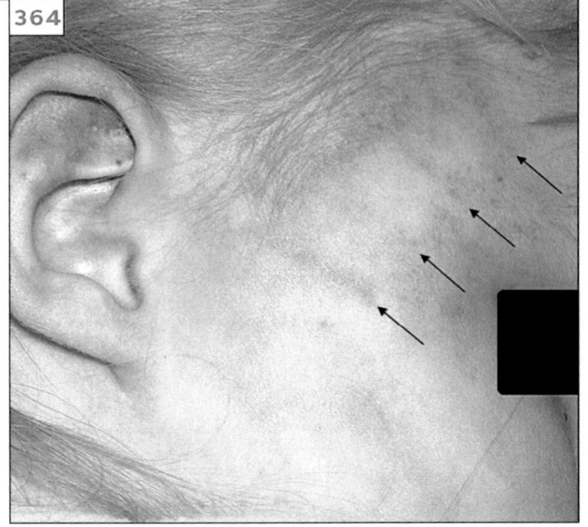

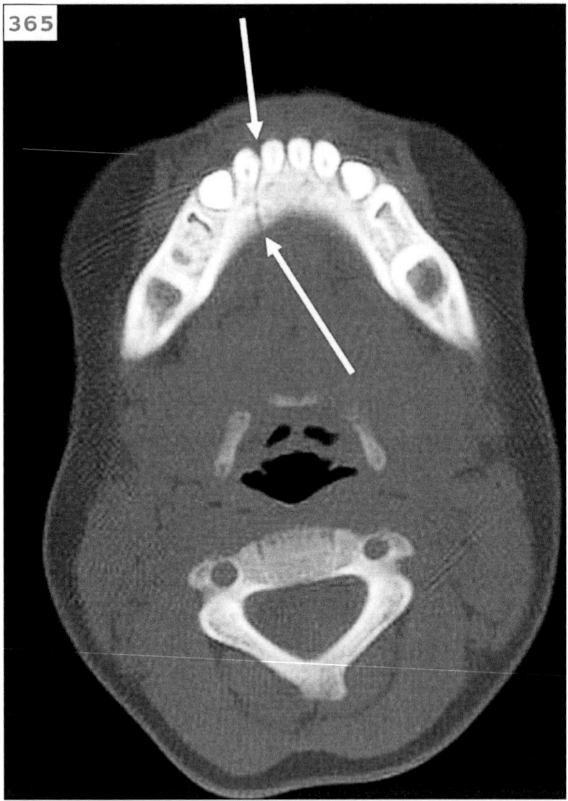

364 A 2-year-old with significant bruises of the face and right ear; no explanation was offered. Note the subtle linear aspects of bruising pattern representing fingers of an open-hand slap (arrows).

365 A 3-month-old with mandibular fracture (arrows) and a history of falling from the sofa onto the carpeted floor. Mechanism by history is inconsistent with the extent of injury.

Nose

Accidental injuries to the nose occur in a manner similar to those of the face in general. However, intranasal injuries should be viewed with suspicion (*Table 14*), since these injuries require significant force to produce. Furthermore, whereas it is common for children to insert foreign bodies into their nasal cavities, associated injury to intranasal structures is extremely rare and is a compelling sign of abuse[17]. Findings such as blood clots, recurrent epistaxis, or deviated septum are, as solitary findings, unremarkable, but have more significance within the context of other findings consistent with abuse. A blow to the nose with nasal cartilage fracture and resulting septal hematoma will lead to resorption of the cartilage with perforation and possible nasal deformity if not managed acutely. Therefore, the findings of septal perforation or columella destruction may be sequelae of injuries that did not receive medical attention and, as such, reflect neglect at best. Delay in seeking medical attention should always raise suspicion. Acute management of septal hematoma is surgical incision and drainage. Septal perforations can be surgically repaired, and this is often desirable in order to prevent drying of the edges with recurrent bleeding as a result[18]. In general, the nose does not bruise without direct impact and fracture or pinch. The finding of nasal tip or columella bruising is highly suspicious for intentional injury from pinching these structures.

Table 14 **Abusive injuries of the nose**
Blood clots, recurrent epistaxis
Septal deviation
Septal perforation
Columella destruction
Impaired nasomaxillary development
Foreign body insertion, with internal nasal trauma
Cerebrospinal fluid rhinorrhea

Oropharynx

The oral cavity may reveal signs of abuse (*Table 15*). Comprehensive examination of the oral cavity should document the frenulae, hard and soft palates, gingivae, tongue, floor of mouth, buccal mucosa, posterior pharynx, and teeth, if present (**366**). Severe dental decay should be noted as evidence of neglect (see Chapter 8, Recognition of child abuse by dentists, heath care professionals, and law enforcement). Attempts to silence a crying infant using a hand or other object, such as a bottle, can result in lacerations or tears. A laceration, frenulum tear, or bruising of the palate in a nontoddler (pre-ambulatory) is extremely suspicious for the forcible insertion of an object or blow to the mouth (**367**)[19]. In contrast, this category of injury is not uncommon in the toddler. It is unusual for oral lacerations to require surgical repair because of the excellent local blood supply and local growth factors.

Multiple scars on the lips suggest repeated blows over time. Abrasions or scars at the lip commissures can suggest repeated use of a mouth gag; both should be viewed with much suspicion. The oral cavity is also a common place for manifestations of sexual abuse, with lesions resulting from sexually transmitted diseases. The finding of petechiae or bruising at the junction of the soft and hard palates or on the floor of the mouth may suggest forced fellatio[20]. It is noteworthy that hearing-impaired children are at increased risk for this type of abuse[21].

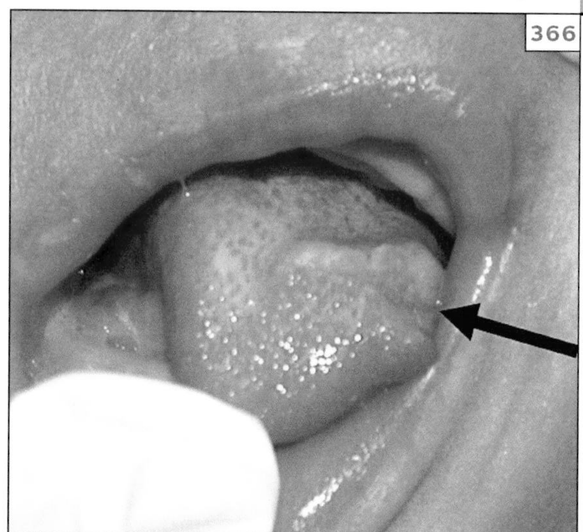

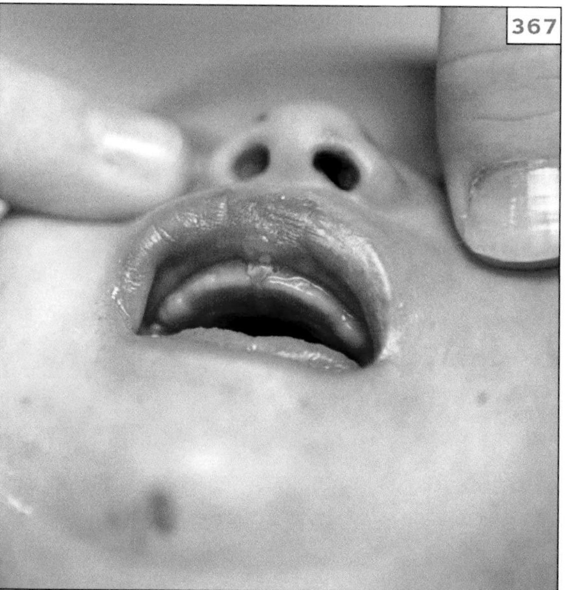

366 A 6-week-old infant with Down syndrome and an unexplained deep tongue laceration (arrow).

367 A 2-month-old infant with small, acute subdural hemorrhage, bilateral retinal hemorrhages, chin bruise, and healing frenulum laceration. The father admitted to shaking the infant and throwing her down onto the bed. He also confessed to forcing her bottle into her mouth during feeding due to her persistent crying just before the abusive head trauma event.

Table 15 **Abuse injuries of the oropharynx**
Bruising of the palate or fauces
Lacerations or evidence of foreign body trauma
Missing teeth in unusual areas
Multiple scars on lips
Burns of lips or oral mucosa
Abrasions or scars at the commissures
Labial frenulum tear
Lesions consistent with sexually transmitted diseases

Skin of the head and neck

Throughout the examination, all exposed skin should be scanned for evidence of bruising, scars, abrasions, lacerations, burn marks, or other abnormalities (**368**). Any mark that has a regular geometric pattern, design, or repeated pattern as may result from blows with a belt or other object, is pathognomonic for physical abuse. Whereas any burn in a child should be considered suspicious, a cigarette burn mark on the head and neck is pathognomonic for abuse (**369**). The consistency and texture of the soft tissues should be observed, since abuse can result in fibrosis or edema of the soft tissues without obvious asymmetry or discoloration. Subcutaneous emphysema can present as 'crackly' skin in an irritable infant due to associated discomfort, and is pathognomonic for intentional injury (**370**)[22,23]. A comprehensive examination should include meticulous documentation, including detailed description of findings and photographs[24]. The historical tale that sounds plausible at first may need to be re-evaluated if a routine screening examination includes all skin and the entire body of the child (**371, 372**).

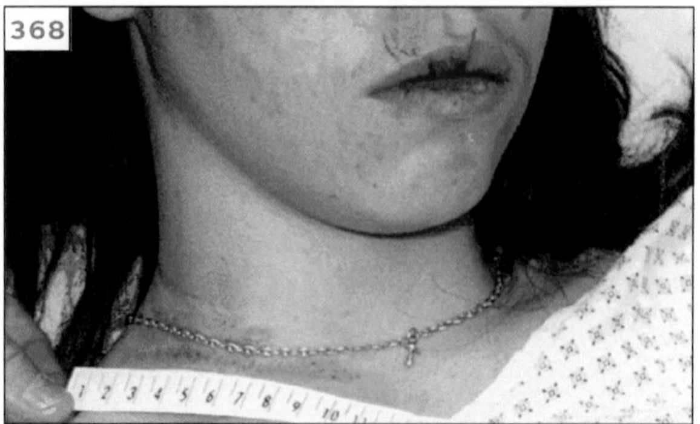

368 A 16-year-old who sustained injuries during an altercation with her mother. Peri-oral facial injuries and neck contusions due to attempts to grab her by the neck can be seen.

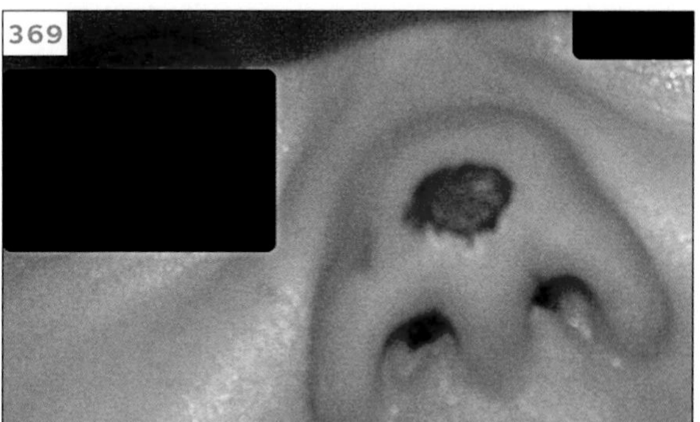

369 A 3-month-old infant with multiple fractures, small acute subdural hemorrhage, and eschar of nasal tip that measures 8 mm in diameter (demonstrated here), consistent with a cigarette burn.

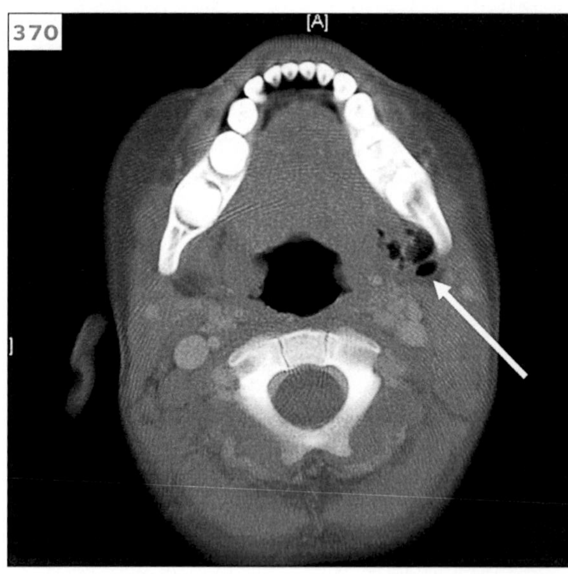

370 A 2-year-old with failure to thrive noted to have external bruising and no plausible history of injury. Computed tomography of the neck demonstrates parapharyngeal soft tissue emphysema (arrow). Such injuries can arise from oral foreign body trauma and even from violent shaking.

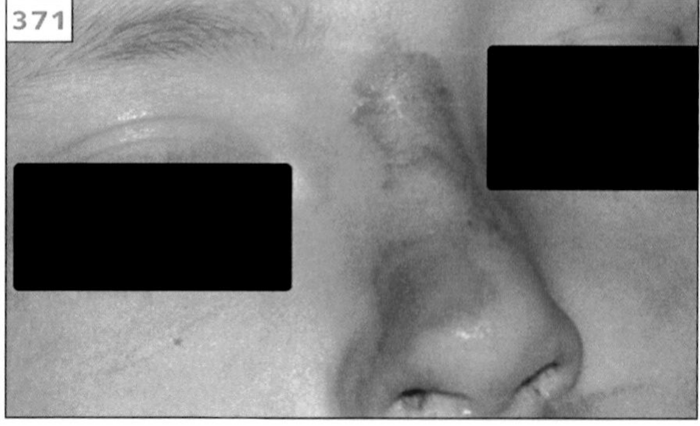

371 A 3-year-old with a history of falling onto a carpeted floor. A diffuse area of nasal abrasion is shown which is inconsistent with the mechanism by history.

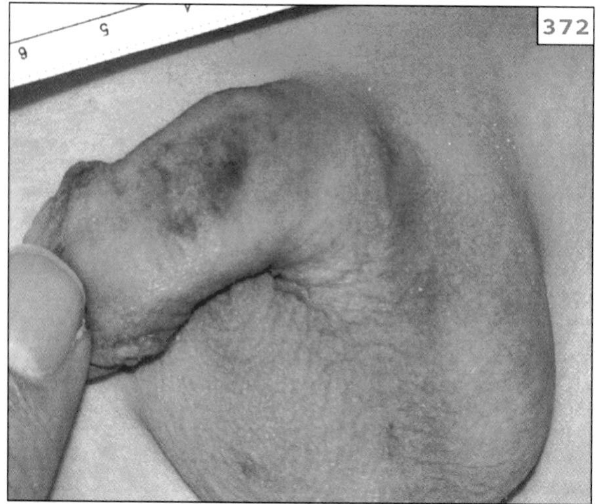

372 The same patient as shown in 371 with additional findings consistent with physical abuse. This case emphasizes the importance of a thorough screening examination to uncover hidden injuries.

Teaching points

- Nearly 75% of physically abused children will manifest injuries of the head and neck.
- Screening for abuse and neglect must be incorporated into the routine pediatric ear, nose, and throat examination.
- Be alert for the injury that is not consistent with the provided history or is inconsistent with the child's level of development, a changing or evolving history, or a delay in seeking medical care.
- Strive to continue treating the entire family with respect and courtesy, and consider that one's suspicions may be incorrect.

Chapter 8

RECOGNITION OF CHILD ABUSE BY DENTISTS, HEALTH CARE PROFESSIONALS, AND LAW ENFORCEMENT

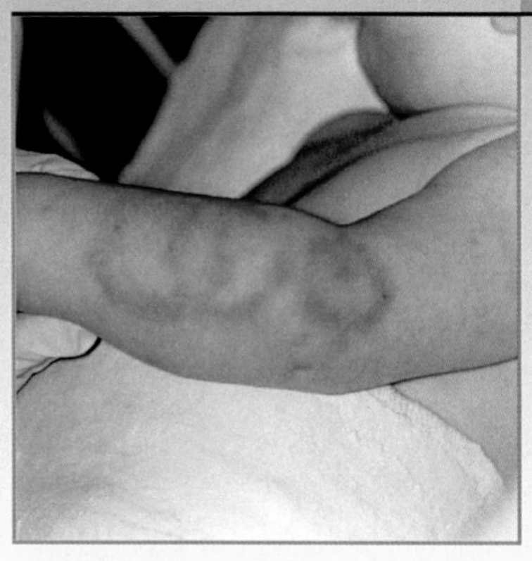

Pamela Wallace Hammel DDS, DABFO

Child abuse is rarely a single isolated event. Rather, it is a steadily escalating pattern of physically assaultive behavior that can end in the death of the child. It is important not to separate child abuse from domestic violence, of which it is a part. There is a strong connection between child abuse, partner abuse, and elder abuse. Abused children often have abused parents, battered women have battered children, and abuse of the elderly does not occur in previously nonviolent families. Intrafamily violence is intergenerational, and a large component of mental abuse and intimidation are integral parts of the violence. Abusive caregivers are often victims of family violence themselves and from families who react to stress with violence. The key for the dentist is awareness, recognition, and referral[1].

Introduction

Family violence tends to occur in a cycle, which essentially has three phases: tension build-up, acute battering episode, remorse, and reconciliation[2,3]. Tension increase is characterized by verbal abuse and minor physical abuse, such as pushing or shoving. Once the tension exceeds the abuser's ability to cope, anything can spark a fully fledged attack. The acute battering episode is the uncontrollable discharge of tension, and often alcohol or drugs play a part at this point. Abusers use drugs as an excuse to sanction their behavior, while victims believe it is the cause. The tension-relieving aspects of the attack may actually encourage an abuser to attack; lowering the tension, i.e. the attack 'feels good.' In the third phase, remorse, the abuser soon learns he controls the victim, and not much effort needs to be put into remorse. Child abuse, as with other forms of violence, is about dominance and control. Abusive caregivers use corporal punishment routinely, and tend to increase the force of the attack if they feel the behavior is not corrected. Dr James Garbarino, a national expert on emotional abuse, states that emotional abuse is a 'persistent chronic pattern of abuse that erodes and corrodes a child[1].'

Children with increased risk for oral–dental abuse are:

- Male
- Premature or handicapped (who are physically abused at twice the rate)
- Newborn to 3 years (newborns because of their crying and wakefulness; toddlers because of pre-verbal frustration, feeding times with bottles, spoons, and high chairs, and toilet training).

Recognizing inflicted injuries

Dentists and physicians have important ethical responsibilities in recognizing inflicted injuries[2–9]. Approximately 65% of child abuse injuries are to the head and neck, clearly visible to the dental team or knowledgeable observers, such as teachers, social workers, health care professionals, or law enforcement. Head trauma is the most frequent cause of morbidity and death in abused children. The head and face are attacked because they represent the sense of 'self' of the child, the center of communication and nutrition. The mouth is often injured due to the abuser's desire to silence the child. The dentist and physician should consider non accidental injuries when there are one or more of suspicious injuries present (*Table 16*). In general, the child should be observed for age-inappropriate behavior, fear of adults or authority, flinching at space infringement, lack of appropriate crying, or excessive crying. Observations should include the location, severity, and whether there are injuries in various stages of healing[10–12].

Abusive peri-oral injuries are widely distributed, the lips and labial frenum being the most common areas injured. There may be contusions of the tongue, buccal mucosa, gingiva, hard and soft palate, and lingual frenum. Fractures of the facial bones, jaws, or teeth are suspicious, as are teeth that are displaced or avulsed. Teeth that are discolored due to pulpal necrosis can indicate previous abuse. Oral and peri-oral injuries may be inflicted with instruments, such as eating utensils, feeding bottles, pacifiers, fingers, hot or caustic liquids. A recent systematic review of labial frena found nine studies documenting torn labial frena in young children and abuse fatalities[13]. Only a direct blow was substantiated as a mechanism of injury. Two studies noted potential accidental mechanisms, both from intubation. Other abusive intra-oral injuries were widely distributed to the lips, gums, tongue, and palate, and fractures were seen with intrusion and extrusion of the dentition, bites, and contusions.[14]

Table 16 **Injuries which are suspicious for abuse**
Soft tissue bruising, i.e. cheeks, neck, buttocks, abdomen, calves, lower back
Pattern injuries, such as bite marks, handprints, finger or nail marks, belts; injuries with identifiable shapes from cords, belts, irons, etc.
Bruises or fingernail marks on the pinna of the ear
Traumatic alopecia
Any fracture, including fractured teeth
Lacerations of the mouth, injuries to the corners of the mouth due to gags
Bilateral injuries
Burns
Circumferential tie marks around the wrist or ankles from ligatures
Genital injury
Failure to thrive
Retinal hemorrhages

Bite marks

Teeth marks are patterned injuries, essentially tool marks that can exhibit highly individual characteristics of the biter's teeth. Teeth are weapons and have always been used as such. Bite marks are found on the living and the dead, perpetrator and victim, and sometimes, both. Bite marks occur frequently in violent assaults, child abuse being no exception. Bite marks are under-reported because they are not always recognized, or if recognized, dismissed as having little significance. They are often thought to be incidental bruises, but there may be teeth marks around the periphery, and swabbing for salivary DNA is possible, and often desirable, in an unwashed bite mark wound.

Individual teeth marks and arch form can provide valuable data for the forensic odontologist to associate or relate to the teeth of a suspect (**373, 374**). In child abuse, there is usually a small group with access to the child, so it may be possible to rule in or rule out the teeth patterns of those who have had contact with the child. When evaluating an injury pattern as a possible bite mark, be suspicious of all annular lesions that would approximate arch size or form (**375, 376**). Usually both arches will mark, creating elliptical or ovoid marks with a central ecchymosis from tissue crushing.

The clearest bite marks exhibit linear interrupted abrasion patterns consistent with tooth size. Incisors mark as rectangles, canines mark as triangles, and premolars leave a single or dual triangular mark (**377–379**). Subcutaneous bleeding may follow tissue planes or the path of least resistance, so the ecchymoses may not correspond to the point of dental impact. Bite marks may also be vague contusions, lacerations over bony prominences, or tissue avulsion (**380–384**). If bite marks are considered as a frequent injury in child abuse, they will be recognized. Almost half of bite

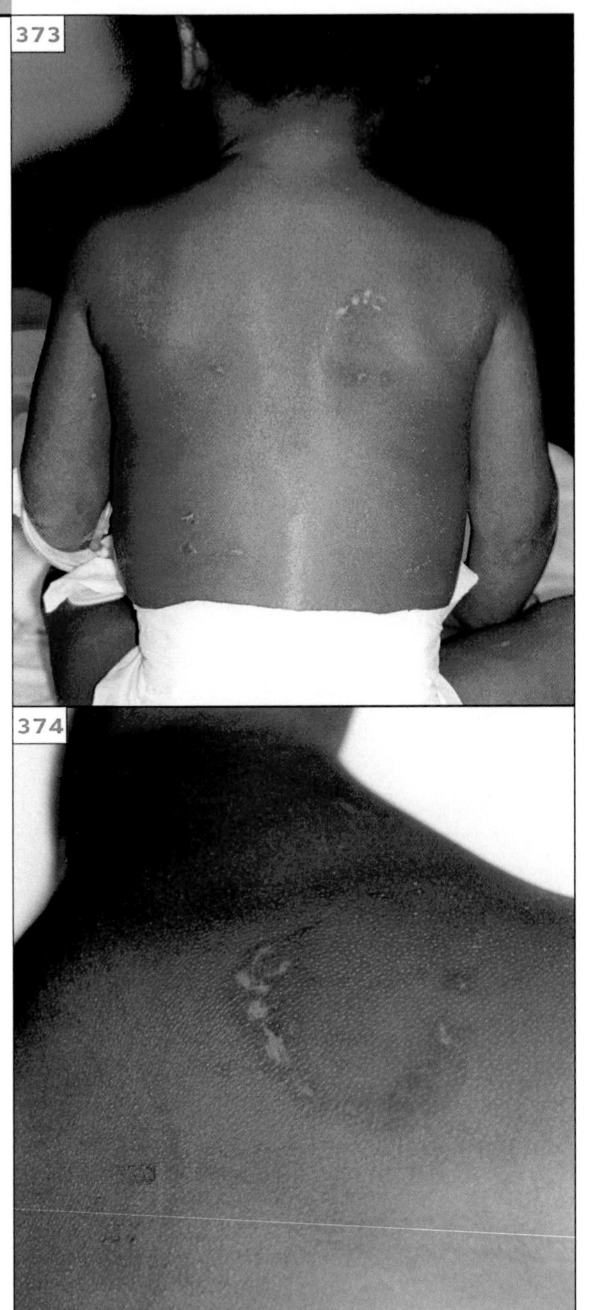

373, 374 A large, adult human bite mark on a child's back. 374 is a close-up depicting an almost complete human mouth pattern, with some hypopigmented scarring.

marks are on the head and neck, and when one is found, there is often another on a remote area of the body. When a bite mark is recognized, a full body examination is indicated, without the diaper/nappy in place (**385**). Children often exhibit bite marks on their hands and feet, fingers and toes (**386–396**). Their small hands and feet will almost entirely fit in the biter's mouth, frequently leaving sequential (in rows) bite mark patterns. When tooth marks are discovered, make certain the dorsal and ventral surfaces of the extremity are examined as well, since the teeth of both dental arches may leave marks.

Distinguishing pediatric from adult bites can be difficult. Generally, the distance between canine teeth in adults is 3 cm and the bite mark has a more ovoid shape (**397–400**). Pediatric bites have an intercanine distance of less than 2.5 cm and a somewhat flatter ovoid pattern, with diastemas distinguishable between the anterior teeth. Distinguishing animal from human bites is easier, as animals do not have the same dental formulae as humans. Humans have four incisors, two canines, four premolars, and three molars. Dogs and cats have six incisors, long curved canines, two premolars, and three molars. Differentiation can be made on the size and shape of the bite as well. Human bite marks are ovoid and superficial with an abrasion pattern; animal bites demonstrate deep punctures with tissue tearing and laceration. Animals have a long arch form, with a short, straight anterior segment. It is not possible to date bruises or bite marks with certainty, although there are some patterns of healing that can help with age estimation[15–17].

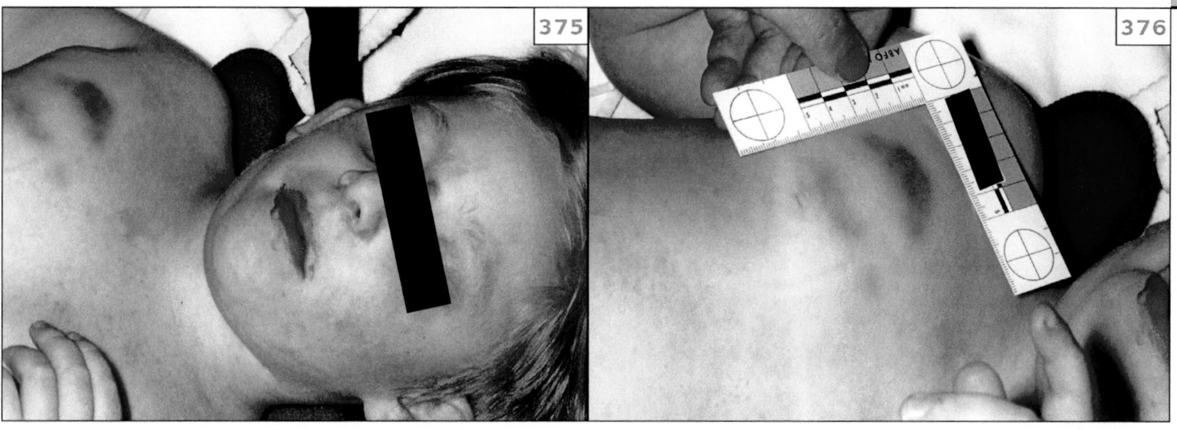

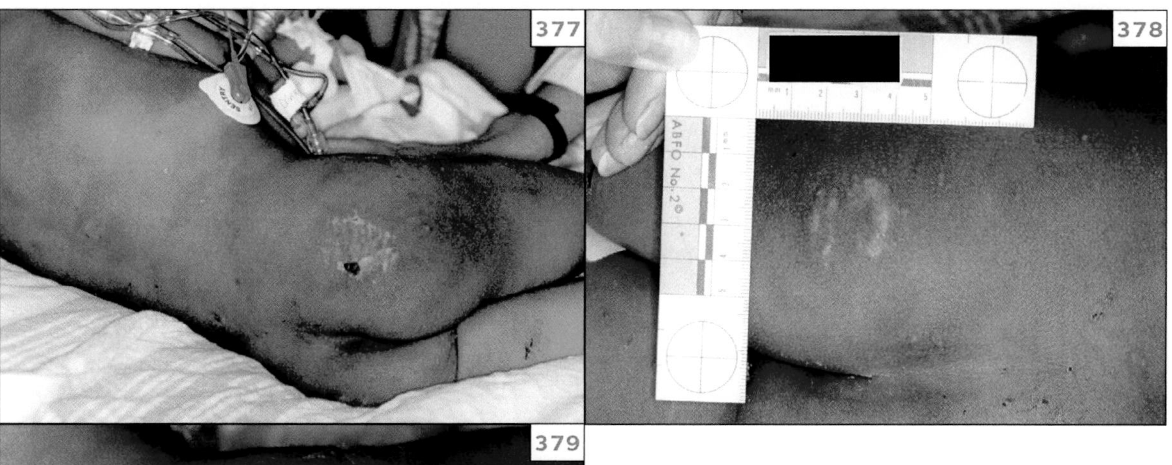

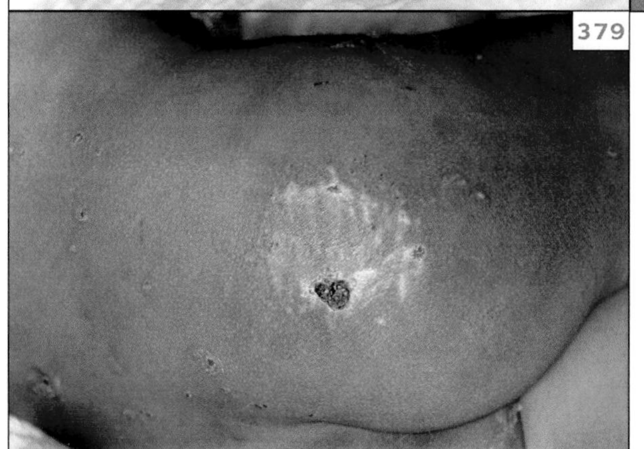

375, 376 Older child with bite pattern bruising which is more diffuse and in which specific teeth marks are harder to discern.

377–379 Bite mark noted on the buttock; 378 is an old, healed bite mark on the buttock of a previously abused child. 379 shows a human adult bite with tissue perforation by the lower arch.

380

381

382

383

384

385

380–384 Infant with multiple bruises over the vertebral column from being dragged. 384 shows a straddling injury to axilla from being hung from a fence.

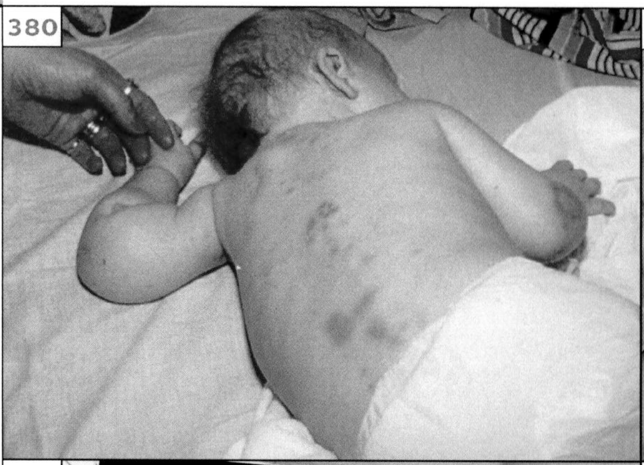

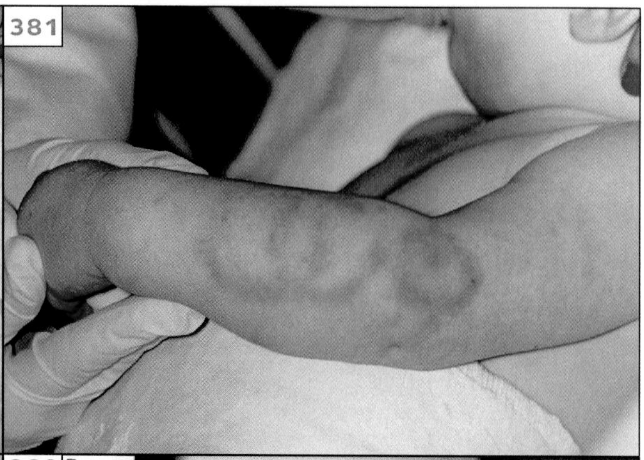

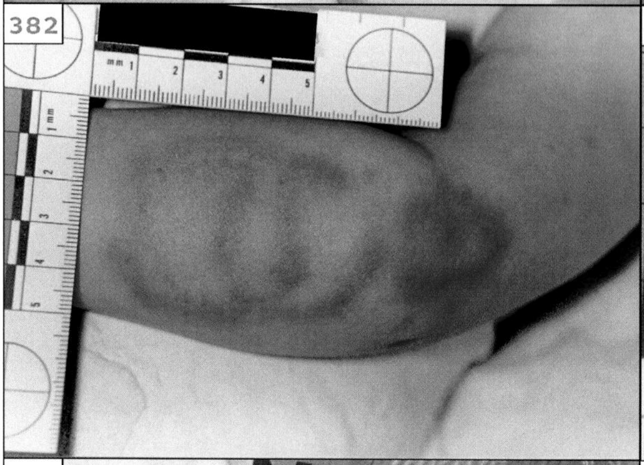

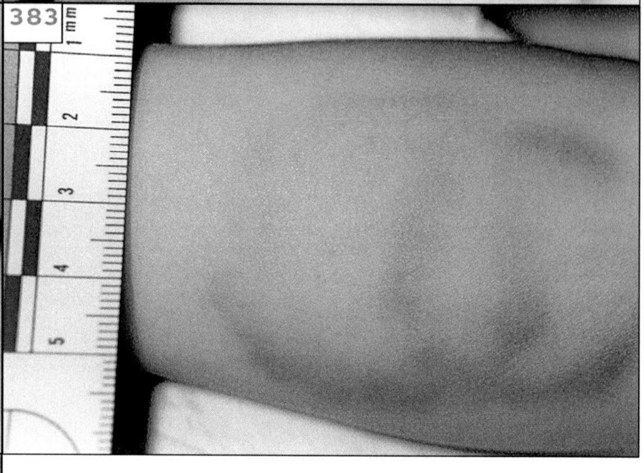

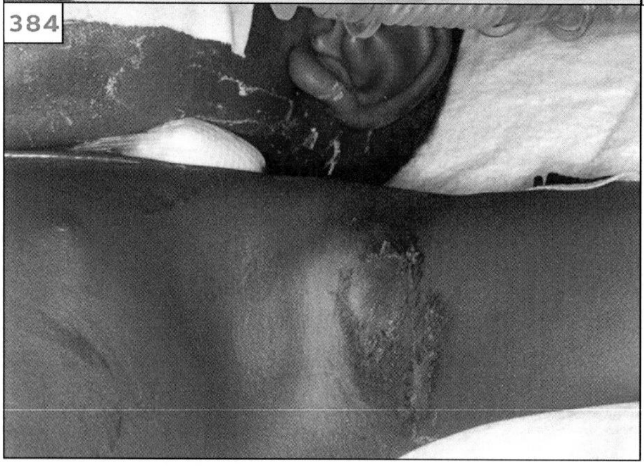

385 Healed scarring from teeth marks on the penile shaft.

386–393 Infant with several small, incomplete bite marks on the buttock, leg, hand, and foot. Note symmetric marks on the palm and dorsum of the hands (394–396).

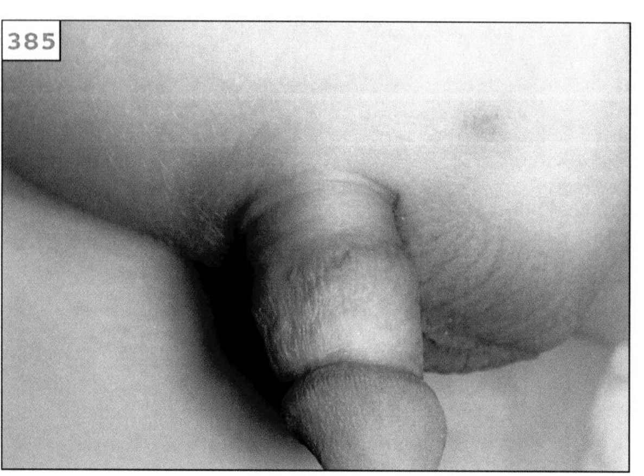

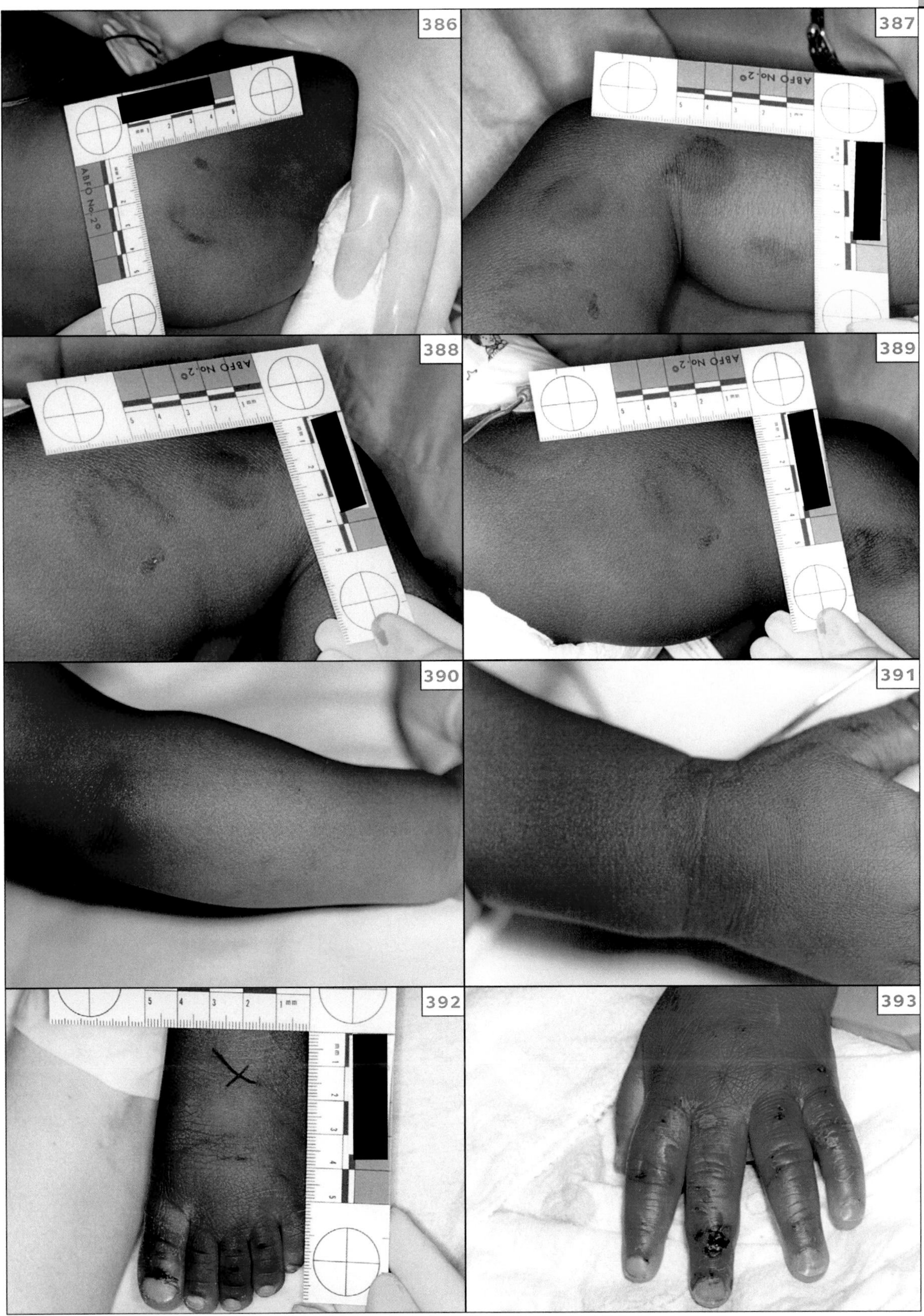
386
ABFO No. 2
387
ABFO No. 2
388
ABFO No. 2
389
ABFO No. 2
390
391
392
393

394

395

396

397

398

399

400

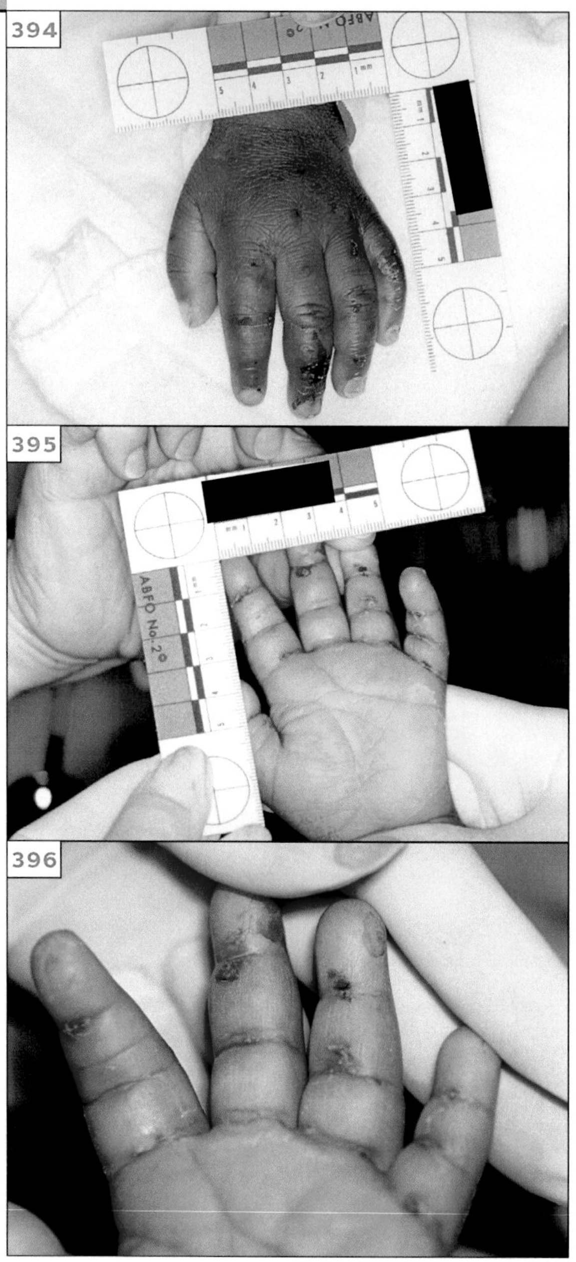

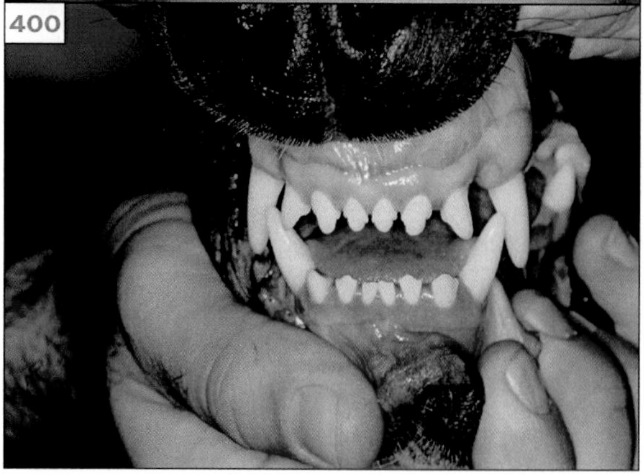

394–396 Infant with multiple bite marks on the buttock, leg, hand, and foot (386–393). Note opposing marks on palm and dorsum.

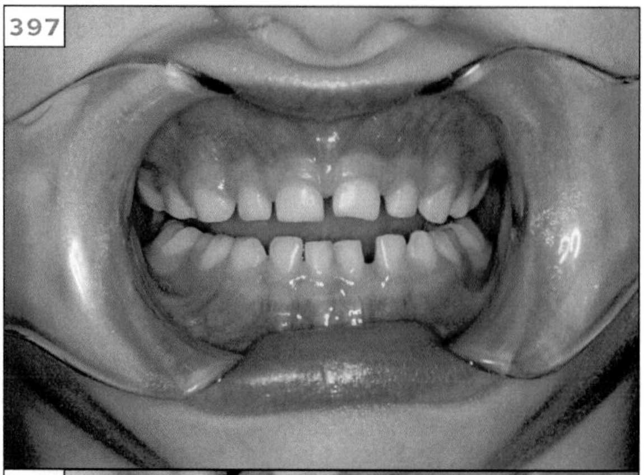

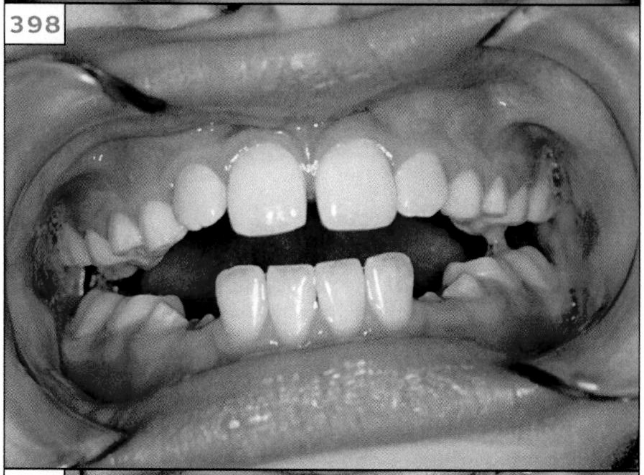

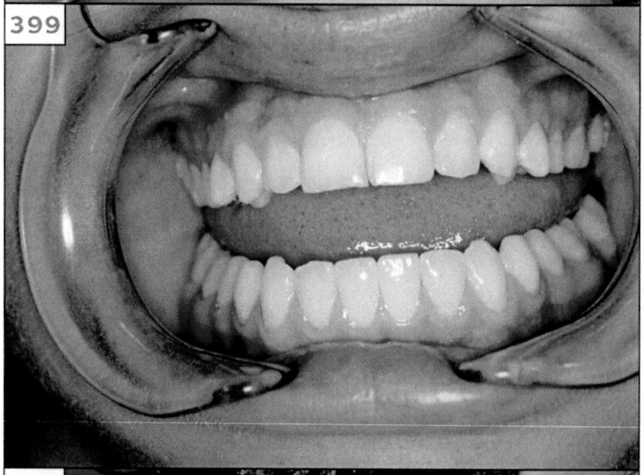

397–400 Pediatric dentition of a 6-year-old child (397). Mixed pediatric and adult dentition of a 9-year-old child (398). Adult dentition (399). Contrast this to the sharper and longer teeth on a dog (400), which would cause more tissue tearing and a different bite pattern.

Oral manifestations of sexual abuse

The oral cavity is a frequent site of sexual abuse in children[18]. Unexplained erythema or palatal petechiae at the junction of the hard and soft palate could indicate forced fellatio[19]. Bite marks may also be noted on the genitals, extremities, or trunk (401–403). Certain sexually transmitted infections in the mouth or pharynx are pathognomonic of sexual contact. The most common sexually transmitted infection in child abuse is gonorrhea; there may be mucosal or pharyngeal lesions that are generally asymptomatic. Condylomata acuminata (genital warts) and syphilis also manifest with oral lesions. Detection of semen in the oral cavity is possible for several days after exposure. Swabs should be taken from the buccal mucosa and tongue (Chapter 10, Anogenital findings and sexual abuse).

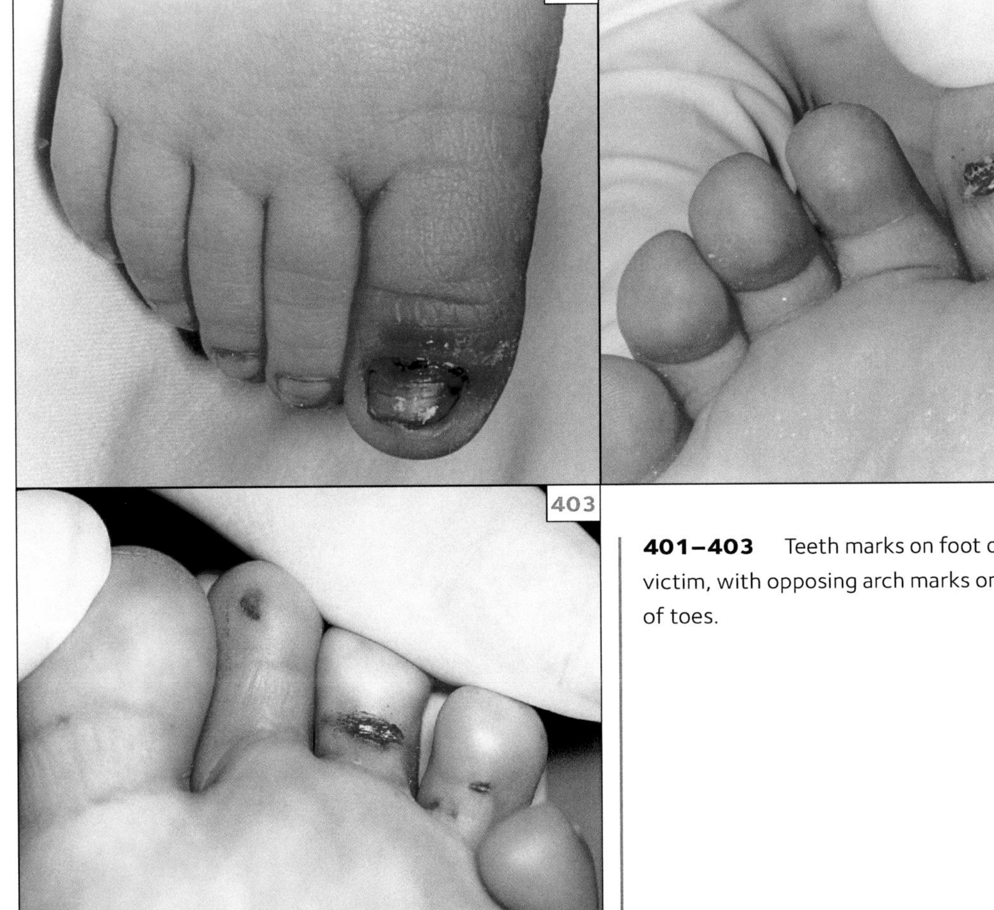

401–403 Teeth marks on foot of sexual assault victim, with opposing arch marks on both sides of toes.

Dental neglect

Neglect is the chronic failure of a parent or guardian to provide a child under the age of 18 with basic needs: shelter, clothing, food, medical and dental care, and supervision. As defined by the American Academy of Pediatric Dentistry[20], dental neglect is 'the willful failure of a parent or guardian to seek and follow through with treatment necessary to ensure a level of oral health essential for adequate function and freedom from pain and infection.' Most often physical and dental neglect occur simultaneously; therefore the oral cavity of the neglected child should be examined by a dentist. Both aspects of neglect affect the child's ability to perform basic functions of attending school, playing, or working. Dental infections can cause chronic pain, life-threatening abscesses, retard a child's growth and development, and make routine eating difficult or impossible.

Documentation

All physical signs and symptoms of abuse and neglect should be documented, including location, degree, and severity, and whether there are wounds in various stages of healing. It should be determined whether the injuries are compatible with the explanation. If possible, the child should be interviewed in a sensitive, nonjudgmental manner, and the answers recorded in quotation marks. 'Why' questions generally elicit more information than 'who' or 'how'. Where possible, the wounds and dentition should be recorded photographically. There are several guidelines that can be of help[21].

Good photographic technique preserves the evidence in a form suitable for analysis and maintains a permanent record of the injuries. A good rule in photographing injuries is that you cannot take too many photographs. These should be exposed in both color and black and white, varying the F-stop, and using a 50 mm macro lens. Adequate documentation includes positive identification on and in the photograph, orienting the photograph in relationship to a known anatomical landmark, and close-up photographs, with and without a scale in place. The scale should be a linear measure with a circular reference. Ideally, the American Board of Forensic Odontolgy scale (ABFO2) should be used[21]. This scale is a metric scale with a circular reference, and has a gray scale. It is designed so that the photographs can be rectified for distortion. The case number/name, date, and your initials should be marked on the scale. If the ABFO scale is not available, a metric scale and a circular coin can be used. The scale should be placed in the same plane as the injury, and adjacent to the wound.

Reporting and referral

The key to the interruption of the cycle of family violence is the awareness and recognition of inflicted injuries, including bite marks. Dentists are mandated reporters of child abuse and they have done a remarkably poor job of reporting abuse[22]. The level of awareness in those who have contact with injured children must be increased; only this will lead to proper intervention and referral to the appropriate agencies and disruption of the pattern of ongoing family violence.

Teaching points

- Oral and dental findings are seen in a large number of abused children, and the dentist is an important member of the health care team who can identify injuries and protect children.
- Bite marks are often found on victims of abuse and there are several characteristics that can aid the examiner in determining the potential source.
- Certain injuries and infections in the mouth, gums, and palate should be recognized and reported as potential physical or sexual abuse.
- Proper documentation can assist in preserving evidence of the injury for the investigators and the courts.

Acknowledgments

This chapter is dedicated to Ryan, Terrell, Derrick, Brian, Malik, Dakota, Sherrell, Alex, and all the others. With thanks to my daughters, Holly, Sandra, and Amanda, for their love, patience, and support.

Chapter 9

ABUSIVE ABDOMINAL TRAUMA

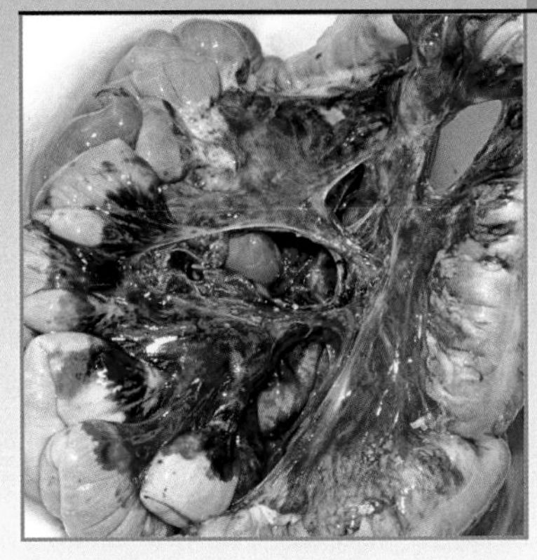

Colleen M. Fitzpatrick MD and Scott Langenburg MD, FACS, FAAP

Severe intra-abdominal injury caused by child abuse is a relatively rare occurrence. However, the morbidity and mortality of such injuries can be devastating. This requires a high level of vigilance and keen diagnostic skill in those caring for battered children.

Epidemiology

In a series of victims of blunt abdominal trauma, child abuse represented 11% of patients involved[1]. However, major abdominal trauma with visceral injury accounts for only 0.5–2% of all cases of abused children[2–4].

Children who sustain intra-abdominal injury from abuse tend to be young. The mean age of the abused child is 2 years as opposed to 6–7 years for accidentally injured children[1–3]. In one report, abuse was the cause of abdominal trauma in 44% of patients under the age of 4 years[1]. Another series cited an incidence of 0.9 cases of abuse per million children per year; however, this number rose to 2.33 cases per million children per year when limited to children of less than 5 years of age. In that study, the average age of patients sustaining abdominal injury from abuse was 3.7 years as opposed to 9.7 years for victims of motor vehicle collisions and 10.4 years for those who fell[5]. In a third series of 79 children suffering from abdominal trauma, 19% had been abused, none was over 5 years old and 73% were under the age of 3 years[6]. In many instances, the families are already known to social services for previous episodes of abuse involving either the patient or siblings[2].

Pathogenesis

Abusive abdominal injuries are due to direct blows to the abdomen. Younger children have prominent abdomens with wide costal margins and minimal abdominal musculature. This results in more frequent injuries to the central upper abdomen[7]. Abused children are more likely to have injury to the duodenum, duodenal–jejunal junction, and jejunum than are accidentally injured children[1]. Additionally, the anterior–posterior diameter of young children is small[7]. This allows for compression of the viscera against the spinal column. In cases of fluid-filled loops of bowel, this can result in perforation[2]. Shear forces against points of mesenteric fixation can also result in avulsion of the gut from its mesentery[3,7].

Injuries to solid organs also occur from direct blows over the liver, spleen, and kidneys which can result in contusions and lacerations. Lacerations may also be the result of associated rib fractures.

Clinical history

Obtaining a reliable and accurate history in cases of child abuse can be a daunting task. Often the person bringing the child to the emergency department is not the abuser and may not be able to provide details of the event[1]. The information provided by the caregiver may be inaccurate and inconsistent as there may be fear of self-incrimination. The abused child may be too young or too frightened to provide further information[2].

The history provided for abusive abdominal injury usually does not provide adequate explanation for the magnitude and distribution of injuries. Falling down the stairs has been reported as the most common history given in instances of bowel perforation. Falling down the stairs, however, is an unlikely mechanism to cause bowel injury[8]. Other frequently cited histories include falls from the bed and couch, 'stopped breathing', and 'sick and vomiting'[1]. Inaccurate histories can delay appropriate diagnosis in a significant proportion of patients[6].

Furthermore, there is often a delay from the time of injury to presentation at the hospital. Average delays of 13–24 hours have been reported[2,6] and it is due to this delay that about 50% of patients are critically ill at the time of presentation[6]. In contrast, 91% of accidentally injured patients are likely to be brought directly to the hospital from the scene of injury[1].

Physical examination

The diagnostic work-up and evaluation of the abuse victim is identical to that of the accidentally injured child[9]. Standard trauma protocols should be followed.

The airway and breathing must be established first. Assessment of the circulation may reveal tachycardia and hypotension in cases of significant blood loss. Aggressive fluid resuscitation may be warranted in such cases. A thorough neurologic examination is necessary to exclude concomitant injury to the central nervous system. The patient is fully exposed for complete examination. Often signs of previous abuse, such as burn scars, bruising, or abrasions will be present[1].

Inspection of the abdomen may reveal abdominal wall bruising (**404**). While this sign may be pathognomonic of abuse, it is rarely present[2,5]. The presence of abdominal distension should also be noted on inspection. The abdomen should then be palpated in a systematic fashion to elicit tenderness or signs of peritonitis, including rebound tenderness, guarding, or in advanced cases, rigidity. Such advanced cases may represent patients with a significant delay in presentation. These patients may also be moribund with evidence of significant blood loss[1].

Once the physical examination is completed, adjuvant studies should be obtained. Blood should be sent for complete blood counts, electrolytes, and liver function studies. A urinalysis for occult blood should be obtained. Standard radiographic studies include cervical spine, chest, and pelvic roentograms. A full skeletal survey should be obtained to look for evidence of associated or old fractures consistent with an abuse pattern. The need for additional imaging studies, such as abdominal computed tomography (CT) scan, should be guided by the findings on physical examination (see Chapter 5, Imaging child abuse).

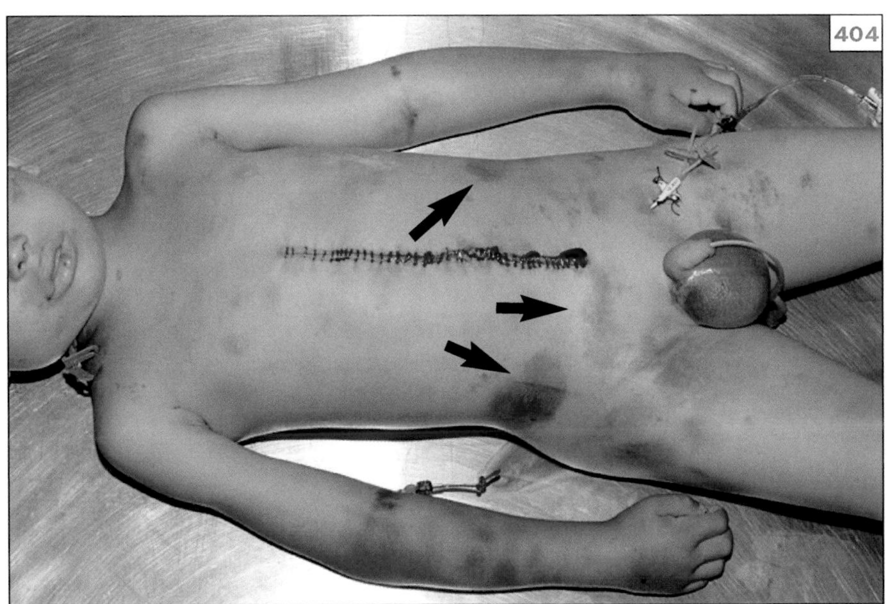

404 Multiple bruises and contusions are readily apparent over the abdomen of this abuse victim (see arrows). While abdominal bruising is rarely seen, it is pathognomonic for nonaccidental trauma.

Differential diagnosis

The patterns of injury seen in abuse differ from those in accidental trauma. In one series, patients with accidental trauma had an 8% rate of visceral injury, as opposed to 65% of abused patients. Abuse was more likely to produce upper abdominal, midline intestinal perforations. In contrast, accidental injury was more likely to be seen in the lower abdomen[1]. In another report, injuries to the gut were seen in 55% of abuse cases, compared to 21% of motor vehicle collisions and 10% of falls. Conversely, solid organ injury was seen in 60% of abuse cases, 67% of motor vehicle collisions, and 85% of falls[5].

Despite the differences between accidental and nonaccidental trauma, injury to any of the intra-abdominal organs can occur in cases of abuse. Lacerations and contusions of the liver and spleen can occur. These injuries may be associated with overlying rib fractures. Frequently bleeding from these types of injuries will stop spontaneously. However, in severe injuries, patients may present with hemoperitoneum and hemodynamic instability. Injury to the kidney should be suspected in the presence of hematuria. Frequently, these injuries are contained within Gerota's fascia.

Traumatic pancreatitis is rare in children. However, when it does occur, it is most likely secondary to abuse[7]. Pancreatic pseudocyst can also be a manifestation of child abuse, especially in younger children where an accidental mechanism (such as falling on bicycle handlebars) is unlikely[10]. The mean age of presentation has been reported as 27 months[11].

In abused patients, injury to the bowel must be suspected. Possible injuries include intramural hematoma, perforation, or injury to the mesentery, including hematoma or avulsion (**405–407**). Significant peritonitis on examination is highly suggestive of an advanced injury to the bowel with contamination of the peritoneal cavity.

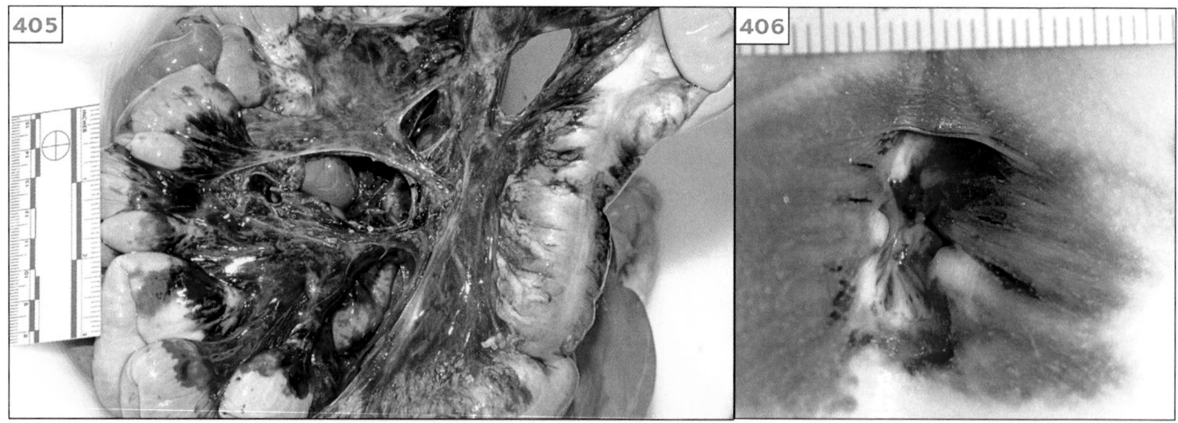

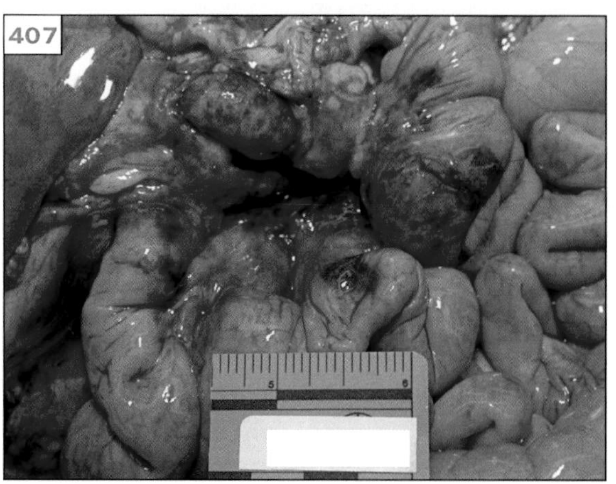

405, 406 Significant injury to the mesentery of the small bowel and colon. The mesentery is torn in several locations, associated with hemorrhage and ischemic compromise of the bowel. There is also evidence of peri-anal bruising and anal trauma from sexual assault (406).

407 Injury to the mesentery of the colon. The segment was excised in the operating room and both ends of the colon were brought together primarily.

Investigations

Basic laboratory data, such as a complete blood count, chemistries, and liver enzyme tests should be obtained. Low hemoglobin or hematocrit levels are indicative of significant acute or ongoing blood loss. Leukocytosis is nonspecific; however, it may reflect significant intra-abdominal contamination from a perforated bowel. Electrolytes should be checked as well. A low albumin may reflect a state of chronic malnutrition associated with neglect.

Serum aspartate transaminase (AST) and alanine transaminase (ALT) have proven useful in detecting occult hepatic injury. Of 49 patients with no evidence of abdominal injury, three of four patients with elevated transaminases were ultimately found to have liver lacerations. These laboratory values normalized in 24–48 hours. In general, the levels of AST and ALT in abused patients are not as high as those seen in accidentally injured patients. This may be a function of delayed presentation[12]. Routine screening of amylase has not proven to be useful, likely due to the infrequent occurrence of pancreatic injury. Nonetheless, this value is likely to be elevated in cases of traumatic pancreatitis or pseudocyst[10].

Urine should be sent for urinalysis to assess for renal injury. Gross hematuria is clearly indicative of significant injury. Microscopic hematuria warrants further imaging studies to investigate the possibility of occult injury.

Various imaging modalities can be used in the evaluation of child abuse. Plain radiographs are useful for obtaining the standard cervical spine, chest, and pelvis images. Additionally, plain films are used to obtain a full skeletal survey.

Ultrasound (US) can be used to perform a focused abdominal sonography for trauma (FAST) examination in the resuscitation room. This can be performed by the evaluating surgeon or emergency department physician and allows rapid assessment for free fluid within the peritoneal cavity. The presence of free fluid may assist in the decision to perform a CT scan of the abdomen. Additionally, more detailed ultrasound studies by a radiologist may be warranted and are most useful in assessing solid organs. If a significant ileus is present, the overlying bowel gas may limit the utility of ultrasound.

Computed tomography scanning has become the most versatile study in the evaluation of injured patients. CT scans adequately visualize both the peritoneal cavity and the retroperitoneum and provide information on vascular integrity. While a recent article reviewed its importance in imaging the pancreas[13], CT is not sensitive for evaluating injuries to the hollow viscera.

Angiography can be used for further evaluation of the vasculature. Angiography can be used for both diagnosis and treatment; angioembolization of active sites of hemorrhage can be performed[4].

Contrast radiograph studies may be used to evaluate the hollow viscera. Filling defects suggest intramural hematomas, while contrast extravasation is diagnostic of a bowel perforation[14]. Duodenal hematoma has a classic appearance on upper gastrointestinal contrast radiograph that was described as an intramural mass with a 'coiled-spring' appearance of the thickened mucosal folds proximal to the hematoma. This classic appearance is seen in the acute phase of disease. Ultrasound of this lesion demonstrates an echogenic mass in the wall of the duodenum with elevation of the overlying superior mesenteric artery[4]. This hematoma is usually confined to the lateral wall of the duodenum. With resolution, the hematoma is resorbed, resulting in smooth nodules in the wall of the greater curve of the duodenum. Thickening of the duodenal folds may be evident. This change in appearance may be significant if there is a delay in presentation[15].

Acute pancreatitis may be visualized with both ultrasound and CT scanning. If pancreatic pseudocyst is present, the stomach may be displaced anteriorly and elevated on upper gastrointestinal (UGI) series. The transverse colon may be displaced inferiorly. US will demonstrate a cystic mass and CT scanning will show the exact location of the cyst[4,13].

For both injuries of the liver and spleen, plain films may demonstrate associated rib fractures. CT scanning is most useful in diagnosing lacerations and hematomas. CT scan is also useful in determining the extent of the injury. Angiography with angioembolization can be performed if there is evidence of active bleeding or pseudoaneurysm formation[4].

CT scanning is most accurate for the diagnosis and extent of injury to the kidneys. The most common injury seen is a fracture or laceration of the renal capsule associated with perirenal hematoma or urinoma. Renal injuries are optimally visualized with administration of intravenous contrast[4].

Prognosis

The mortality rate associated with intra-abdominal injury is higher in abused children than in accidentally injured children. Rates have been reported to be as high as 45–50%[2,6]. In contrast to accidentally injured children who are more likely to die from other injuries, i.e. head trauma, death in abused children older than 3 years of age is generally related to intra-abdominal hemorrhage or sepsis[1]. The highest mortality is seen in children who present with active intra-abdominal hemorrhage[2].

Management

The patient who presents to the emergency department with hemodynamic instability unresponsive to resuscitative maneuvers warrants emergent operative exploration. Management of other patients is dependent on the site of injury.

Injuries to the liver, spleen, and kidneys can be managed nonoperatively in hemodynamically stable patients. These patients are often monitored closely in an intensive care unit for at least the first 24 hours with serial abdominal examinations and serial monitoring of hemoglobin levels (**408**). Patients with hepatic and splenic injuries who remain stable, but have evidence of ongoing bleeding may be candidates for angioembolization. Additionally, patients with evidence of pseudoaneurysm on initial scans may be candidates for embolization due to an increased risk of repeat bleeding. Patients who have ongoing transfusion requirements or who become hemodynamically unstable need to be explored (**409–413**). For patients with splenic injury, spleen salvage should be attempted in an effort to avoid the issues of overwhelming post-splenectomy sepsis.

Traumatic pancreatitis is managed by fasting until the pancreatitis resolves. In severe cases, total parenteral nutrition (TPN) may be needed. In patients who develop a pseudocyst, it is reasonable to observe these patients for resolution of the pseudocyst. If the pseudocyst persists, a drainage procedure may be required.

Patients with free intra-abdominal air and patients with diffuse peritonitis and a rigid abdomen have a perforated viscus until proven otherwise. These patients mandate urgent operative exploration. Patients with an obstructing intramural hematoma of the duodenum or proximal small bowel are fasted and started on TPN support until the hematoma resolves, at which time enteral nutrition can be restarted. Patients with persistent abdominal pain who do not have an identified injury should be fasted. Serial abdominal examinations are performed. Clinical deterioration warrants further investigation, either additional imaging studies or operative exploration if there is a high index of suspicion of occult bowel injury.

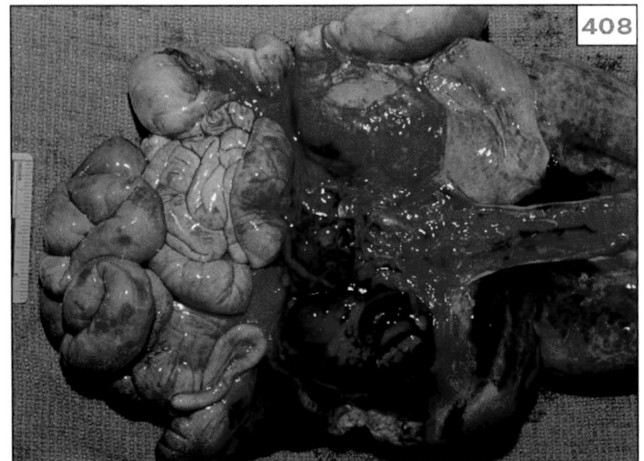

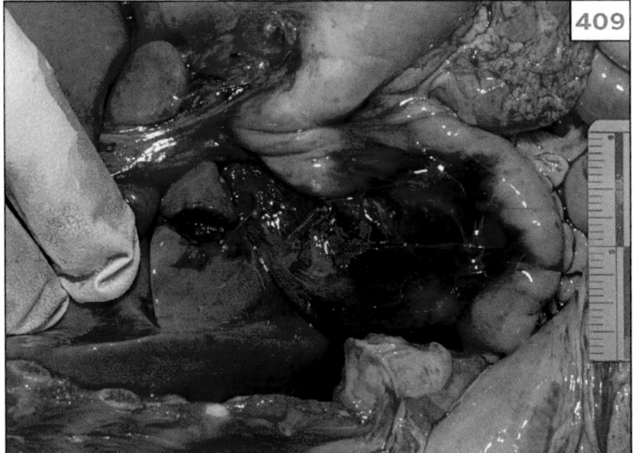

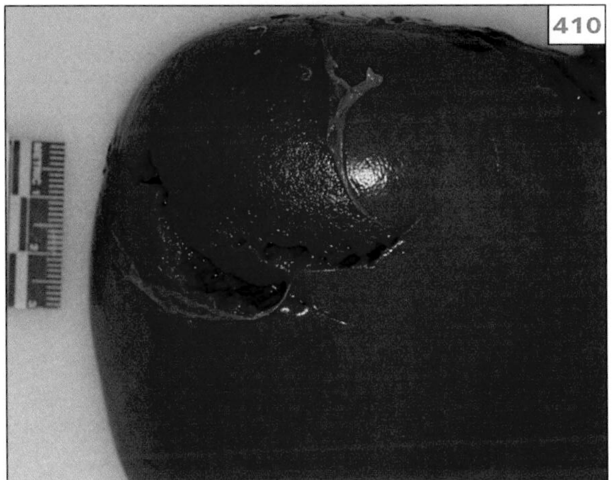

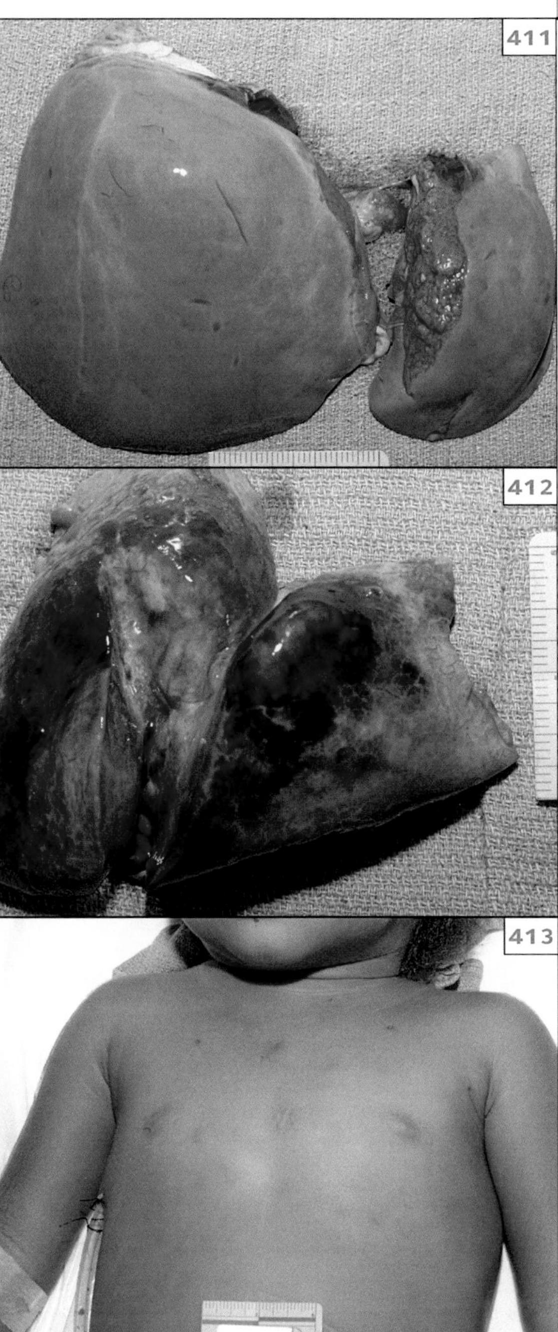

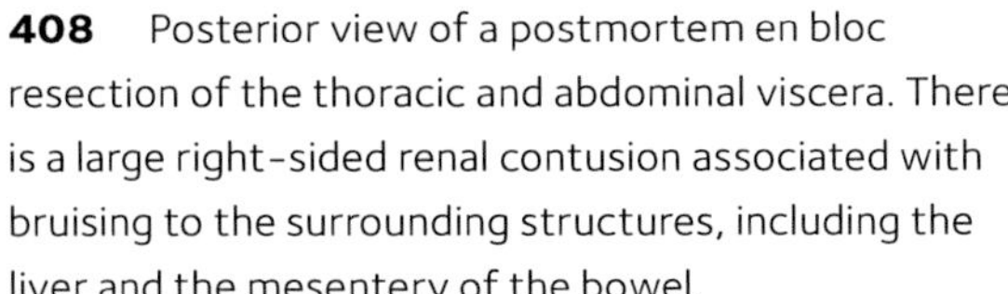

408 Posterior view of a postmortem en bloc resection of the thoracic and abdominal viscera. There is a large right-sided renal contusion associated with bruising to the surrounding structures, including the liver and the mesentery of the bowel.

409 A small liver laceration is present at the tip of the examiner's gloved finger. There is significant contusion of the mesentery of the overlying small bowel.

410 A superficial anterior liver laceration is demonstrated in this image with avulsion of the surrounding liver capsule.

411–413 This abuse victim sustained a liver transection. The left lateral lobe is completely separated from the remainder of the liver. While there are old scars, note the paucity of acute external injury (413).

Teaching points

- Significant intra-abdominal trauma from child abuse is a relatively rare event that generally affects children less than 5 years of age.
- Direct blows to the abdomen usually cause injuries located in the upper, mid-abdomen.
- There is often a delay between the time of injury and presentation to the emergency department for evaluation. Often the circumstances of the event are not known and clinical histories may be vague or misleading. These children need to be evaluated using standard protocols in an expeditious manner.
- Health care providers need to be familiar with the injury patterns associated with abuse.

Chapter 10

ANOGENITAL FINDINGS AND CHILD SEXUAL ABUSE

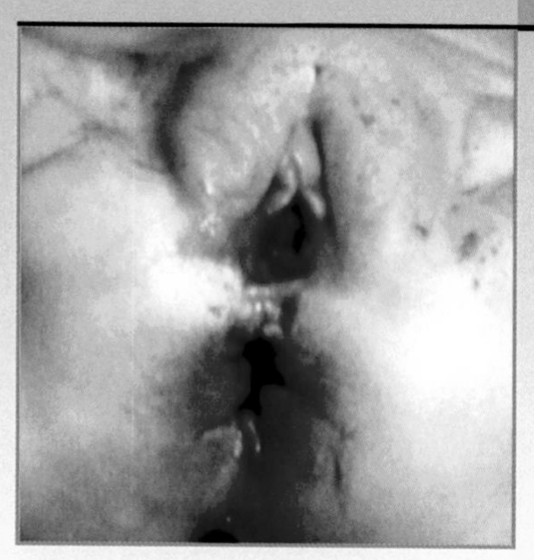

Vincent J. Palusci
MD, MS

The World Health Organization[1] has defined child sexual abuse and exploitation as the involvement of a child in sexual activity that he or she does not fully comprehend, is unable to give informed consent to, or for which the child is not developmentally prepared and cannot give consent, or that violate the laws or social taboos of society. Child sexual abuse is evidenced by this activity between a child and an adult or another child, who by age or development is in a relationship of responsibility, trust, or power, the activity being intended to gratify or satisfy the needs of the other person. This may include, but is not limited to:

- The inducement or coercion of a child to engage in any unlawful sexual activity
- The exploitative use of child in prostitution or other unlawful sexual practices
- The exploitative use of children in pornographic performances and materials.

Introduction

Although precise incidence data are lacking, sexual abuse of children occurs commonly throughout the world. In the United States, it has been estimated that one or more in four females and one in 10 males will be victims of sexual abuse by the time they become adults, and 10% of substantiated reports for child abuse and neglect involve child sexual abuse[2]. Similar or higher lifetime prevalence has been noted in Europe, Africa, and Australia. While males are reported less often than females, the number of male victims may in fact be higher as a result of a reluctance to report cases among males[2].

The medical examination for suspected victims of sexual abuse is but one part of a larger community response[2,3]. Most commonly, the anogenital examination is normal or reveals nonspecific changes that can be seen in normal children, as well as after healed trauma[3–5]. Therefore, the most important determinant for indicating whether sexual abuse has occurred remains witness disclosure, from the child, offender, and others. This chapter will assist the physician in identifying and interpreting physical findings, including those which are normal (which can confuse the examiner), indicative of trauma (in the small number of cases with findings), or unclear or uncertain (based on our understanding of these issues to date).

The medical examination

In most cases of child sexual abuse, the medical examination of the child is normal and few cases have identifiable forensic evidence[3,6,7]. Understanding the relationship of a child victim to a perpetrator may explain why the examination is normal, given that a perpetrator who is known to a child and who victimizes the child over a considerable period of time usually pursues a pattern of behavior to prevent detection. The perpetrator may wish to avoid physical injury to the child, opting instead to engage in repeated events of fondling or genital to genital contact without full penetration past the hymenal opening. To identify abnormal findings, the medical examiner must first therefore thoroughly understand normal female and male genital and anal anatomy and their variations, and guidelines have been published[4,8]. There are several normal, nonspecific, and specific findings seen after sexual abuse, and mandated reporters and investigators should have familiarity with their positive identification, diagnosis, and interpretation.

While the medical examination of a male's genitals may appear to be easier to interpret, the medical examination of a female's genitals is more complex. A female is typically examined while lying on her back in the 'frog-legged position'. The physician separates the labia majora and often applies traction, revealing the hymen and the vaginal opening. A videocolposcope can be used to record well-lighted, magnified images that can be simultaneously viewed by the child, caregiver, and examiner[9]. The child is examined for injuries to the vulva, the hymen, and the surrounding tissue. Penetrating genital injury most often occurs to the posterior vulva and hymenal rim, so these areas require careful inspection. Abrasions, bruising, and bleeding lacerations of the vulva can all be seen in acute sexual assault and should be documented by diagram or photograph. In most cases, the hymen appears very smooth and can have different configurations, most commonly annular or crescentic. Physicians should carefully note the appearance of the hymen, particularly the lower half (commonly described as 3–9 o'clock), for evidence of transections or clefts that extend to the vaginal wall. Abrasions or bruising of the hymen can also occur, and any injury should again be documented by diagram or photograph. Physicians should culture any vaginal discharge, if noted, to determine if there is a sexually transmitted infection. Most findings are likely normal variants, such as bumps, incomplete clefts, hymenal asymmetry, and rolled hymenal edges. Contrary to popular belief, the size of the hymenal opening or the amount of hymenal tissue is not predictive of the likelihood of sexual abuse.

In performing an anal examination in children, the examiner carefully notes the symmetry and tone of the anus when the buttocks are separated. In addition to symmetry, the physician should note the presence of tags, fissures, or scars[4,10]. With the exception of a bleeding laceration after a report of sodomy, the presence of tags, bumps, and scars may be nonspecific findings that do not confirm whether a child has been sexually abused unless they can be positively related to previously identified acute findings. Documented anal injury after a child sexual assault is distinctively uncommon, and any injuries that do occur can heal quickly and often without visible residua[5,6].

Normal variants

There are a number of normal variants which are present at birth and which have been confused with potentially concerning findings (*Table 17*). The size of the urethral opening is quite variable and can vary widely in normal children without neurologic or urologic disease (**414**). Peri-urethral bands (**415**) are supportive ligaments extending from the urethra to the labia; they can be confused with post-traumatic scars or injury. Note the smooth edges and lack of epithelial changes in these bands that denotes their nontraumatic nature. These can also be seen extending from the hymen to the labia. As one inspects the visible vagina, it is common to see intravaginal ridges or columns (**416–419**), which also represent supportive ligaments in this location. As these extend to the genital outlet, it is not uncommon to note hymenal bumps or mounds (**420–423**) at their insertion points. The examiner should carefully note that these hymenal finding reflect extension of the intravaginal column. Their smoothness and lack of epithelial changes on the hymenal surface reflect their nontraumatic nature. As the examiner looks externally, a linea vestibularis (**424**) is sometimes present in the midline where the labia join posteriorly. Also called a 'linea alba', this white, smooth linear change reflects a congenital lack of pigmentation at a presumptive fusion line, which is not related to healed trauma (**425**). Similarly, hyperpigmentation of the labial or peri-anal tissues can be congenital and unrelated to trauma (**426, 427**).

Historically, it is only over the past 25 years that we have recognized that there are several normal hymenal variants in prepubertal females. These undergo predictable developmental changes through infancy, childhood, and adolescence and should not by themselves raise concern of sexual trauma. Infants are most often noted to have annular hymenal openings with residual hormonal effects from estrogen *in utero*. Estrogen can cause thickening and elongation of hymenal tissues, which can be described as redundant and floppy (**428–430**). By definition, an annular hymen extends completely around the opening to the vagina (**431**). When such tissue is incomplete, generally with a lack of tissue anteriorly near the urethra, we describe the hymenal tissue as crescentic, or in the shape of a crescent (**432–434**). Many females have a crescentic hymenal opening during childhood and this is thought to be a part of normal development. Hymenal notches, clefts, and lack of anterior tissue between 10 and 2 o'clock in the supine position should not be interpreted as reflecting trauma. Any abnormal findings should be confirmed in the knee–chest position (**423**). During embryogenesis, the cloacal membrane normally undergoes perforation that results in a single opening. However, a significant proportion of females have more than one opening, defined by the presence of a hymenal septum or septa (**435–438**). Small hymenal notches can also result from prior septa insertion and/or colocation of bumps or mounds from intravaginal ridges or columns. When present, hymenal septa should be positively identified by their smooth insertions on the hymenal rim and lack of extension internally. Such extension may indicate the important congenital condition of vaginal duplication. This may require imaging to assure normal internal anatomy. Hymenal septa can dehisce from their insertions spontaneously as they regress during development, and their separation can also be accelerated by hygiene practices, insertion of tampons, and sexual trauma. The cause of acutely dehisced septa can be difficult to determine based on examination alone. Another derangement of anogenital development can result in a lack of genital opening or imperforate hymen (**439**). Females with imperforate hymen generally have few physical symptoms and this finding goes undetected during infancy and childhood unless that female is examined for other reasons. Current experience suggests that a significant proportion of females with imperforate hymen have spontaneous perforation during late childhood and puberty as the hymenal tissues undergo developmental changes. This knowledge often results in 'watchful waiting' before puberty starts, with the plan for re-examination and gynecologic treatment as menarche approaches to prevent potential secondary complications of hematocolpos, scarring, and infertility.

As with hymenal and urethral opening size, the anal opening size also varies based on a number of normal and pathologic conditions. A small number of children are born with failure of midline fusion in which the external peri-anal epidermis appears to be more mucosal than cornified epithelium. This lack of epidermal fusion is generally asymptomatic, but can be confused with trauma. A congenital absence of muscle tissue in the posterior and anterior midline has been called diastasis ani. This can result in apparent soft tissue defects that have erroneously been attributed to trauma. Diastasis ani is not associated with problems in defecation and is usually identified as a normal variant on examination when epithelial tissues are normal and no evidence of overlying scarring is seen. Many normal infants and children are found to have anal fissures, which often present after painful defecation and bleeding related to stooling, but which can also be found after sexual trauma (**440**). It is interesting also to note that children with multiple anal procedures have been noted to have few or no anal findings despite repeated, documented medical instrumentation. When present, most fissures are superficial and heal quickly without residua. A small number of children may have skin tag formation, associated with fissures, constipation, or both (**441**). Such tags should be differentiated from venous protrusions, such as hemorrhoids, which are more swollen, vascular, and more concerning for increased intra-abdominal venous pressure. The duration and progression of tags, if any, are not well understood, and many are found in normal children without visible fissure or recent injury.

Table 17 **Physical findings after child sexual abuse**[a]

I. Findings documented in newborns or commonly seen in nonabused children. The presence of these findings generally neither confirms nor discounts a child's clear disclosure of sexual abuse	Periurethral or vestibular bands
	Longitudinal intravaginal ridges or columns
	Hymenal tags
	Mounds, bumps on hymenal rim
	Linea vestibularis
	Notch or clefts in superior half of hymen (3–9 o'clock, patient supine)
	Superficial notch or cleft in inferior rim
	External hymenal ridges
	Congenital variations in hymenal opening shape, including septate and others
	Failure of midline fusion (perineal groove)
	Diastasis ani
	Perianal skin tag
	Increased labial or peri-anal pigmentation
	Dilation of urethral opening
	Thickened hymen
II. Indeterminate: Insufficient or conflicting data from research studies. These findings support a disclosure of sexual abuse if one is given, and are highly suggestive of abuse even in the absence of a disclosure, unless a clear, timely plausible description of accidental injury is provided by the child and/or caregiver	Acute laceration or extensive bruising of labia, penis, scrotum, peri-anal tissues, or perineum
	Fresh laceration of the posterior fourchette
	Scar of posterior fourchette or peri-anal tissues (difficult to assess without seeing prior injury)
III. Specific findings that are diagnostic of trauma or sexual contact	Laceration of the hymen (acute)
	Ecchymosis of the hymen
	Peri-anal lacerations extending deep to the external sphincter. Hymenal transection (healed)
	Missing segment of hymenal tissue
	Confirmed gonorrhea, syphilis, *Trichomonas, Chlamydia,* HIV (without congenital or transfusion transmission)
	Pregnancy
	Sperm on or in child's body

[a]Modified from Adams JA, Kaplan RA, Starling SP, *et al.* (2007). Guidelines for medical care of children who may have been sexually abused. *Journal of Pediatric and Adolescent Gynecology* **20**: 163–172.

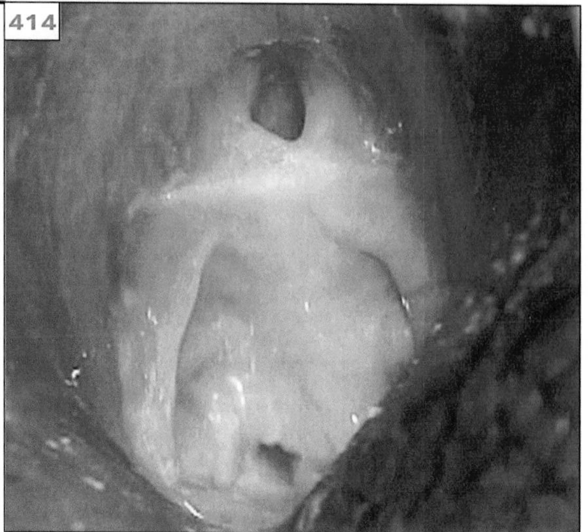

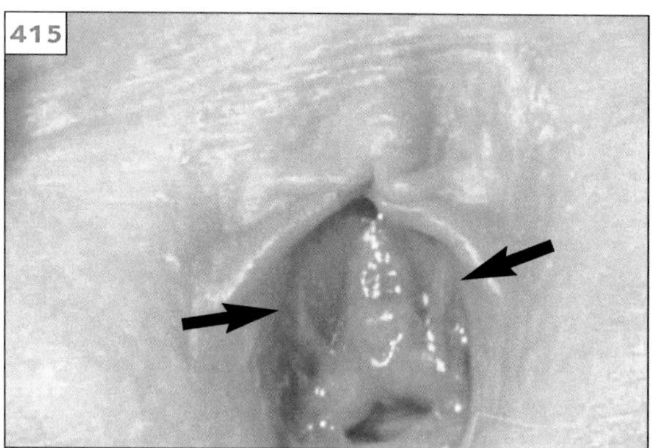

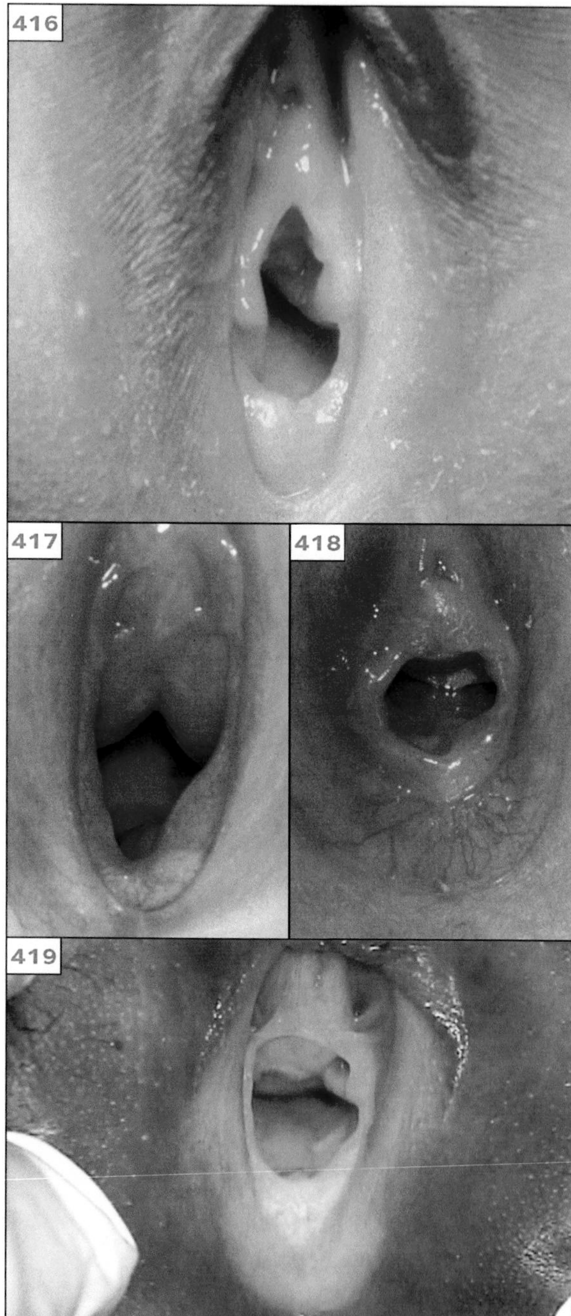

414 Urethral dilation. Widening of the urethra in this prepubertal female is an incidental finding.

415 Peri-urethral or vestibular bands (urethral). This child has bands of tissue (arrows) surrounding the urethra and connecting to the hymen and labial tissues. These should not be confused with scars.

416–419 This child has intravaginal columns at 3 and 9 o'clock (416). This child (417) has an intravaginal ridge inserting onto the hymen at 4 o'clock. This child (418) has a similar ridge, but the hymen is more erythematous and thickened. In this child (419), intravaginal ridges are visible with insertions into the hymen at 2 and 6 o'clock.

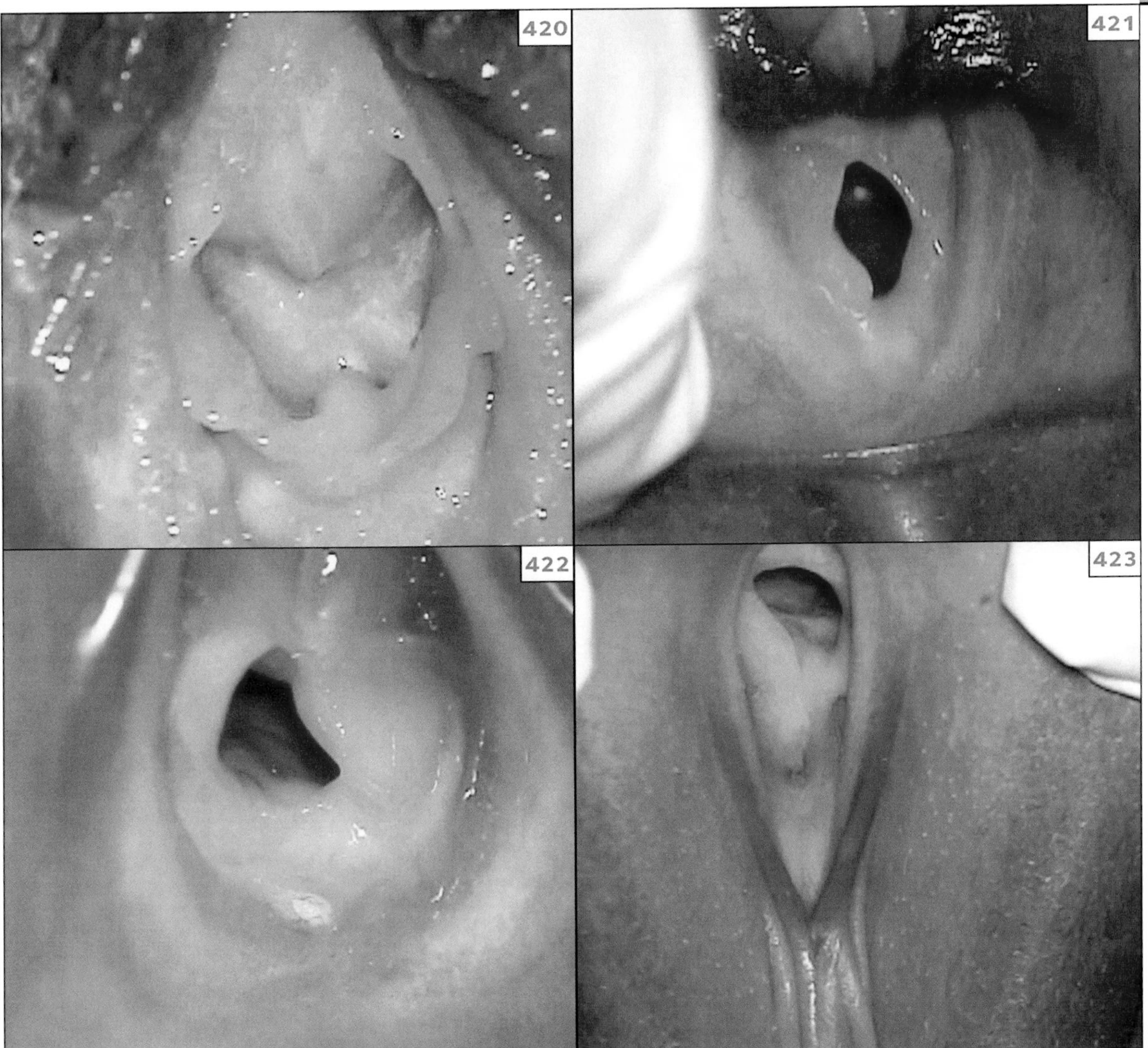

420–423 Hymenal bumps or mounds. Bumps are depicted in several locations, including 6 o'clock (420) and 8 o'clock (421, 422) with peri-urethral bands. This child has a potential bump in supine position that is actually not present when examined in the knee–chest position (423).

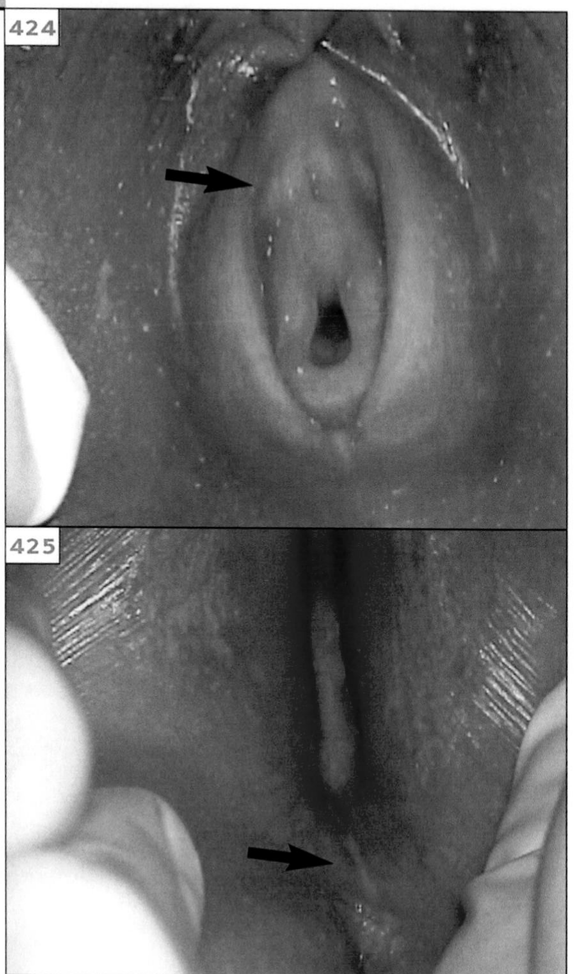

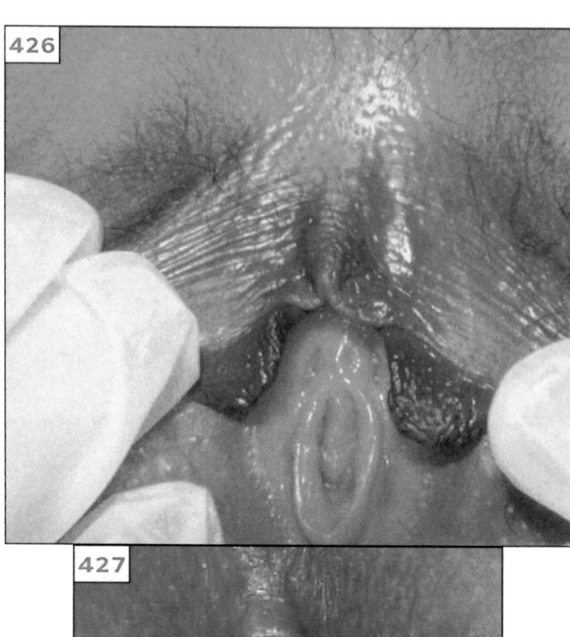

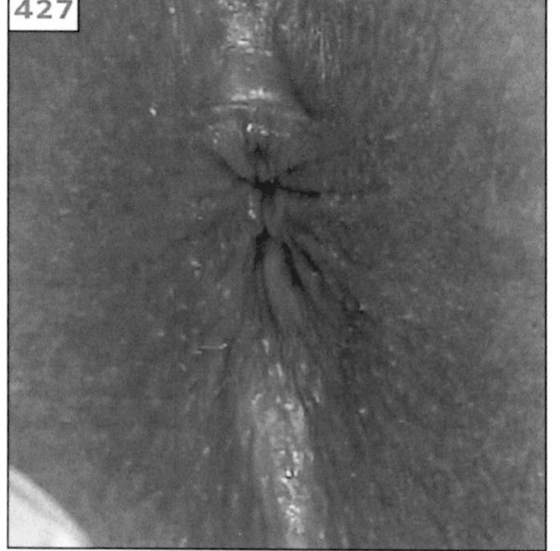

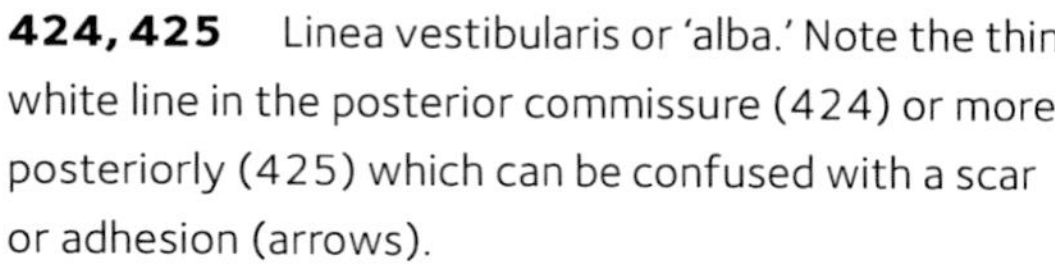

424, 425 Linea vestibularis or 'alba.' Note the thin white line in the posterior commissure (424) or more posteriorly (425) which can be confused with a scar or adhesion (arrows).

426, 427 Labial hyperpigmentation (426). This child (427) has peri-anal hyperpigmentation and flattening of the peri-anal muscles both anteriorly and posteriorly (diastasis ani).

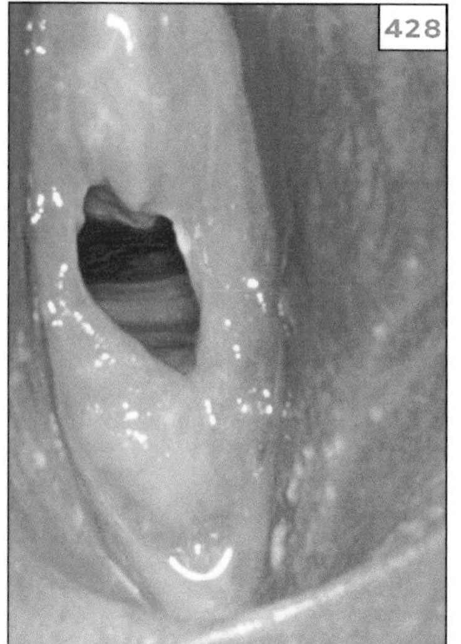

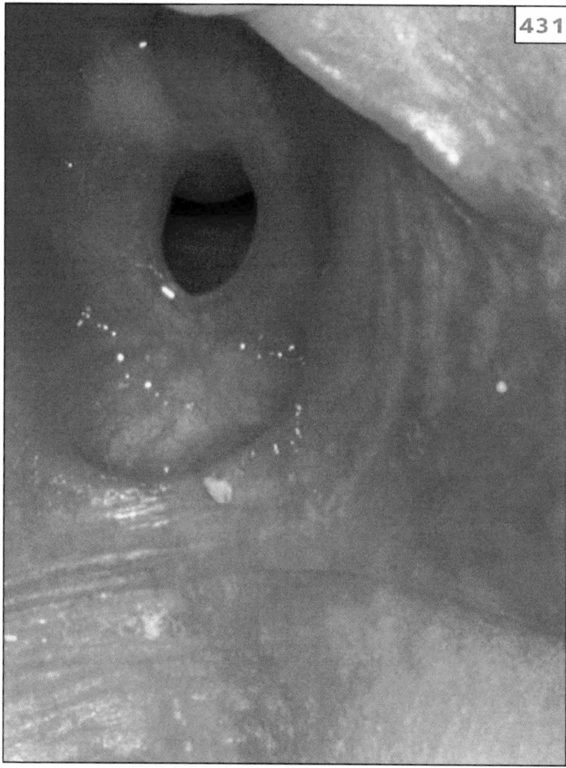

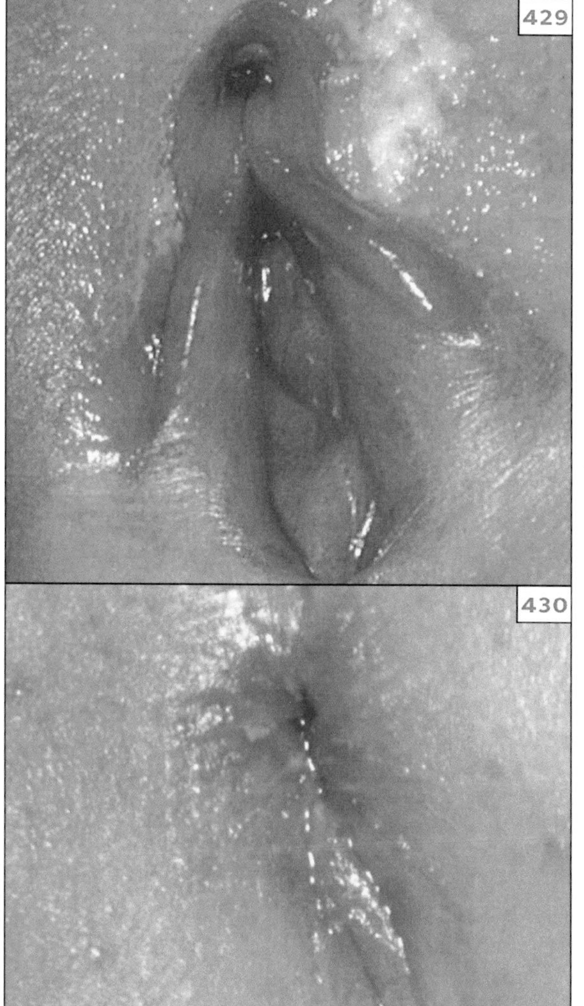

428–430 (428) Estrogenized hymen. This teenaged female shows tissue swelling, erythema, and scant white physiologic discharge associated with puberty. Redundant hymen (429, 430). This newborn female has marked evidence of maternal estrogen effect, with redundant hymenal (429) and peri-anal tissues (430).

431 Congenital hymeneal variants: annular. This child has hymenal tissue completely surrounding the genital opening.

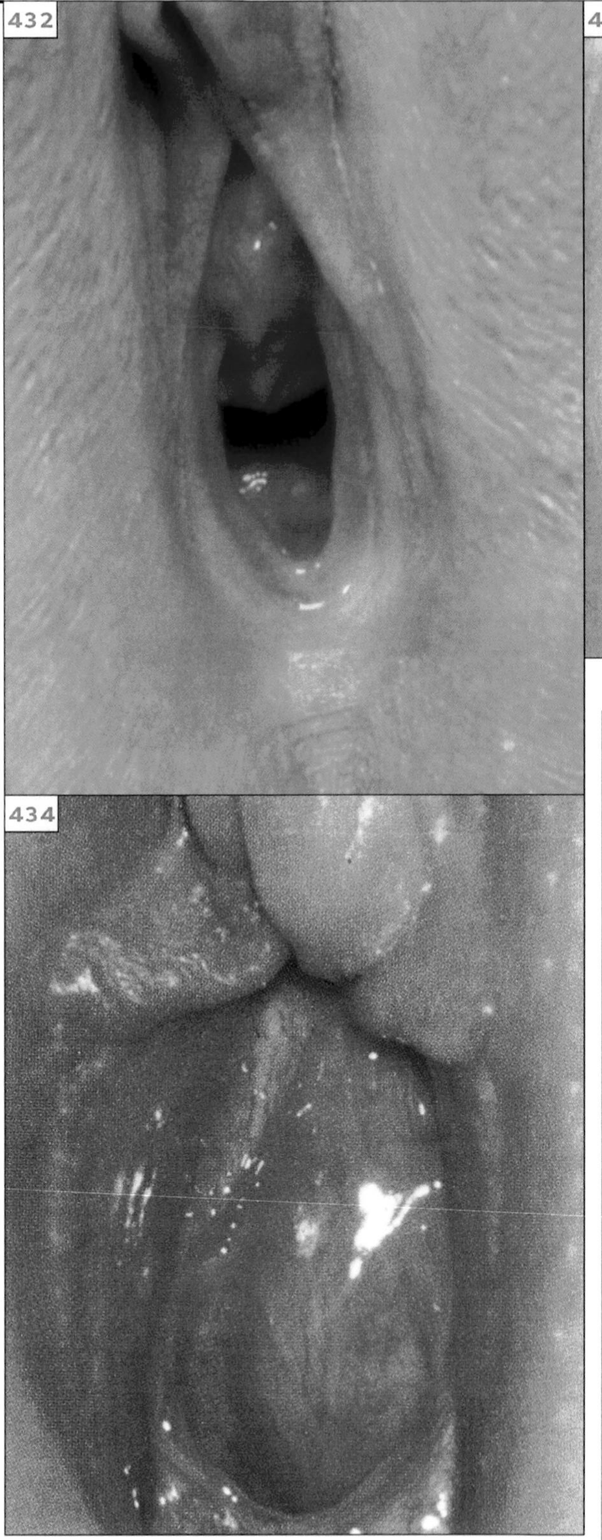

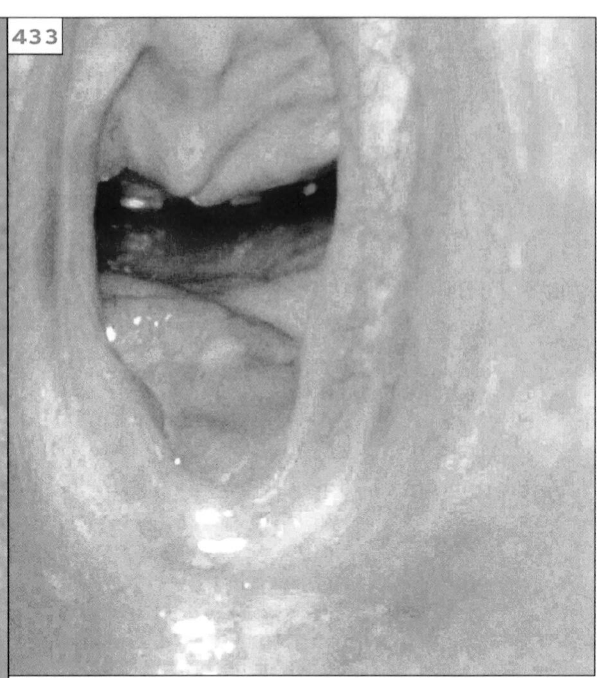

432–434 Crescentric hymen. This child has a classic crescentic hymen, here photographed using a hand-held close-up camera (432). The same child viewed with a colposcope with binocular lenses (433). This variant of a crescentic hymen, the posterior rim, shows absence of a significant part of the anterior hymen, but has smooth edges and otherwise normal hymenal tissue (434).

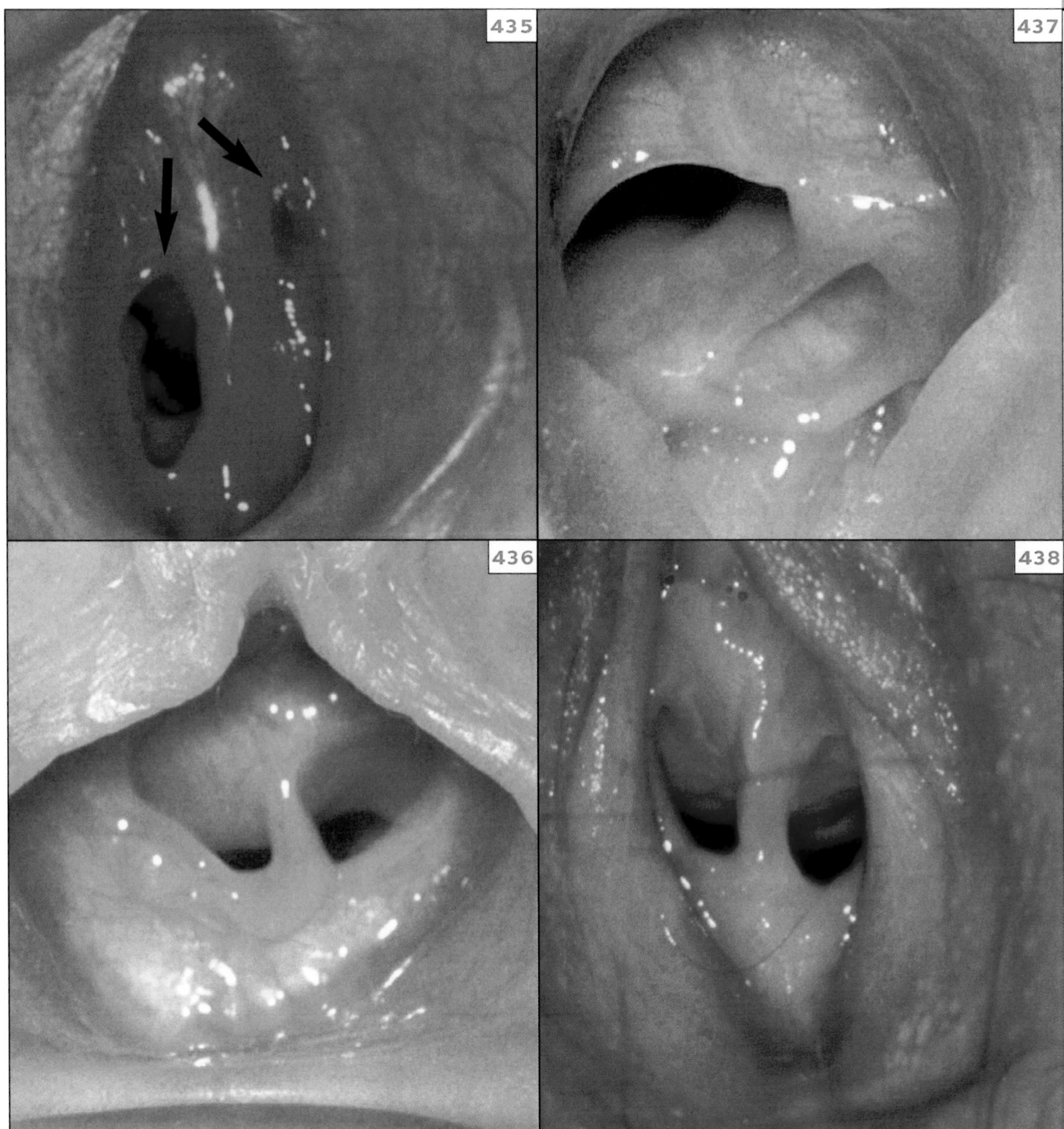

435–438 Septate hymen. This child has an intact hymenal septum with two distinct openings (435). This child has a more asymmetric septum, visualized in the supine (436) and knee–chest positions (437). This teenaged female has a persistent, thick septum without vaginal duplication (438). Reproduced with permission from the American Academy of Pediatrics (1998). *Visual Diagnosis of Child Sexual Abuse*. Author, Elk Grove Village, IL.

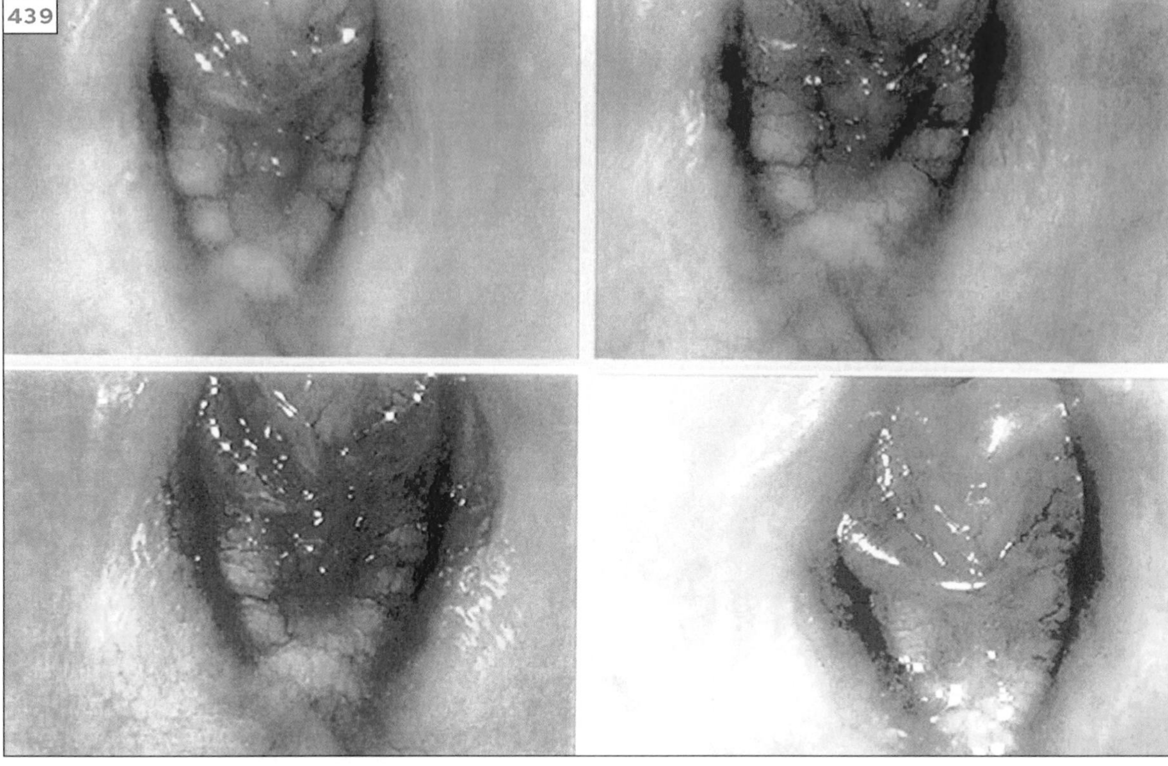

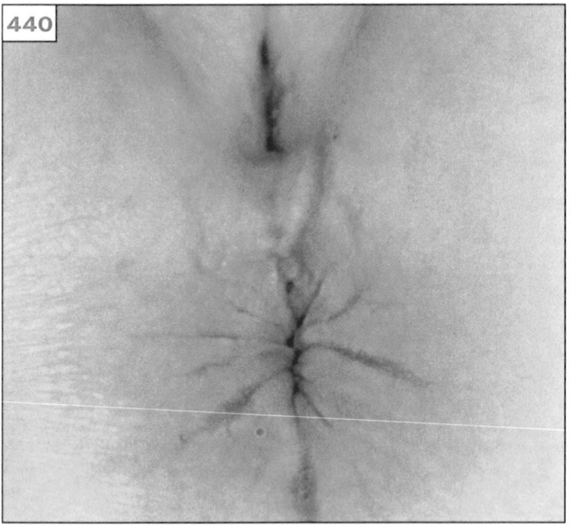

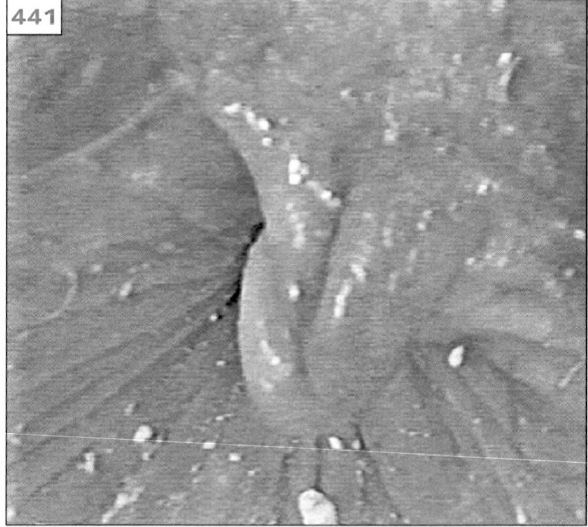

439 Imperforate hymen. These four views (one with green filter) show a thin, hymenal membrane covering the opening, with some erythema. This imperforate hymen shows no evidence of genital discharge or bleeding and may resolve spontaneously at puberty.

440 Anal fissures. This child with lichen sclerosis also has superficial peri-anal fissures.

441 Peri-anal skin tag. This child has a large tag without hemorrhoid because of chronic constipation. There is no underlying fissure or scar visible.

Other medical conditions

There are several medical conditions that, while not present at birth, have low or little association with trauma and are generally not thought to be indicative of sexual trauma (*Table 17*). Erythema of the vestibule, penis, scrotum, or peri-anal tissues (**442, 443**) and increased vascularity (**444**) generally reflect tissue irritation and inflammation associated with poor hygiene, chemical effects (urine, chlorine, stool, medications), self-manipulation, or nonsexual trauma. Vulvovaginal irritation is best classified as vulvitis (inflammation of the vulva usually from poor hygiene), vaginitis (inflammation of the vaginal mucosa with discharge usually from hormones or infection), or vulvovaginitis (a combination of both). These conditions are generally not related to sexual trauma unless a specific sexually transmitted infection can be identified. Yeast, for example, can cause significant swelling and inflammation, but monilial vulvovaginitis has no association with sexual trauma in prepubertal females (**445**). Peri-anal venous congestion or pooling (**446–448**) and flattened anal folds (**449**) are now considered to be findings which are normal or associated with constipation, and while they are often noted during examination, are not indicative of sexual abuse.

In prepubertal females, irritation, coupled with the relative thinness of tissues, can lead to friability of the posterior fourchette or commissure (450) and labial adhesions posteriorly, anteriorly, or both (451–456). Labial adhesions have been noted in 5–10% of nonabused females and are generally asymptomatic, although a small proportion of females may have urinary obstruction and vulvovaginitis when the genital opening is significantly (> 75%) reduced. Labial adhesions are usually identified as thin, symmetric fusion lines in the midline with little or no irregularity at the labial border. Labial adhesions may require treatment, and successful dehiscence is generally achieved with topical application of estrogen or steroid creams for limited periods (< 2 weeks). Most cases resolve spontaneously during puberty or with dehiscence during routine examination or activity, and only a few require manual or physical separation when urinary tract infection or significant physical symptoms are present. Sexual trauma may result in irregular labial fusion lines that deviate from the midline, but it is very difficult to differentiate sexual trauma versus nontraumatic causes of labial adhesion based on examination alone.

Genital bleeding in prepubertal females can be due to a variety of causes, many of which are nonsexual, such as infection, straddle injury, urethral prolapse, or labial adhesion. The urethra can spontaneously prolapse in a small number of females and this is generally of little clinical importance until urinary infection or bleeding is noted (**457, 458**). Little or no intervention is required in prepubertal females other than reassurance and improved hygiene. A specific prepubertal dermatologic condition of the vulvar and peri-anal tissues, called lichen sclerosis et atrophicus (LSA), has been associated with easy tissue breakdown and genital bleeding (**459–461**). This occurs because the epithelium is poorly supported. Symptoms can be improved with topical high potency steroid cream for short periods of time; estrogen cream can help for bothersome symptoms, but testosterone creams are no longer recommended for prepubertal females. This condition is also seen in postmenopausal females and is thought to be related to hormonal deficiency in the tissues. Also seen in males, LSA improves remarkably at puberty. Straddle injury (**462**) causes replicable patterns of labial bruising and/or laceration over bony prominences and at ligamentous support points, with crushing and stretching of tissue. These injuries can be positively identified during examination and are generally linked to a history of specific accidental trauma and no delay in seeking medical care.

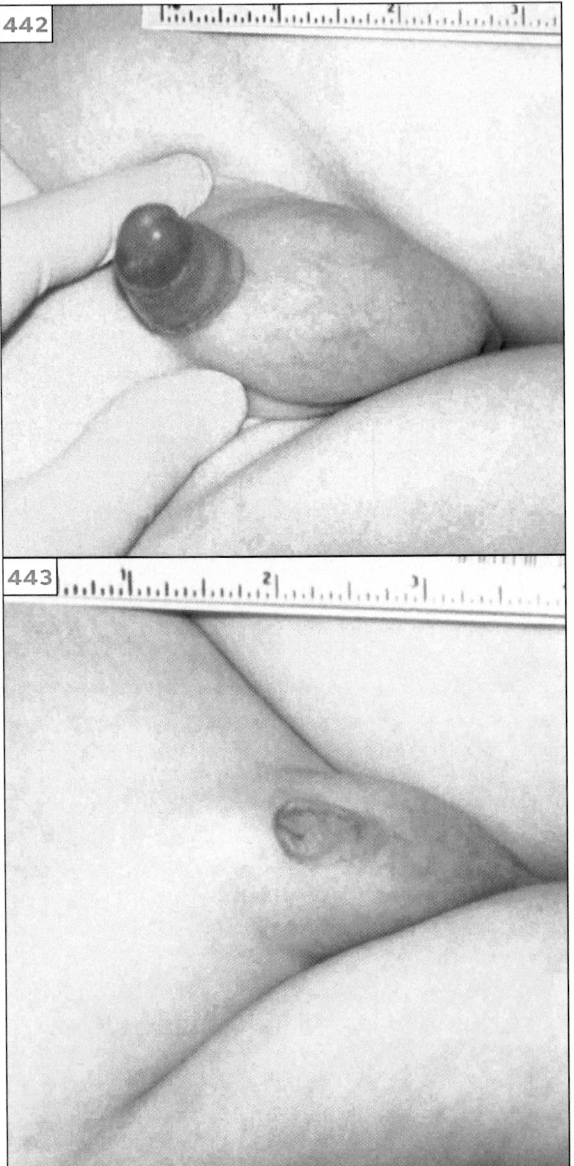

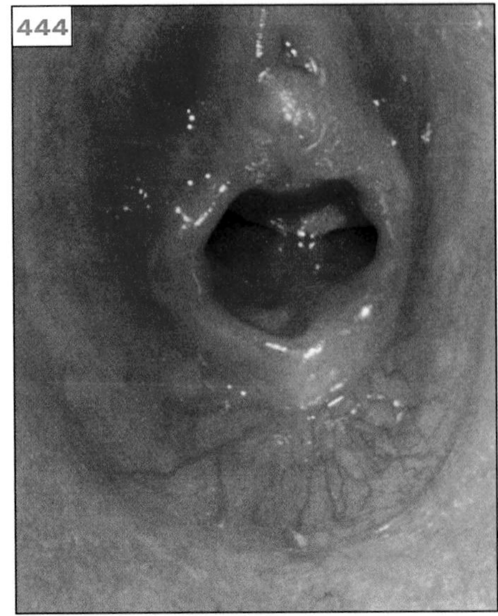

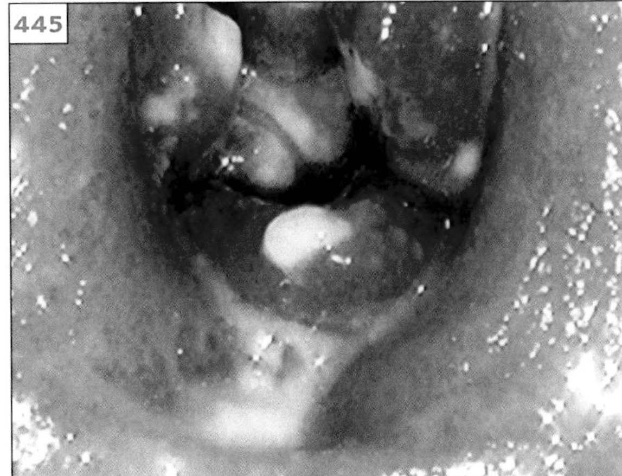

442, 443 This obese male was presented for care because of concerns of an 'absent' penis (443). With gentle manipulation, the penis was coaxed from its pubic fat pad (444). Erythema of the glans and shaft was likely related to poor hygiene and obese habitus.

444 Increased vascularity and thickening of the hymen.

445 Healed hymenal transection or complete cleft. This teenaged female has a healed complete hymenal cleft at 4 and 8 o'clock and monilial vulvovaginitis.

446–448 Venous congestion or pooling, peri-anal. This young male has marked venous pooling (446). Another child with central venous hypertension has labial erythema and perineal venous distension that was initially mischaracterized (447, 448).

449 Flattened anal folds. This young male alleged recurrent digital anal fondling and has flatted anal folds and erythema.

450 Friability of the posterior fourchette or commissure. This teenaged female has friability and easy tissue breakdown in the posterior commissure because of poor hygiene.

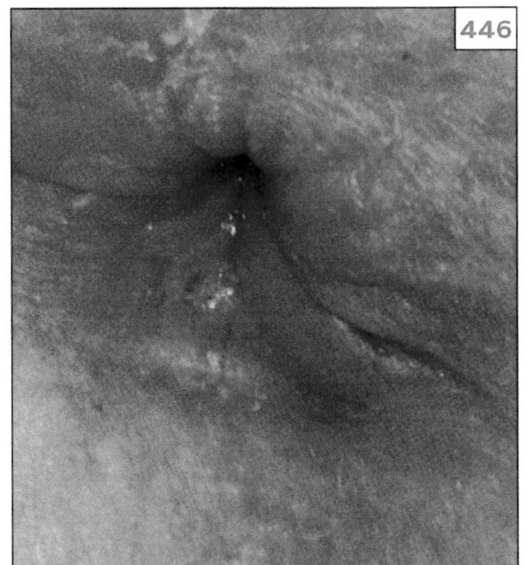
446

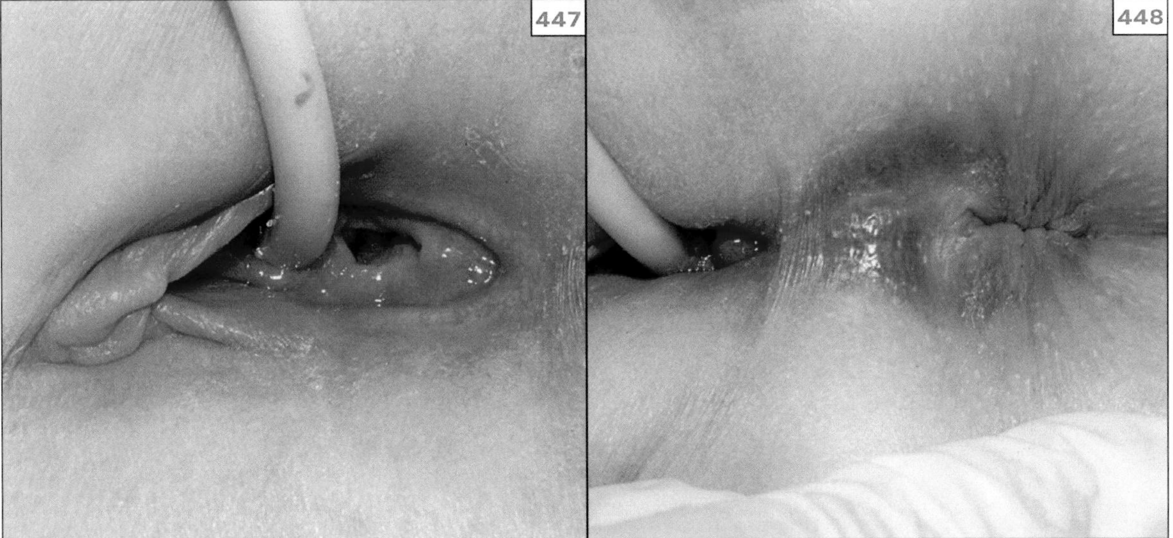
447
448

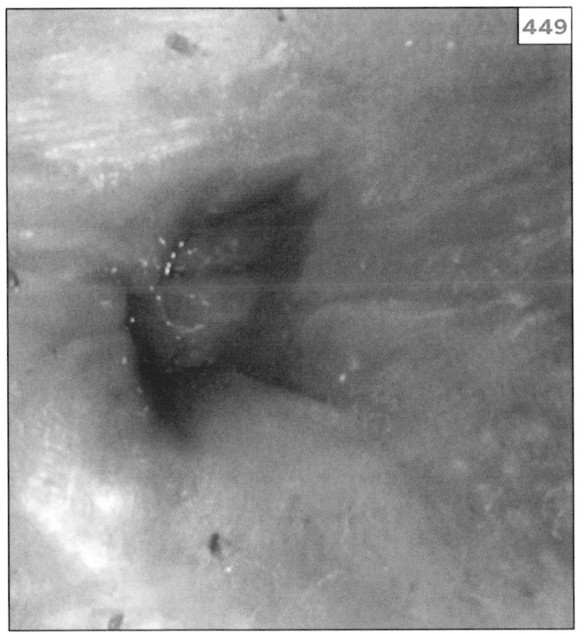
449

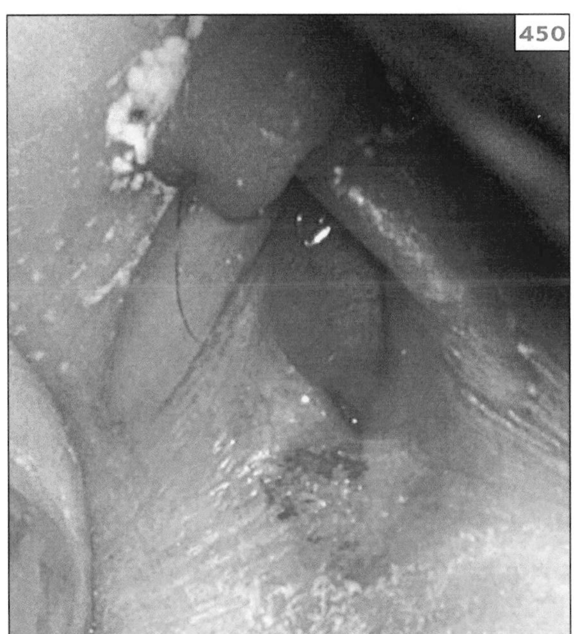
450

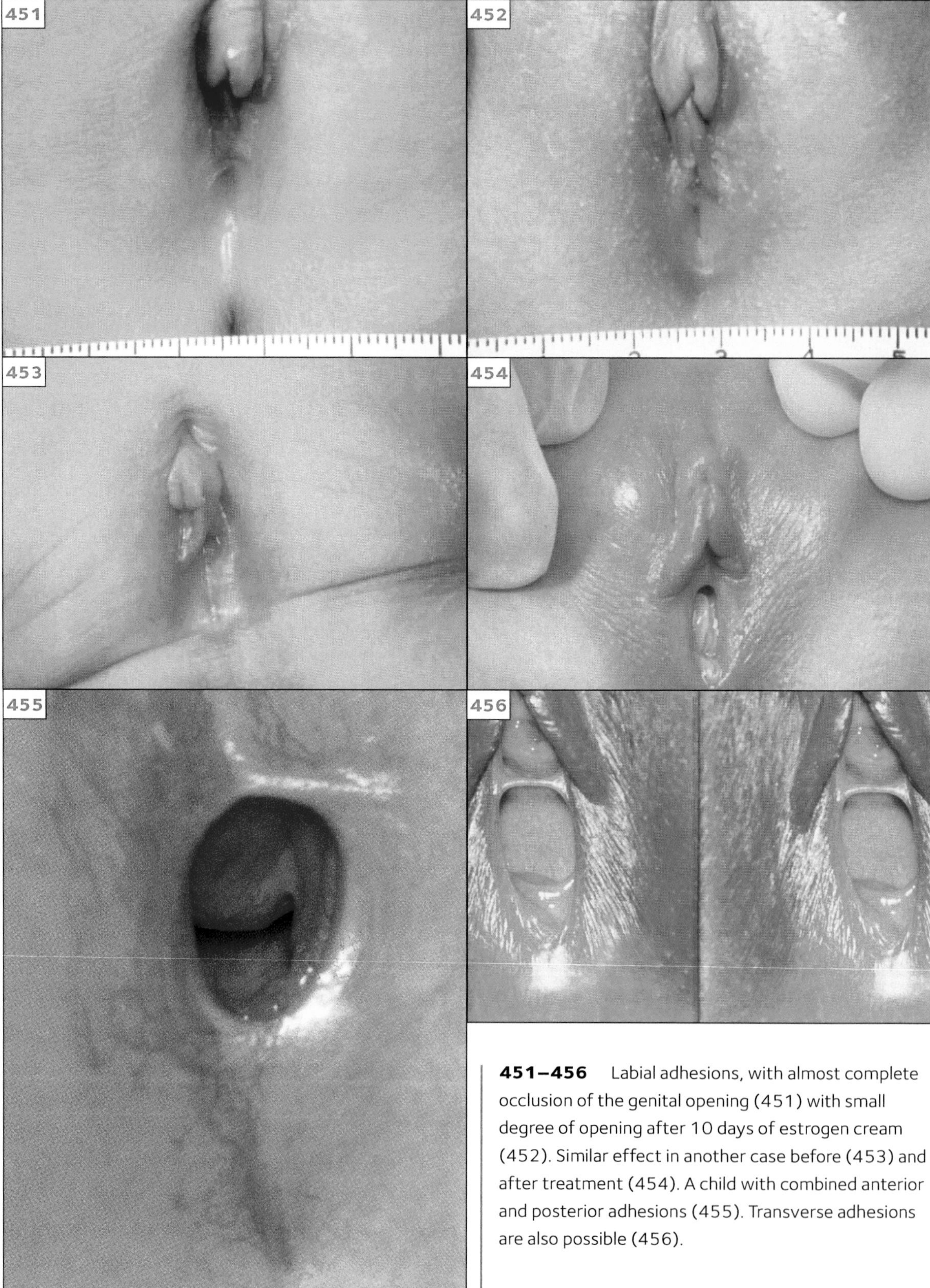

451–456 Labial adhesions, with almost complete occlusion of the genital opening (451) with small degree of opening after 10 days of estrogen cream (452). Similar effect in another case before (453) and after treatment (454). A child with combined anterior and posterior adhesions (455). Transverse adhesions are also possible (456).

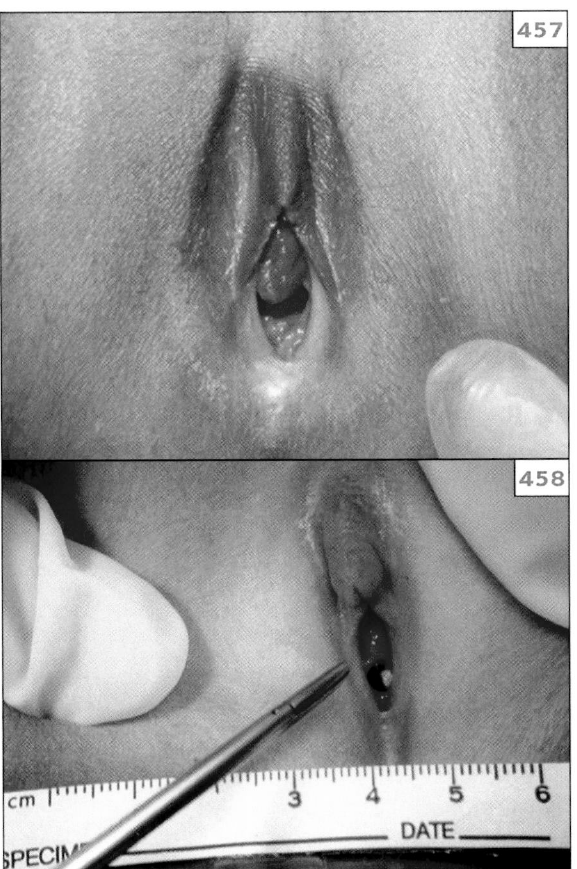

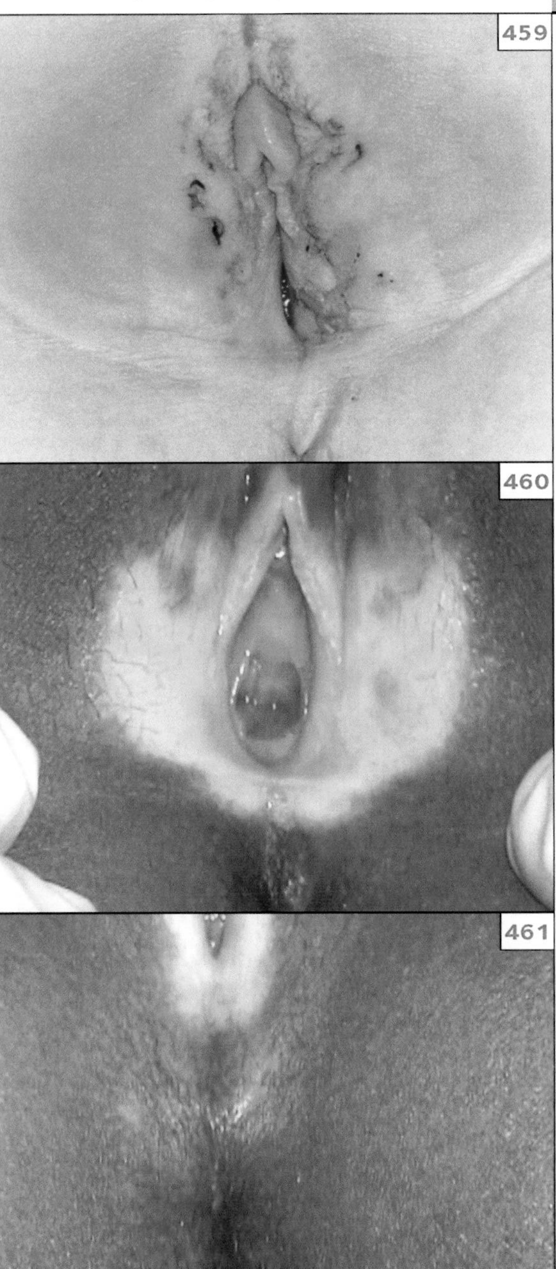

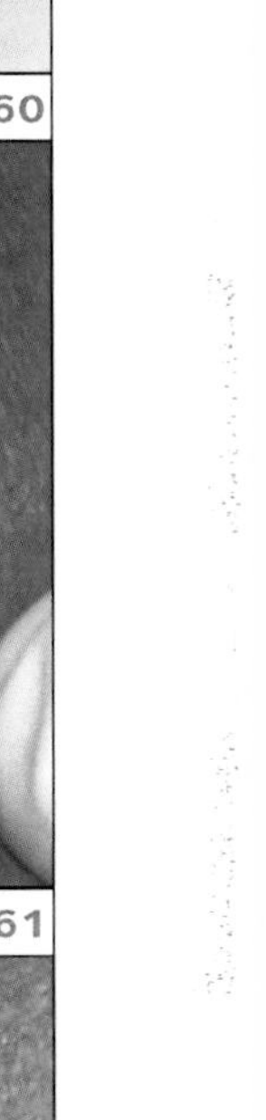

457, 458 This child (457) has prolapsed urethral mucosa that is easily distinguished from hymen tissue. There is no evidence of bleeding at this time. Another child has a vaginal foreign body (cotton) that was removed using the forceps depicted (458).

459–461 Lichen sclerosis et atrophicus. This young female has intra-epithelial bleeding and hypopigmentation on the labia (459). Another child (460) shows classic hypopigmentation with no anal involvement (461).

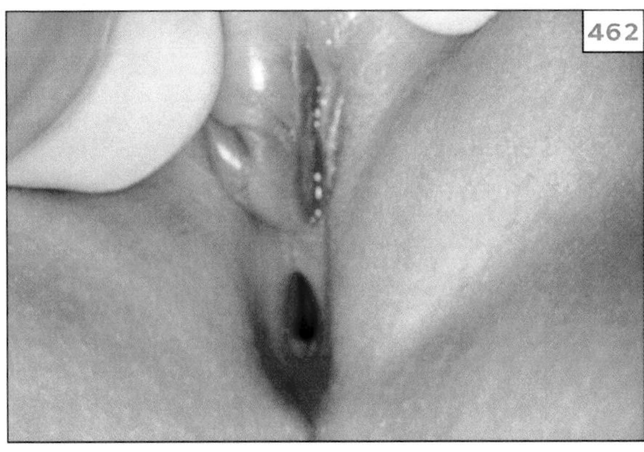

462 Straddle-type injury. This child had blunt genital trauma when her 80 lb (36 kg) dog jumped on her and landed on her vulva. There are acute interlabial lacerations on both the left and also the right sides of the clitoral hood. Note the incidental finding of labial adhesions unrelated to trauma. Reproduced with permission from the American Academy of Pediatrics (1998). *Visual Diagnosis of Child Sexual Abuse.* Author, Elk Grove Village, IL.

Indeterminate findings

There are several findings that are difficult to interpret because there are insufficient or conflicting research findings regarding their link to sexual trauma and abuse (*Table 17*). They may be found in abused children, but are also found in nonabused children, limiting their usefulness in helping to corroborate witness disclosure. For example, while previously thought to be indicative of trauma, deep hymenal notches or clefts in the posterior hymenal tissue are now considered difficult to interpret without knowledge of corresponding previous acute hymenal findings. In adolescents, deep or complete hymenal notches or clefts at 3 and 9 o'clock (**463**) have been described as a normal finding. It is exceedingly difficult to determine the width of hymenal tissue accurately, even with colposcopy and diagnostic quality images, and posterior hymen width less than 1 mm wide (**464**) has been labeled an indeterminate finding. Genital or peri-anal wart-like lesions (**465–474**), or vesicular lesions or ulcers (**475–478**) are also difficult to interpret unless positive identification can be made of human papillomavirus (HPV) or herpes simplex virus (HSV). Steps should be taken to differentiate HPV from molluscum contagiosum, syphilis, and other known wart-like lesions. Ulcerative lesions resembling HSV have been seen with varicella, Behçet's disease, and other conditions. While the size of the anal opening and dilation to less than 2 cm are not thought to be concerning, marked, immediate anal dilation to greater than 2 cm (**479, 480**) without anesthesia, neurologic disease, or stool present in the rectum are concerning, but not specific, for anal trauma. Other injuries to the buttocks (**481**) are concerning to the extent that they are near the genitals but can occur after accidental injuries.

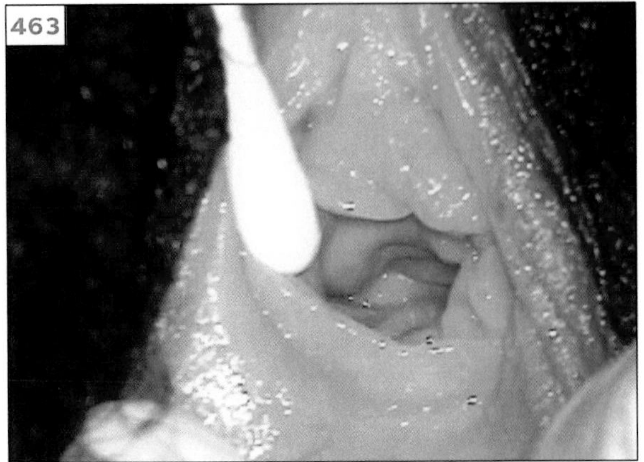

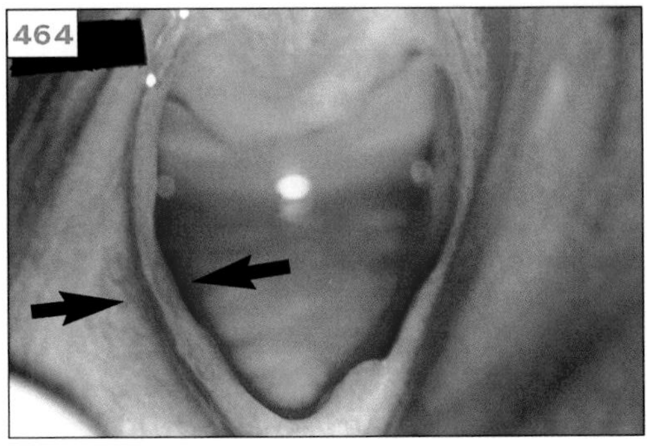

463 Deep or complete hymenal notches or clefts, 3 and 9 o'clock, often seen in adolescents.

464 Hymen less that 1 mm wide, posterior. This teenaged female has a crescentic hymen with thinning of the entire posterior hymen. Arrows display width of the hymen. Reproduced with permission from the American Academy of Pediatrics (1998). *Visual Diagnosis of Child Sexual Abuse*. Author, Elk Grove Village, IL.

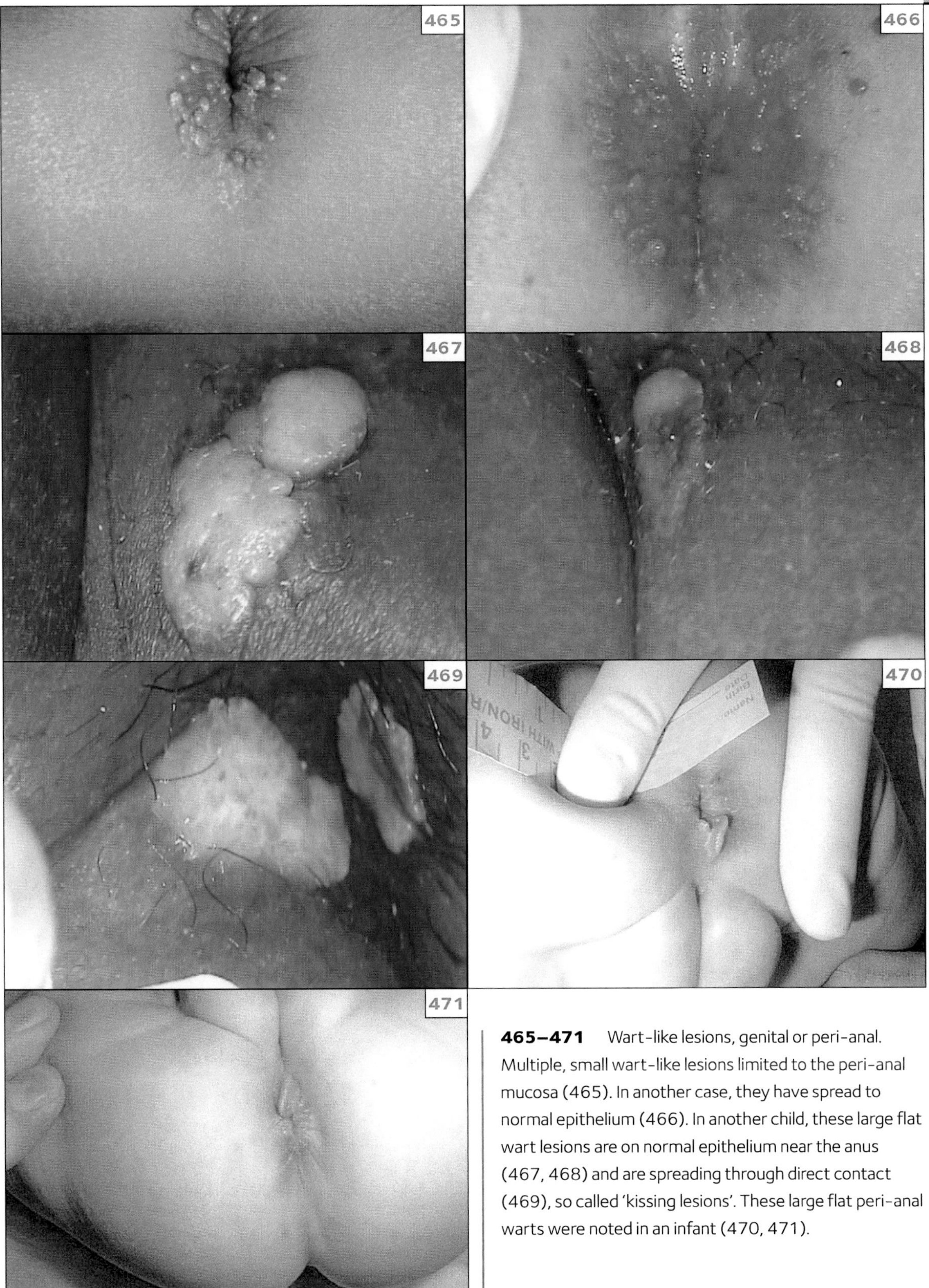

465–471 Wart-like lesions, genital or peri-anal. Multiple, small wart-like lesions limited to the peri-anal mucosa (465). In another case, they have spread to normal epithelium (466). In another child, these large flat wart lesions are on normal epithelium near the anus (467, 468) and are spreading through direct contact (469), so called 'kissing lesions'. These large flat peri-anal warts were noted in an infant (470, 471).

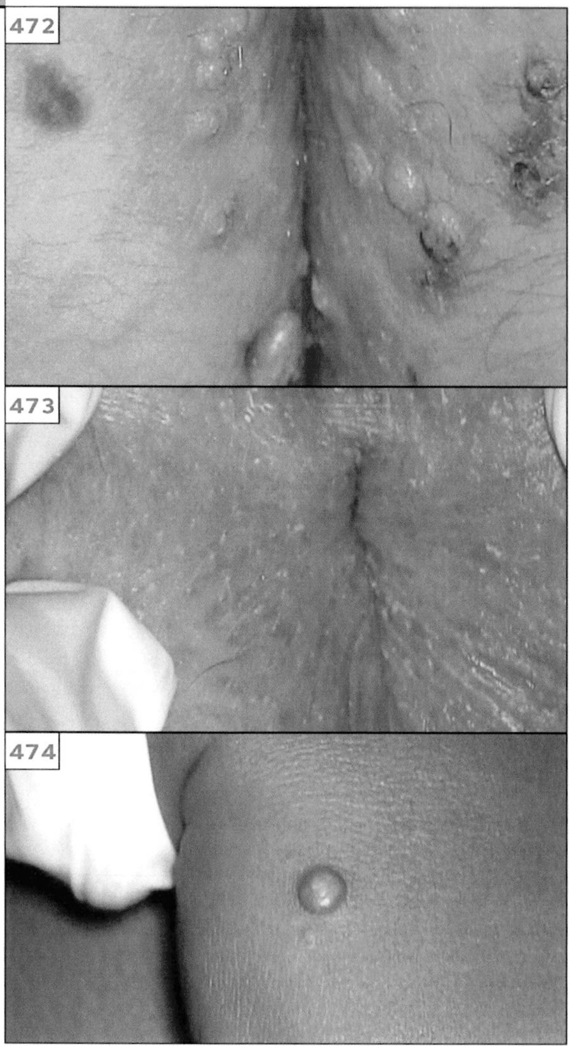

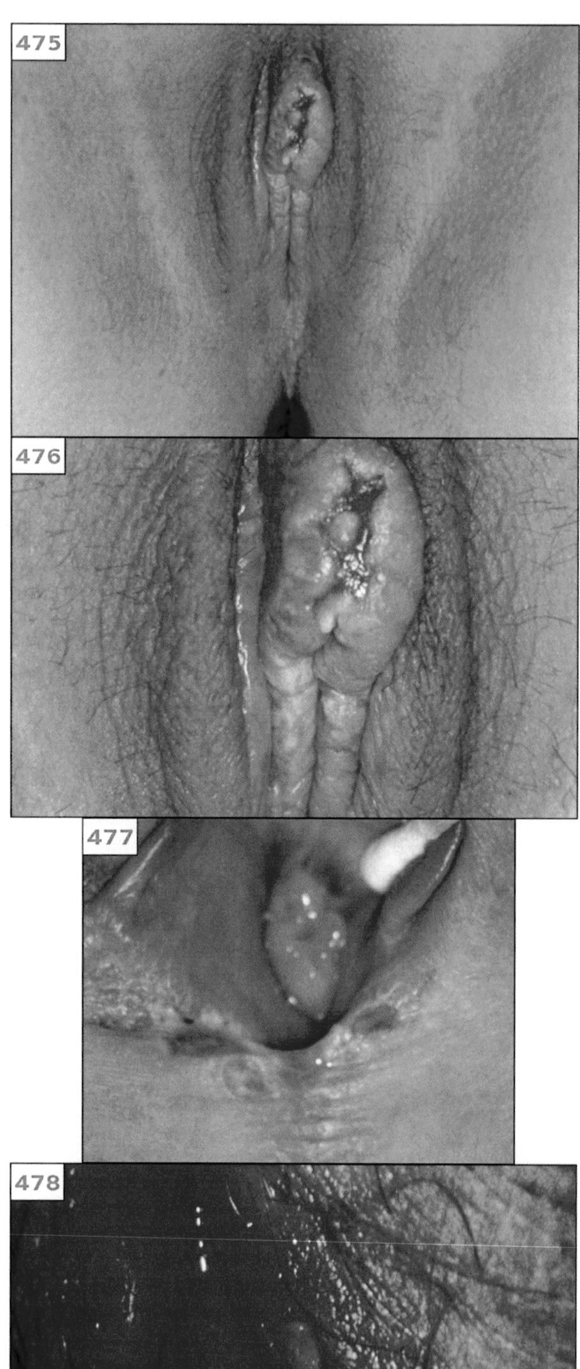

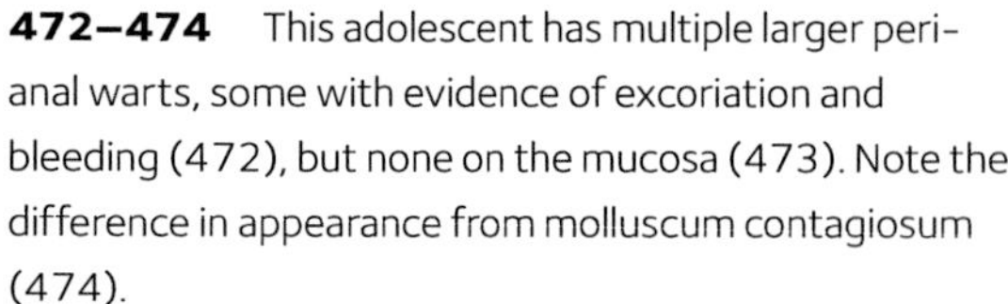

472–474 This adolescent has multiple larger peri-anal warts, some with evidence of excoriation and bleeding (472), but none on the mucosa (473). Note the difference in appearance from molluscum contagiosum (474).

475–478 Vesicular lesions or ulcers, genital or anal. This child has ulcerated lesions over the anterior labia and clitoral hood (475, 476). Here, the lesions cover the posterior labia and commissure (477). A single ulcer (arrow) is seen on the left labium in this teenaged female with Behçet's disease (478). Reproduced with permission from the American Academy of Pediatrics (1998). *Visual Diagnosis of Child Sexual Abuse*. Author, Elk Grove Village, IL.

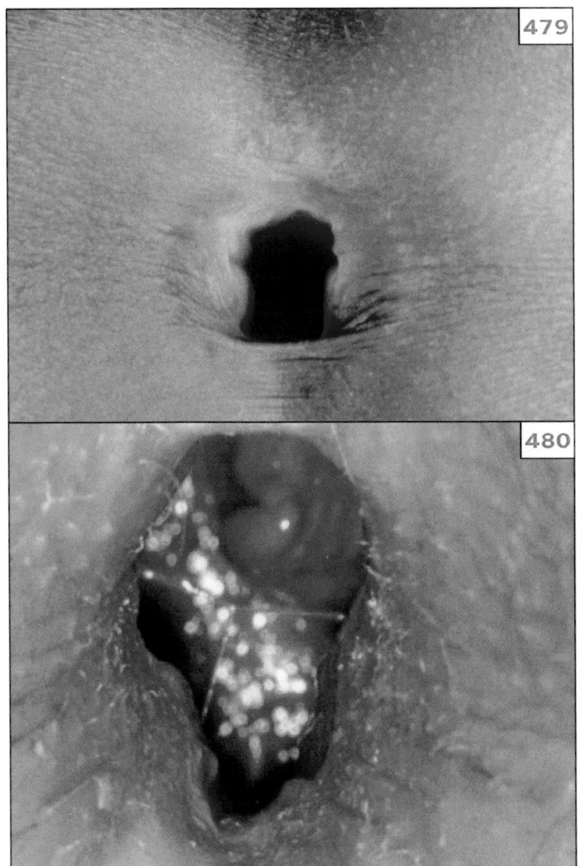

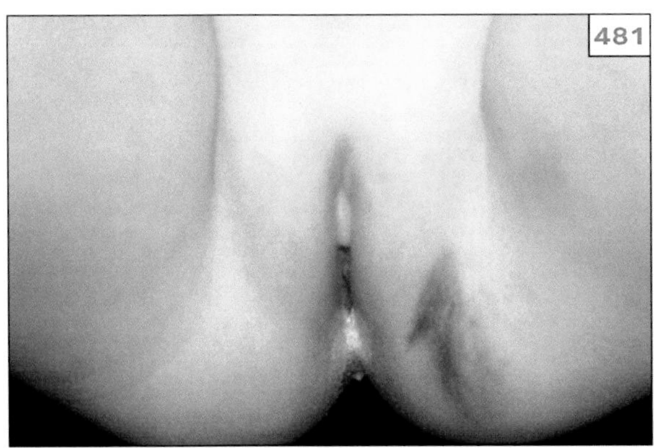

479, 480 Marked, immediate anal dilation to greater than 2 cm without mucosal changes or stool present (479) and with stool present (480). 479 is reproduced with permission from the American Academy of Pediatrics (1998). *Visual Diagnosis of Child Sexual Abuse.* Author, Elk Grove Village, IL.

481 Acute laceration or bruising of labia. This 2-year-old fell on a bed rail and was noted to have a bruise at the labial-gluteal crease over the ischium.

Findings diagnostic of trauma and/or sexual contact

Findings diagnostic for sexual abuse are generally now thought to be limited to acute laceration or bruising of labia, penis, scrotum, peri-anal tissues, or perineum (*Table 17*) (**481–496**). As an isolated finding, fresh laceration of the posterior fourchette or commissure not involving the hymen (**497–500**) is also diagnostic of trauma. Acute hymenal ecchymosis, bruising, or laceration (**501**), when isolated, is thought to be indicative of sexual trauma, but rare case reports with unusual circumstances have been noted with accidental rather than sexual trauma. Similar interpretations have been noted with peri-anal lacerations extending deep to the external sphincter (**487–491**).

A second category of diagnostic findings involves identifying residua of healed sexual trauma. These can be difficult to interpret when the location, depth, and exact nature of the acute injury are not available for comparison. A healed hymenal transection or complete cleft extending to the vaginal wall in the posterior of the hymen is thought to indicate sexual trauma (**445**). Complete or partial healing of such injuries has been noted, but a remaining complete cleft indicates that the primary injury was deep and completely through the hymen[5]. A scar of the posterior fourchette or fossa navicularis or missing segment of the posterior hymen (**502, 503**) are also diagnostic for prior sexual trauma. After associated swelling, bruising and inflammation heal, it is exceedingly difficult to associate these findings with the exact number and timing of traumatic events based on examination alone. This also applies to peri-anal scars.

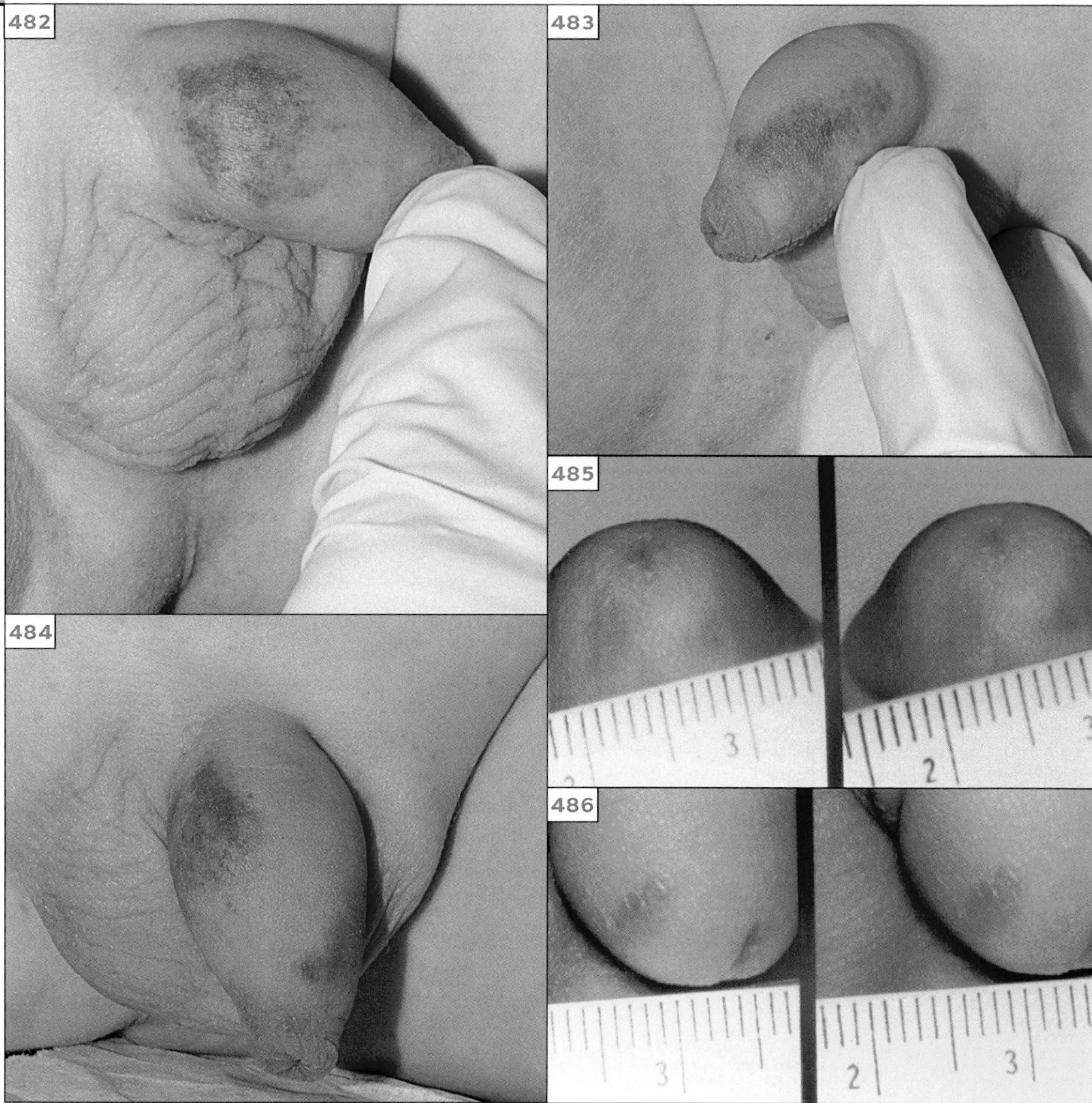

482–486 Acute laceration or bruising of the penis, with symmetric bruises on both sides of shaft, suggesting squeezing (482–484), on both sides of the glans penis (485, 486).

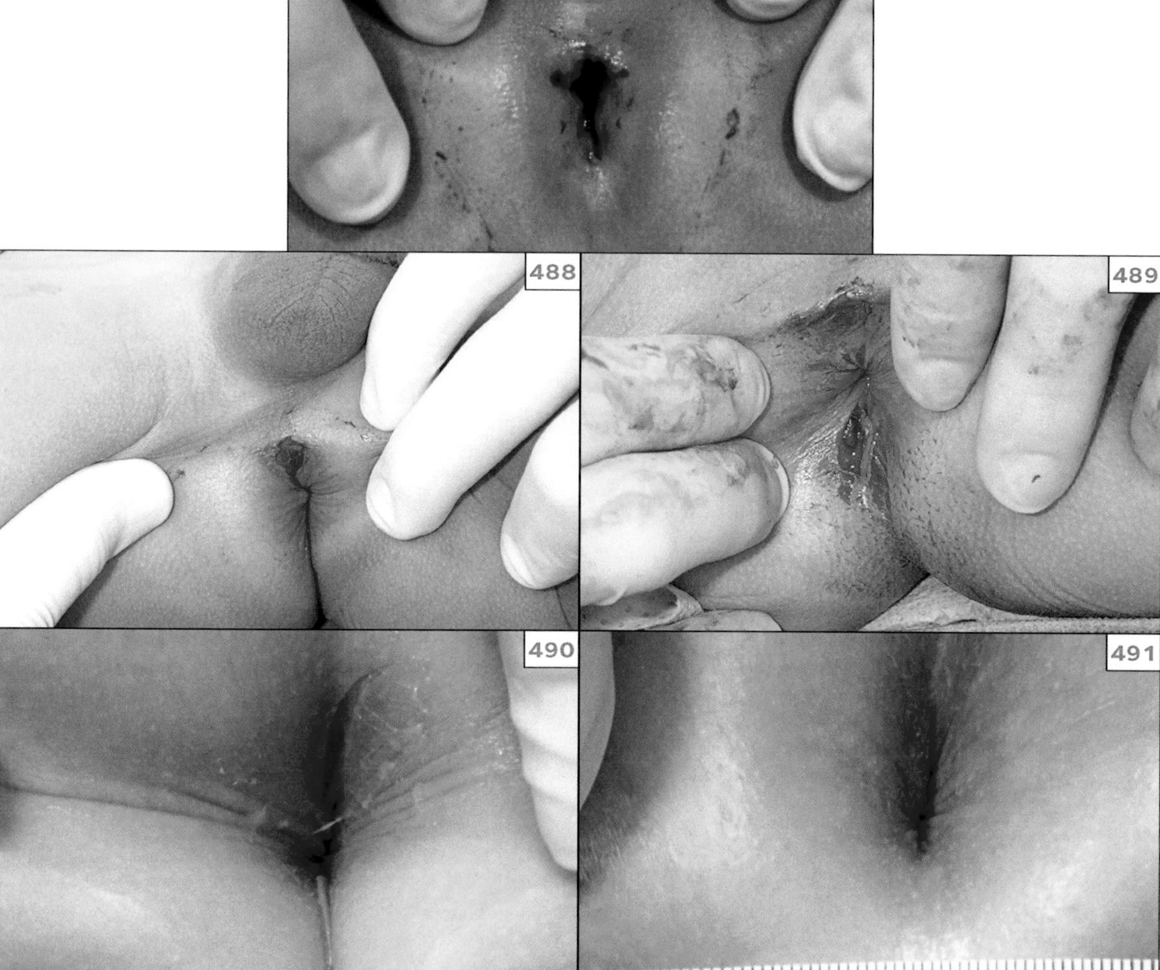

487–491 Acute laceration or bruising of the peri-anal tissues. This deceased child had peri-anal tears and laceration with forensic trace evidence identified (487). Another child has a superficial peri-anal abrasion (488) and another laceration better visualized with gluteal separation (489). This teenaged female had a superficial laceration, seen 2 days after sexual assault (490). Ten days later, there was almost complete healing with little visible residua (491). Genetic material was recovered from the anus.

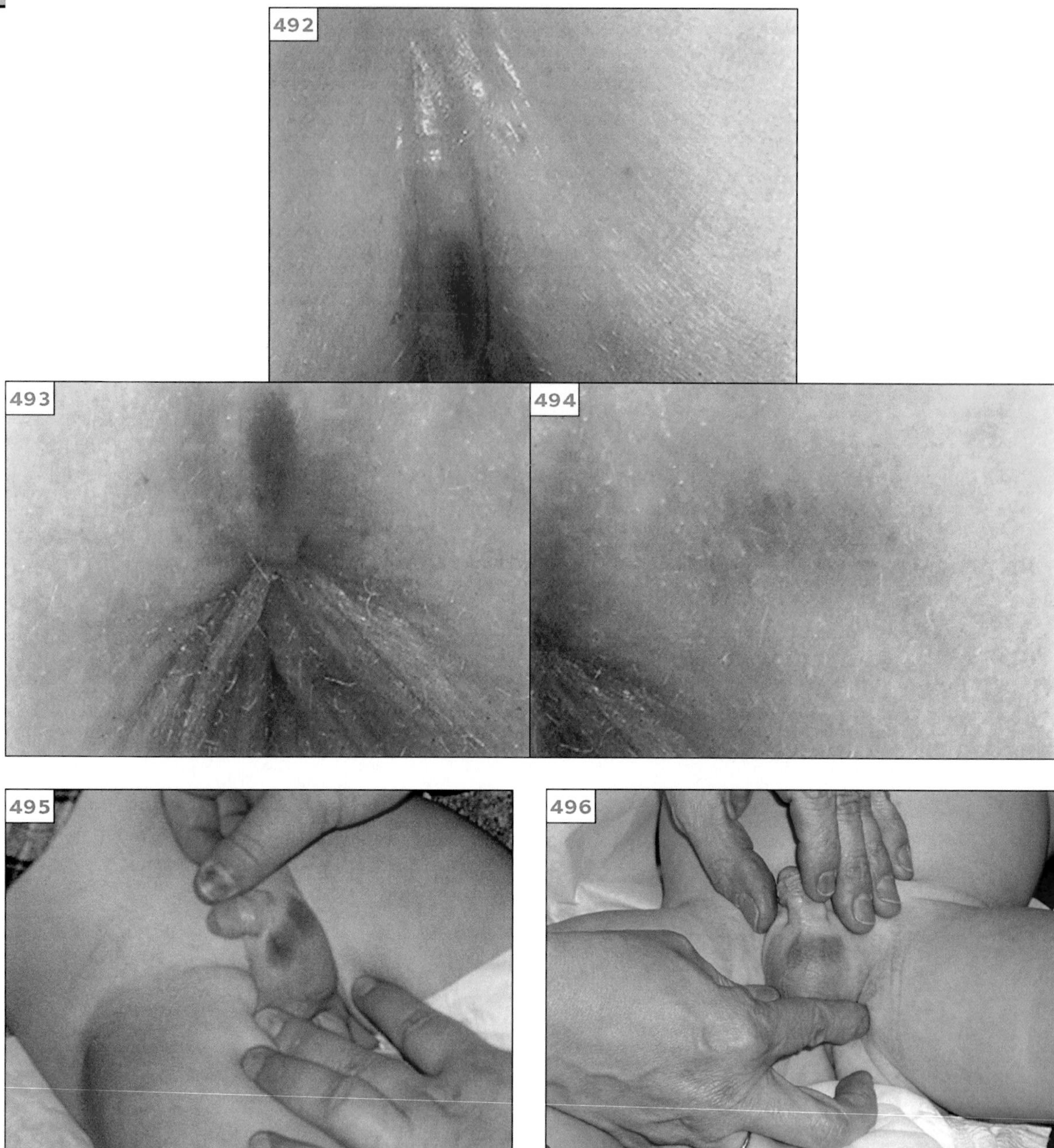

492–494 This child had acute peri-anal bruising in the midline (492–494), as well as on the inner thigh (494).

495, 496 Acute bruising of the scrotum noted in this male, suggesting squeezing or pinching. (Hands shown are the mother's.)

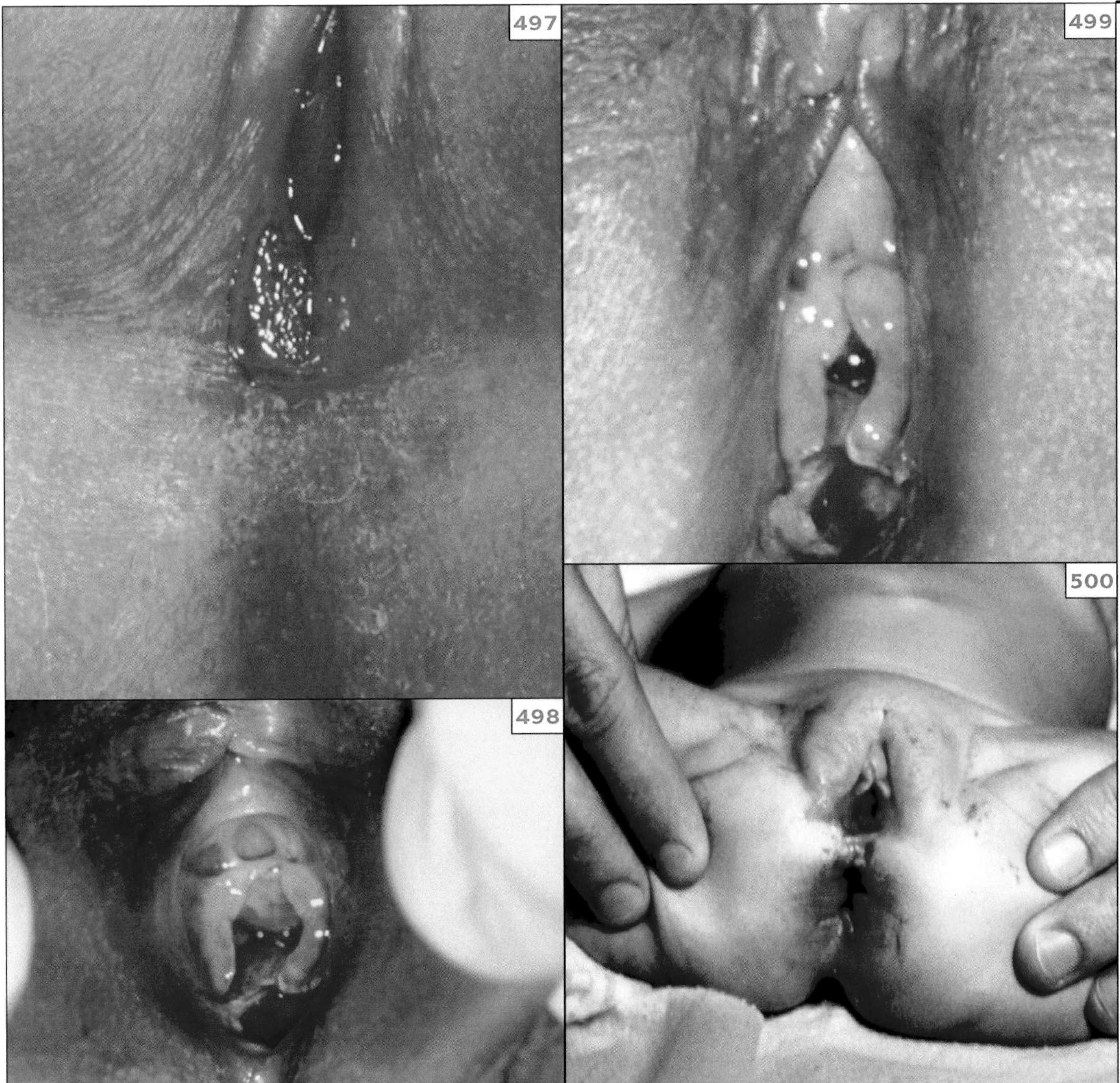

497–500 Fresh laceration of the posterior fourchette or commissure, with superficial tearing at the posterior commissure (497), with additional tearing through the hymen (498, 499). An infant (500) with acute vaginal and peri-anal tears requiring surgical repair after a 14-year-old admitted to sexually assaulting her while intoxicated. Reproduced with permission from the American Academy of Pediatrics (1998). *Visual Diagnosis of Child Sexual Abuse*. Author, Elk Grove Village, IL.

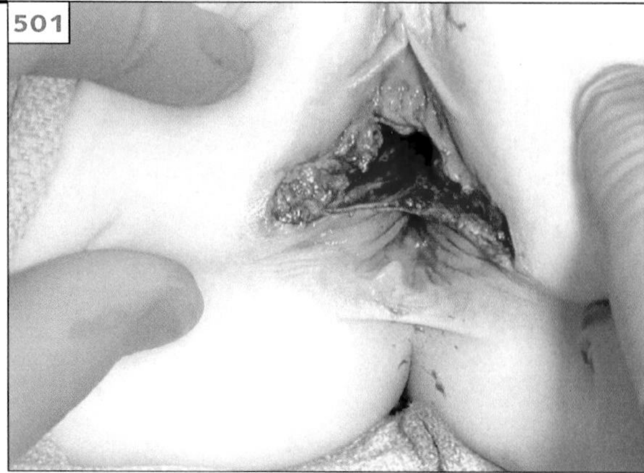

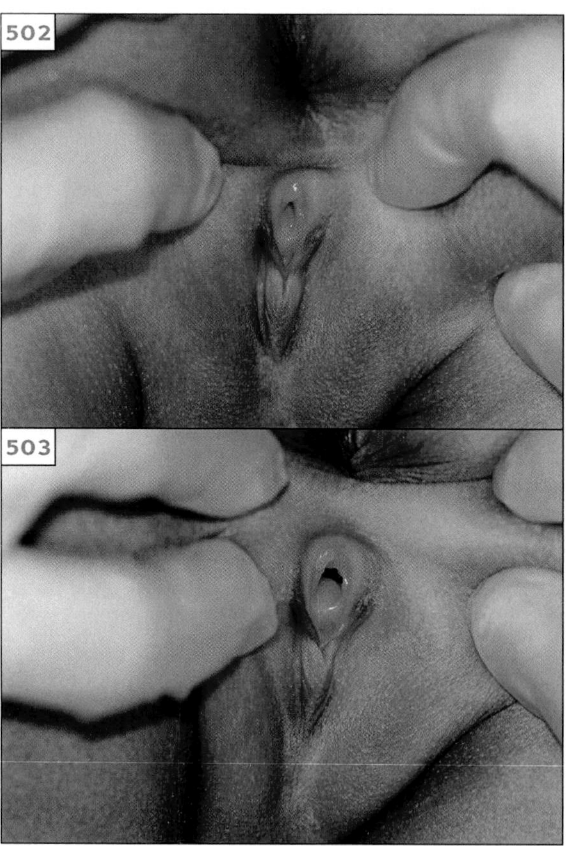

501 Laceration, hymen, acute. This photograph of a young female depicts complete tearing through the perineal body, posterior fourchette, and hymen (501). In the operating room, almost complete vaginal tearing from sexual assault was also noted, although the rectal mucosa was spared. This child has a laceration of the posterior fourchette, hymen, and some vaginal tissue.

502, 503 Missing segment of the hymen, posterior. This child, examined in the knee–chest position, has a cleft in the posterior hymen that is variably seen depending on the degree of labial traction during examination.

Laboratory evaluation

Finding a sexually transmitted infection (STI) in a child who discloses a history of sexual abuse or exhibits behavior worrisome for sexual abuse is supportive evidence of the diagnosis. STIs are uncommonly identified in sexually abused children, as only approximately 5% of victims of childhood sexual assault may acquire an STI from their victimization[10]. The likelihood that an STI represents evidence of sexual abuse is dependent on the specific infection, age of the child, and other factors[11]. There are several gynecologic conditions that can be confused with STI[12]. Some sexually transmitted infections can be vertically passed to a child during routine childbirth. Some pathogens, most notably human papillomavirus (HPV, genital warts) and *Chlamydia trachomatis* (**504**), may have long incubation periods before overt symptoms (warts or discharge) appear[13]. The limit of incubation for perinatally acquired genital warts and *Chlamydia* is unknown, but is generally regarded to be less than 3–5 years. Human papillomavirus and herpes simplex virus (**505, 506**) can also be spread sexually or nonsexually by auto-inoculation or innocent transmission by close household contacts. Although all sexually transmitted infections raise suspicion of sexual abuse, acquired gonorrhea and syphilis are most diagnostic, whether or not there are other corroborating concerns.

In general, the diagnostic test of choice for identification of sexually transmitted infections is culture. Newer tests, such as nucleic acid amplification tests (NAAT) for gonorrhea and *Chlamydia*, are acceptable methods for postmenarchal adolescent and adult victims, but data regarding use in prepubertal children are limited, and they may have unacceptable numbers of false-positive tests[11]. Since most children without symptoms of an STI (vaginal or penile discharge or pain) are unlikely to have a sexually transmitted infection, universal screening for STIs is not necessary, but instead should be selectively performed based on the history and other factors (*Table 18*)[10,14]. When an STI is identified, there are certain criteria for reporting to child protective services.[10] Gonorrhea, syphilis, HIV and *Chlamydia* are all diagnostic and should be reported to Child Protection Services, if not perinatally or hospital acquired. *Trichomonas* is highly suspicious, and condyloma and herpes are suspicious for abuse and should also be reported.

Rates of recovery of forensic evidence from prepubertal children evaluated for sexual assault vary from 6 to 42%[7,15,16]. This has been associated with the age of the child, the gender and age of the offender, and the nature of the sexual abuse. Unlike adult rape, the likelihood of obtaining forensic evidence directly from the prepubertal child's body diminishes greatly after the first 24 hours following an assault. After 24 hours, there may still be a possibility of recovering forensic evidence, but the evidence usually comes from the analysis of bed linen, the child's clothing, or the child's underwear present at the time of the assault. The likelihood of recovering any physical evidence diminishes further after the first 72 hours. In one study, recovery of forensic evidence within 72 hours of assault was best predicted by positive examination findings (such as hymenal transections, abrasions, or bruises, vaginal lacerations, or anal lacerations or bruises), victim age older than 10 years and having reached puberty, and older offenders (age greater than 15 years)[7]. In order to increase the yield of forensic evidence, the Wood's lamp has had limited use for identifying areas of the body with potential traces of semen[17], but several bodily fluids fluoresce, as do food, creams, and other potential confounders (**507**).

In addition to STIs and forensic trace evidence, the physician should consider laboratory and radiologic testing for sexual abuse victims who can have injuries distant from the genitalia, including bruises (Chapter 2, Bruises), bite marks (Chapter 8, Recognition of child abuse by dentists, health care professionals, and law enforcement), abdominal injuries (Chapter 9, Abusive abdominal trauma), and fractures (Chapter 5, Imaging child abuse)[18].

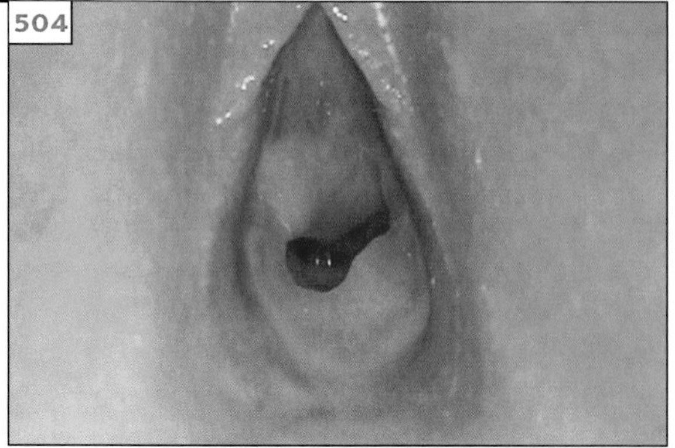

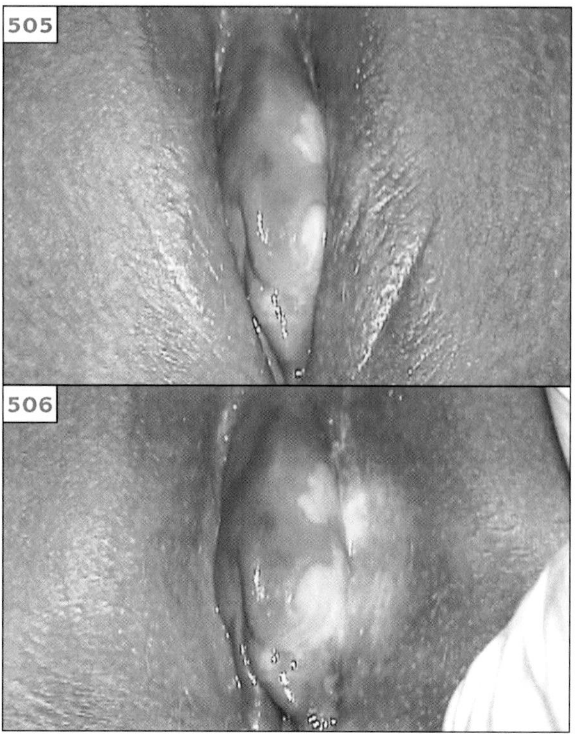

504 Moderately swollen hymen with thin, creamy discharge in a child who was culture positive for *Chlamydia trachomatis*.

505, 506 Genital ulcerations from Herpes simplex virus over the clitoral hood and labia minora. 506 shows lesions with gentle separation.

Table 18 **Indications for STI testing**[10]
Any child with a documented STI or signs or symptoms of an STI or an infection that can be sexually transmitted, such as vaginal discharge or pain, genital itching or odor, urinary symptoms, or genital ulcers or lesions
Any child whose suspected assailant is known to have an STI or be at high risk for STIs
Any child with a sibling, another child, or adult in the household or child's immediate environment who is known to have an STI
Physical evidence of genital, oral, or anal penetration
Any child or parent who requests testing
Any child who is post-menarchal (has started having menstrual periods)

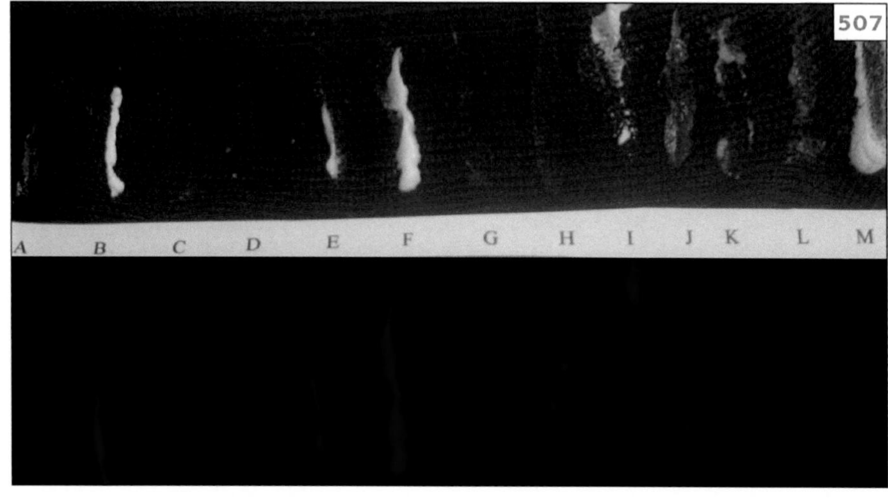

507 The upper panel depicts several body fluids, common creams and food materials and their fluorescence under a Wood's lamp in the lower panel. Semen (H) has a speckled appearance and fluoresces less brightly than other materials.

Teaching points

- Ultimately, in most cases of suspected sexual abuse, a physician will encounter an examination with normal or nonspecific anatomical features of the genitals and anus.
- There are relatively few findings diagnostic of sexual abuse without a corresponding disclosure.
- The reasons for a nondiagnostic examination in suspected victims of sexual abuse are several. The anal and hymenal tissues heal extremely quickly, and findings may disappear within days of an assault.
- Sexually transmitted infections are uncommonly identified in sexually abused children and recovery of semen from a child's body is unlikely after the first 24 hours following an assault.
- Physicians should be knowledgeable about the variety of normal and nonspecific physical findings and the appropriate use of STI and forensic evidence testing to best evaluate children with suspected child sexual abuse.

Chapter 11

CHILD MALTREATMENT FATALITIES

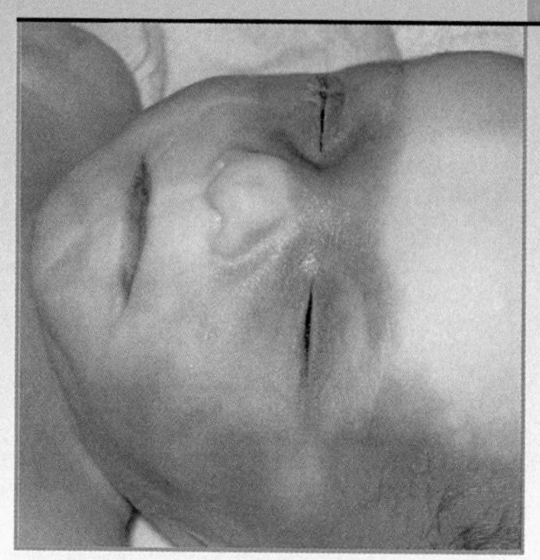

Carl J. Schmidt MD, MPH

Forensic pathology is thought of as a specialty far removed from clinical practice, but relies on the same informational framework as clinical medicine. The clinical history is the information gathered from the scene of death. The autopsy is analogous to the physical examination. It uses antemortem laboratory results if available, but commonly relies on postmortem body fluid testing. The diagnostic impression is the cause of death. There is an additional term, the manner of death, which is used to categorize the context in which the death occurred. This chapter describes mainly deaths that occur in the context of accident or homicide.

Introduction

It can be argued that there are few truly accidental deaths, since many, if not most pediatric accidents, after careful review of the events leading up to them, are the result of neglect. Many of those incidents of neglect are not willful, but rather the result of ignorance or lack of common sense. Conversely, willful neglect constitutes homicide.

Because of the often conflicting stories or simply lack of information that accompanies a child's death, forensic pathology relies on patterns of injury and their distribution to arrive at a cause of death. The lack of a pattern of injury can be equally informative. The descriptions of injuries are among the most important aspects of the practice of forensic pathology, because their comparison with the story of how they arose is key to determining whether it is true or not.

Sudden infant death

It is easy to cause the death of an infant without leaving a pattern of injury. Most sudden infant deaths result in autopsies with no findings, including many that are homicides[1,2]. More thorough scene investigation and increased understanding of the circumstances in which infants are found dead have also resulted in a diagnostic shift away from sudden infant death syndrome (SIDS), where by definition there is no pattern of injury, to a cause of death that more accurately reflects how the infant was found[3–5]. Hence, asphyxia and its variants are being used more frequently to certify an infant's death, depending on how an infant was found. In many instances, especially where the infant was sharing a sleeping surface with an adult, the cause of death is simply certified as unknown rather than as SIDS, but this depends on the certifier, and individual practices vary[6–8].

In the absence of a pattern of injury, the answer to a more accurate certification of death lies in scene investigation and re-enactment of how the infant was placed to sleep and, most important, how the infant was found. This can be carried out with a doll. Documentation of the infant's health history, including the maternal obstetrical history, is part of this investigation. There are efforts in the United States to standardize infant death investigation. The Sudden Unexpected Infant Death Investigation (SUIDI) form is one of the results of these efforts and is especially useful in those jurisdictions that do not see many cases.

It is now clear that unsafe sleeping practices are responsible for many cases that used to be considered idiopathic, or SIDS, and are probably the most common reasons for sudden infant death[3,9–11]. These patterns of unsafe sleep are identified with re-enactment of the scene with a doll. Perhaps the most common form of unsafe sleep is placing an infant in bed with an adult. Sometimes the infant is placed between two adults, and there are examples of situations where there were three or more people, usually a mix of children and adults, sharing a mattress on a floor. A deeply sleeping adult may place an extremity on top of an infant, or push the infant away, preventing excursion of the chest by the offending extremity or by wedging the infant into the space between a bed and a wall. Many people fear their infant will be cold, so they place many blankets on top of the infant, sometimes covering its face. **508** demonstrates how an adult placed an infant to sleep next to him on a soft mattress. During deep sleep, the adult lay on top of the infant, resulting in asphyxia. **509** shows the re-enactment of an infant who was held by an adult while sitting on a couch. The adult fell asleep; the infant rolled over to the adult's side, and was compressed by the adult's thigh against the armrest. **510** shows an analogous event, except that the infant was pushed by a deeply sleeping adult into the space between the bed and the wall, compressing the infant's chest.

Infants are frequently placed on soft bedding. **511** shows the re-enactment of an infant found with its head pressed against soft bedding in an adult bed. Similar findings are seen in cribs and bassinets where the infant is placed on soft bedding, or where objects such as soft animals are placed along with the infant. There is reason to think that some infants are unable to shift their head position and maintain a clear airway with softer sleep surfaces[12].

We have found that most adults are truthful regarding the circumstances in which they find a dead infant. Sometimes, however, they are not and it can be difficult to determine what happened. One of the most important findings on an infant's body is the lividity pattern, because this is the only

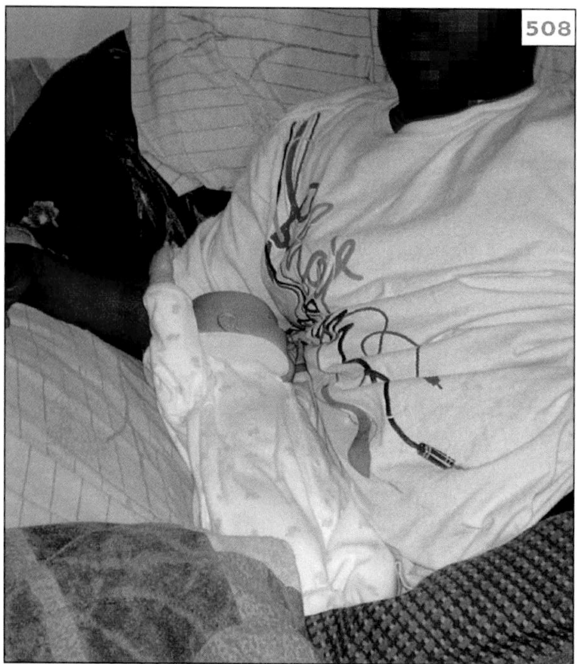

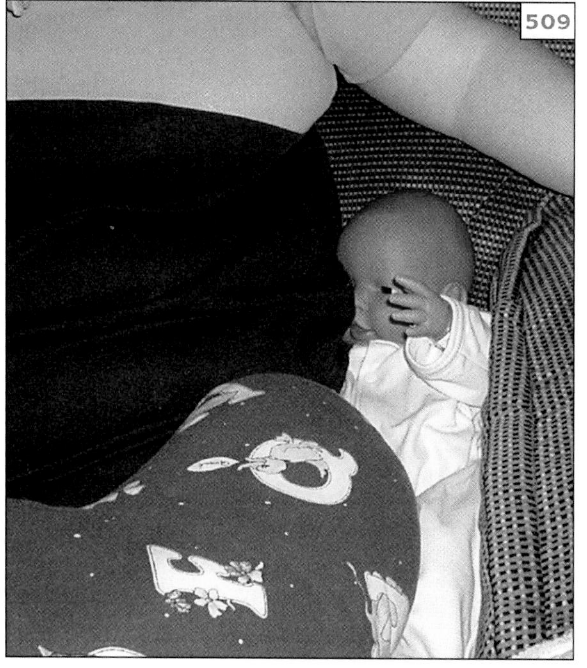

508 Re-enactment of infant placed next to an adult on a soft mattress. The weight of the adult has created a trough in the mattress against whose side the infant's chest and airway were compromised.

509 Infant compressed by adult against the armrest of a sofa. The armrest provided a firm surface for compression of the infant's chest.

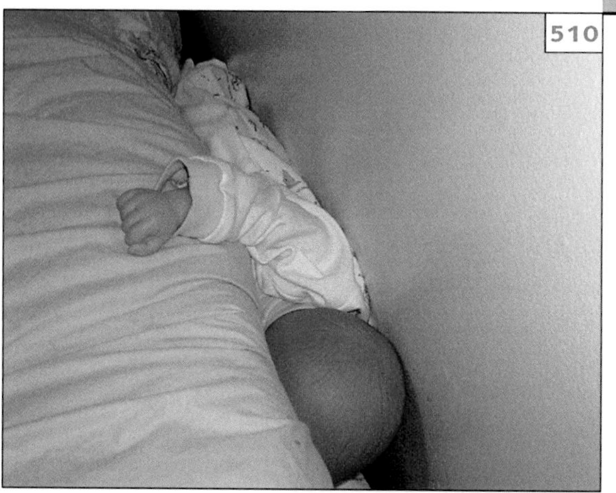

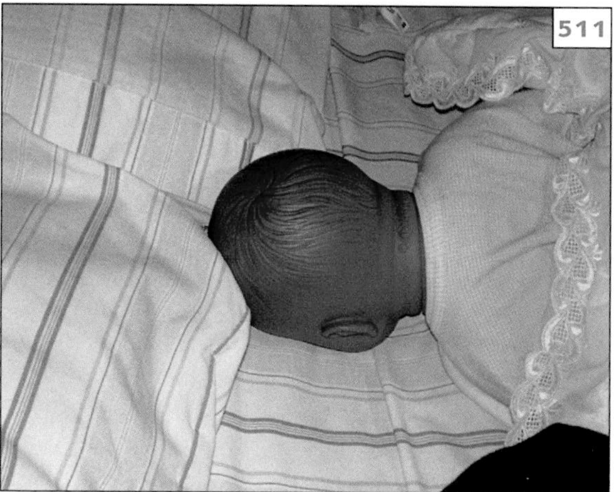

510 Re-enactment of an infant wedged between a mattress and a wall. The narrow space prevented adequate respiratory excursion of the infant's chest.

511 Infant with head pressed against soft bedding in an adult bed. The soft bedding effectively obstructed the infant's airway.

objective sign that indicates the position in which the infant was found[13]. It is important that emergency room staff be aware of this because many infants are taken there even if they have no vital signs, and that is the time to take a photograph. Sometimes, before lividity has fixed, an infant will remain in a hospital for several hours before being picked up by the medical examiner or coroner. Since bodies are placed supine, the lividity can shift posteriorly erasing this potentially useful finding. **512** illustrates the lividity pattern in an infant found prone, in a photograph taken shortly after the body arrived at the hospital.

The lividity pattern can be used to confront the caregiver if the infant was thought to be found in a different position. **513** shows a re-enactment as originally described by the daycare provider in whose care this infant died. After confrontation with the lividity pattern, the child was placed as it was really found, on an adult bed with a soft sleeping surface which could mold around the infant's face and result in airway obstruction, as seen in **514**.

Sometimes scene re-enactments result in unexpected and tragic conclusions. Although breastfeeding is the ideal way to feed an infant, its techniques are not always intuitive, and in spite of instruction provided in its practice in many hospitals, those lessons are not necessarily absorbed or practiced at home[14,15]. Hence, a mother may fall asleep in bed while breastfeeding, resulting in overlay, or an arm settling on an infant's chest. **515** illustrates an infant who was not latching on properly to the nipple, so the mother pushed the child's face into the breast in an attempt to force it to attach to the breast, completely obstructing the infant's upper airway. We have also seen infants that slipped while being fed in a reclining chair; the mother fell asleep and the child was asphyxiated between the thigh and the armrest.

Scene re-enactments are also useful to assess the possibility of homicide. One of the clues to child abuse is the claim that a child did something he was not yet developmentally able to do. **516** illustrates how a 4-month-old infant was found with a plastic bag over his head. The claim was that the child somehow grasped a plastic bag that was outside the crib, put his head inside it, and was asphyxiated. The caregiver was prosecuted.

There is a class of sudden pediatric deaths which has no distinctive pathologic findings and which needs to be considered in the differential diagnosis of death in ambulatory infants. These are deaths caused by poisoning, often with narcotic analgesics having been prescribed or obtained illegally by an adult[16]. Deaths have been seen due to methadone that was removed from the refrigerator by the child, and we saw a death from a discarded fentanyl patch that was found on the floor by a toddler, who then licked it. The only way to discover these is through toxicologic testing of body fluids, preferably blood or vitreous humor. Not all jurisdictions test comprehensively for drugs, especially fentanyl, so there must be a high index of suspicion that ingestion of this drug occurred.

Many sudden infant deaths are circumstantial asphyxias that are not accompanied by any physical signs, and that happen by obstruction of the upper airway or mechanical compression of the chest. It is clear that it is also possible to asphyxiate an infant by covering its upper airway and that this will leave no physical signs[1,2]. Occasionally, however, a careful search of the body will disclose signs of asphyxia (**517**). On the mandibular region, there are two pairs of roughly parallel erythematous lines, with blanching between each pair, consistent with fingers that were pressed against the child's face during smothering.

Older children are better able to defend themselves and are more likely to display the signs of strangulation readily seen in adults. **518** shows an ecchymosis on the right side of the neck of a 4-year-old child who was strangled. The ecchymoses resulted from intense pressure at that point on the neck. **519** shows the peri-orbital petechiae found after manual strangulation. These petechiae can also be found in the conjunctivae and oral mucous membranes. Because the victim is conscious for a short time during manual strangulation, abrasions and ecchymoses can be found in the arms and legs. These result from attempts by the victim to fend off the assailant.

Accidental circumstances that asphyxiate children, other than unsafe sleep, abound[17–19]. Ultimately, many result from adults who lack common sense. **520** shows the body of a 6-month-old infant who was swaddled in an 'Ace' wrap that was wrapped tightly around the body, impeding adequate chest excursion. The erythematous lines correspond to the edges of the bandage and are an indication of the pressure with which the bandage was applied to the body.

Some asphyxias are ideally re-enacted with the child's body. **521** shows a 3-year-old who was playing in the back seat of a car, was unrestrained, and, while her head was outside the window, her foot activated the window switch, raising the window and compressing the neck. **522** shows how the child's body was placed inside the car door showing that her foot was able to reach the window switch.

Drowning is a form of asphyxia. Most drowning deaths in children do not represent diagnostic problems because they occur in a context in which there is no doubt that that is what happened, such as the child who wanders into an unattended pool. Lack of supervision needs to be considered in such cases. Deaths in a bath can occasionally give rise to diagnostic questions given that the death may have been intentionally caused, related to inadequate supervision, or a true accident. **523** shows the neck organs of a 2-year-old child who was in a bath with running water while playing with his two brothers, one 4 years and the other 8 years old. The esophagus was opened longitudinally, demonstrating a distinct boundary above which tissue is congested at the level of the larynx. A visit to the scene and interview with the children showed that the older child pushed the spigot with running water into the younger child's mouth because he said he was 'thirsty'. **524** shows a spigot in the bath with water flowing. The lungs were filled with fluid.

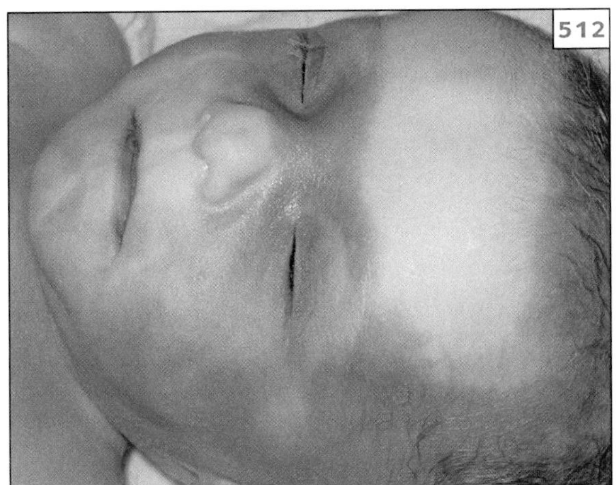

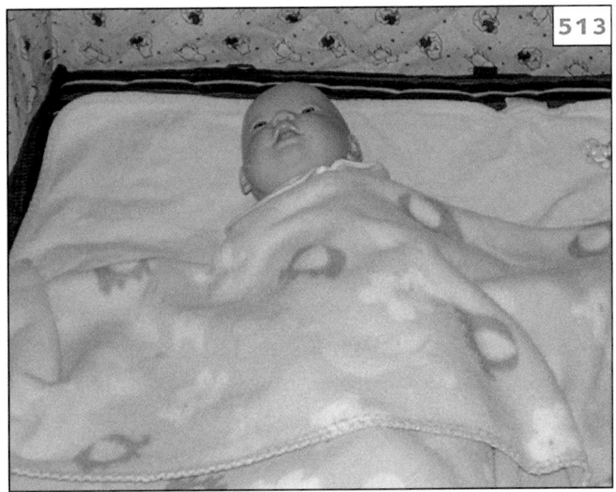

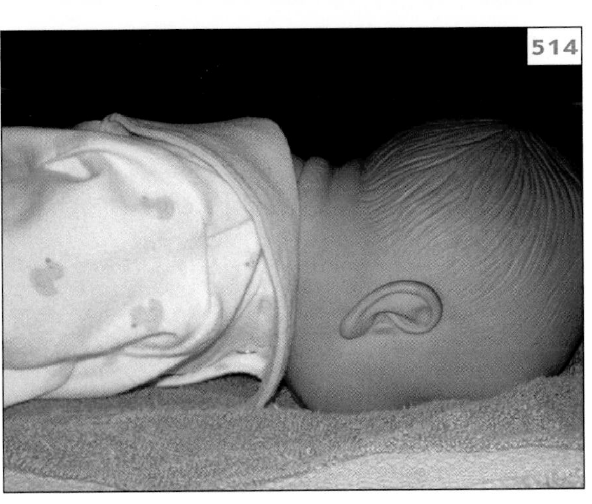

512 Anterior lividity pattern in an infant found prone. This is proof that the infant died with the face compressed against the sleep surface.

513 Re-enactment of a dead infant found in a crib. Finding an infant in this circumstance conforms to the traditional definition of sudden infant death syndrome (SIDS), is unusual and should prompt further questioning of the caregiver.

514 Actual position of the infant originally described as found in 513. Airway obstruction is evident with the soft cloth.

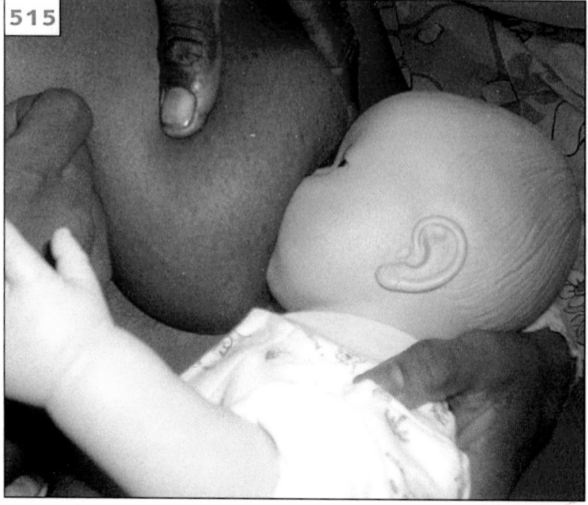

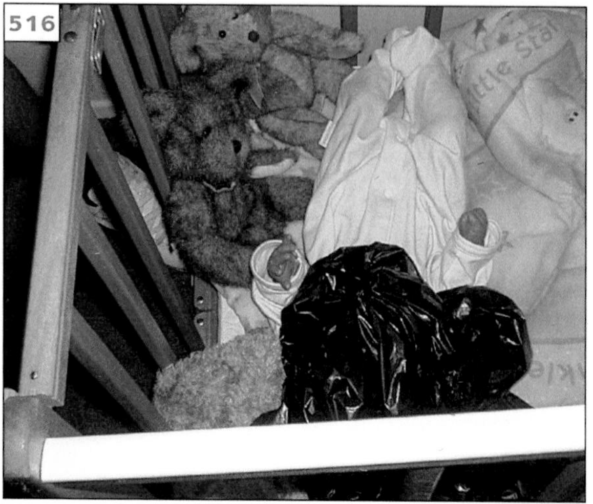

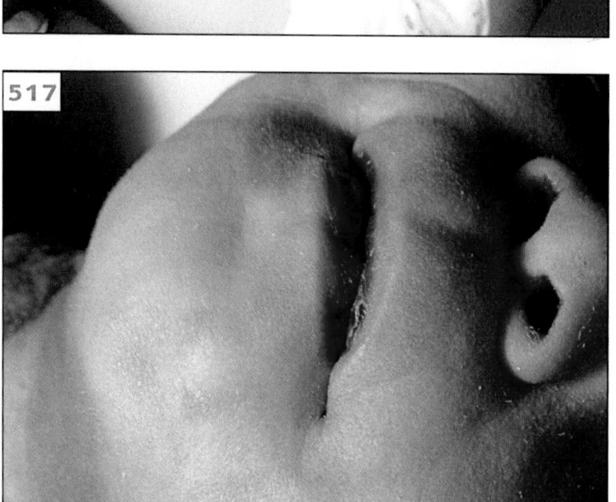

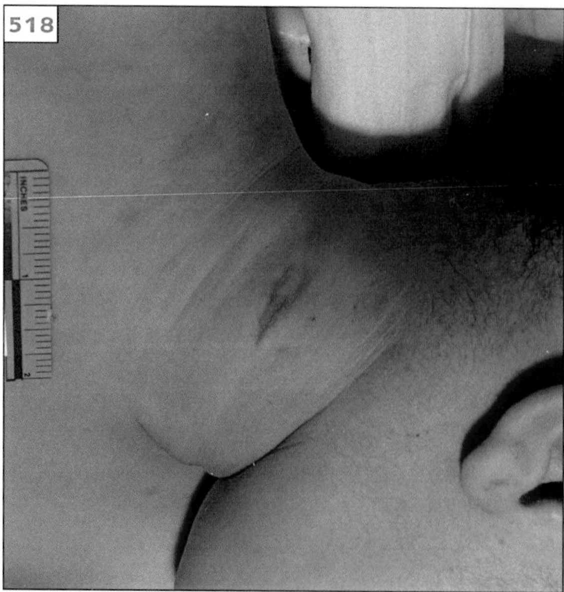

515 Re-enactment of an infant's face pressed against the mother's breast. The flexible subcutaneous tissue and skin was molded around the infant's airway, effectively smothering the child.

516 Re-enactment of an infant found with a plastic bag over its head. Correlated with the infant's likely developmental abilities, it can help assess whether the child was capable of reaching for an object such as this one or confirm the likelihood of homicide.

517 Infant with adult finger outlines on the mandible after smothering. Patterns such as this one rule out accidental explanations for the infant's death.

518 Ecchymosis on the neck of a child who was strangled due to pressure applied at that point. This is a typical finding in homicidal strangulation.

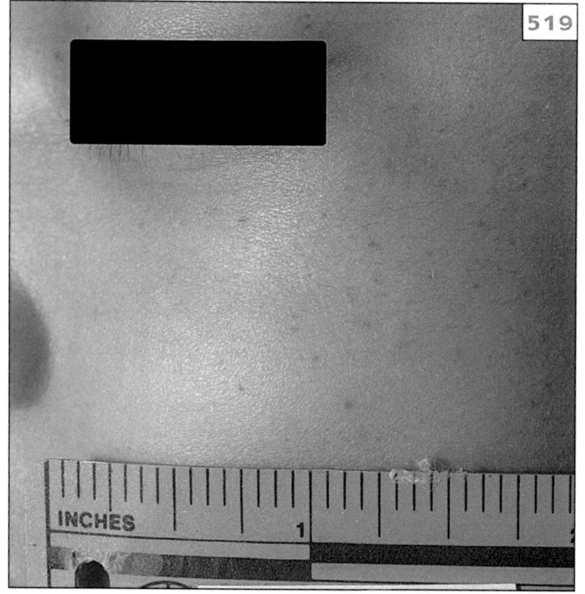

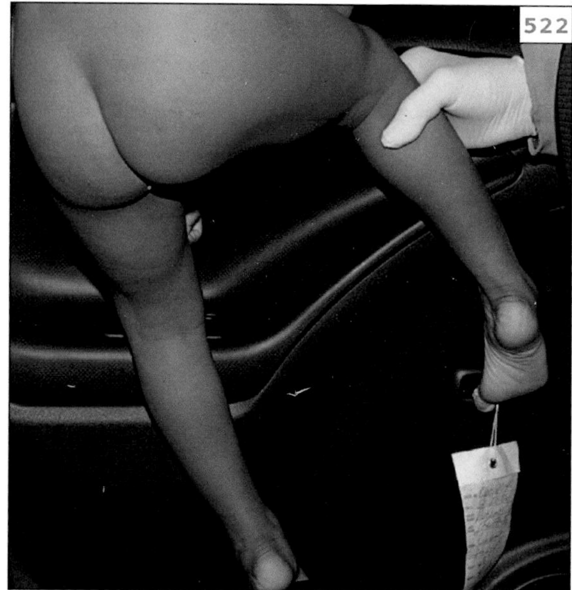

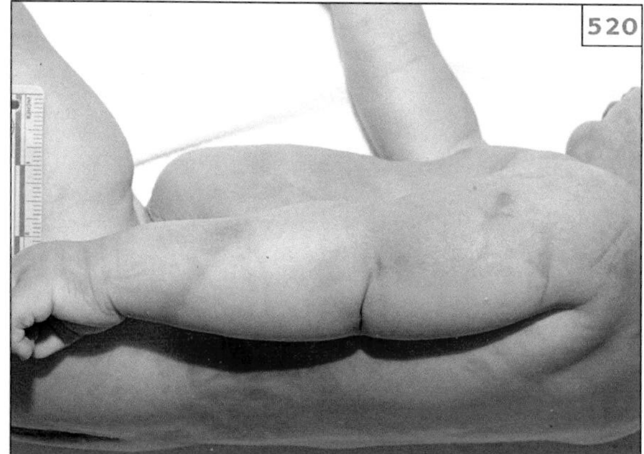

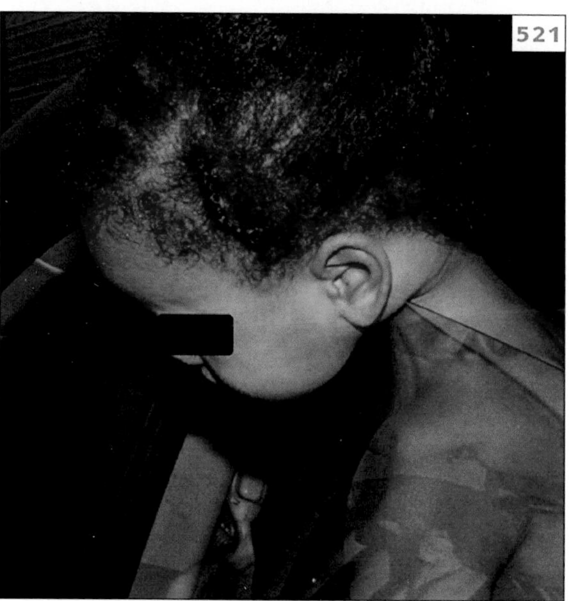

519 Peri-orbital petechiae found after manual strangulation. Another typical finding of strangulation.

520 Bandage markings on an infant's body. The ecchymotic lines help outline the edges of the bandage with which this child's entire body was wrapped.

521 Girl strangled by car window. This demonstrates the usefulness of re-enacting the event with the child's body and the vehicle in which it occurred.

522 Re-enactment of car window strangulation. Using the child's body, it was possible to assess the likelihood that the limbs could reach the car window switch.

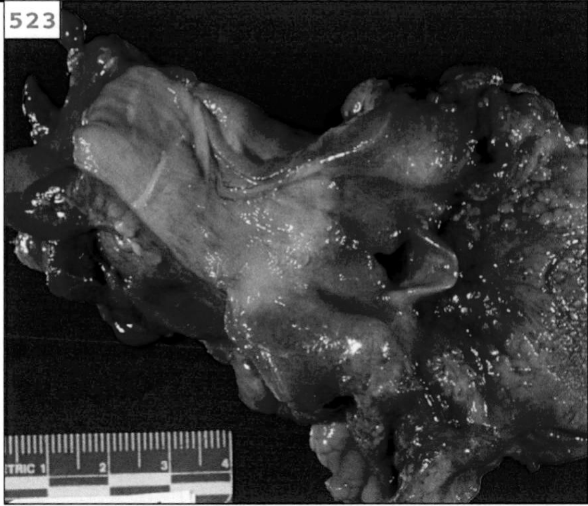

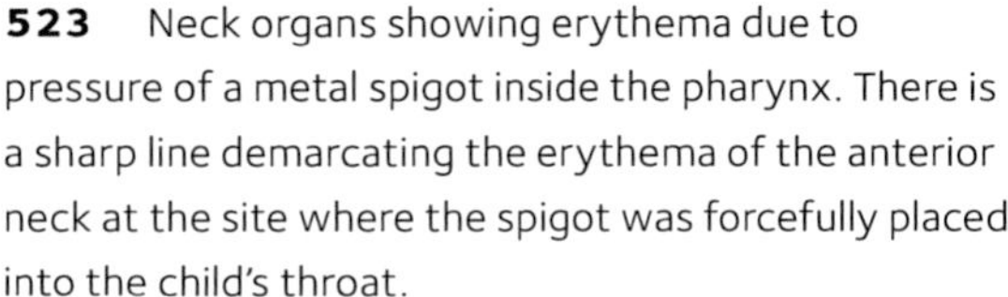

523 Neck organs showing erythema due to pressure of a metal spigot inside the pharynx. There is a sharp line demarcating the erythema of the anterior neck at the site where the spigot was forcefully placed into the child's throat.

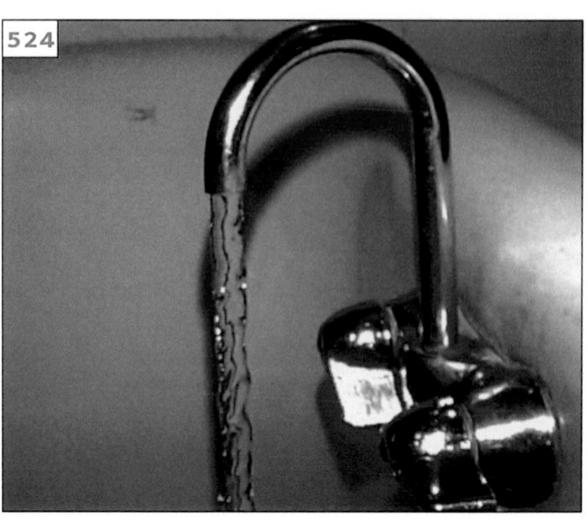

524 Spigot with unaerated water. This was inserted deep into the child's mouth and held there while the water flowed. The solid column of water is evident.

Fatal neglect

Neglect can take many forms. Indeed, many children suffer from some kind of neglect, and it rarely results in the death of a child. When it is fatal, it can have dramatic clinical presentations which depict the later stages of treatable natural disease[1,2,13]. This kind of medical neglect often results from ignorance, or alternative religious or lifestyle views that cause parents to avoid seeking medical care. There is also willful neglect, where the caregiver simply refuses to take a child for medical attention. Children most at risk for this kind of neglect are those with disabilities, since they often are unable to express their needs, and, tragically, the child's death is often a way for the adult to resolve the problems these children pose due to complicated, long-term therapeutic needs. There tends to be a systematic pattern of disregard for the child's well-being. Scene investigation reveals homes that are unkempt and dirty. Food is often not provided regularly. These deaths can be difficult diagnostic problems, because of the paucity of findings. A child fatality can be dehydrated and not show overt evidence of it, especially in older children with fused fontanelles, whose concavity in severe dehydration is a helpful sign in younger infants. Perhaps the most useful test for dehydration are vitreous (eye) electrolytes, i.e. sodium and chloride. Potassium is always elevated after death. Extreme neglect results in malnutrition and dehydration. **525** shows an example of the latter, while **526** shows the face of a child with dehydration. The eyes are sunken into the skull. Instances like these show other signs of abandonment. The lividity was fixed and there are tiny abrasions in this child on the forehead due to postmortem insect activity, indicating the child was dead for some hours before authorities were notified.

527 shows the small bowel of a child who died from dehydration due to diarrhea secondary to an intestinal intussusception. The intussusception is on the left. The middle and right segments of bowel show agonal intussusceptions that are an occasional finding with no diagnostic significance. They can be differentiated from true intussusceptions in the same child, which have significant edema and are more difficult to reduce. The infant's mother had developmental disabilities and did not recognize the significance of the infant's diarrhea. **528–529** are from a child who died from septicemia and dehydration. She had multiple erosions that have a symmetrical pattern evident in the face and the perineum. She also had erosions on both ears, knees, and great toes, some extending to the bone. This child suffered from an unrecognized Lesch–Nyhan syndrome, as did her twin who survived. The parents covered the erosions with gauze and electrical tape and did not seek medical care because of their religious beliefs. It was easy to demonstrate that this child's hands could reach all the affected anatomical regions and could cause the lesions. Another child with this condition is presented in **530**.

Older, functional children can also succumb to willful neglect, sometimes with public health consequences. **531** shows the lungs of a 12-year-old girl who died with miliary tuberculosis. The lesions are extensively consolidated and cavitary. She had been going to school where a teacher noticed her progressive wasting, but attributed it to simple malnourishment. The caregiver had occasionally taken her to a pediatrician who documented the progressive weight loss, but did not comment on it. This girl had episodes of respiratory distress interpreted as asthma, but medication was not regularly obtained. **532** shows the classic granuloma with Langhans-type giant cells, and **533** shows confirmation of the presence of acid-fast bacilli, diagnostic of *Mycobacterium tuberculosis* infection.

Some neglected children are tortured, as is demonstrated in **534** which depicts a child whose malnourishment is evident in his prominent ribs. He was tortured by his caregivers with an electrical device used by police to subdue uncooperative individuals.

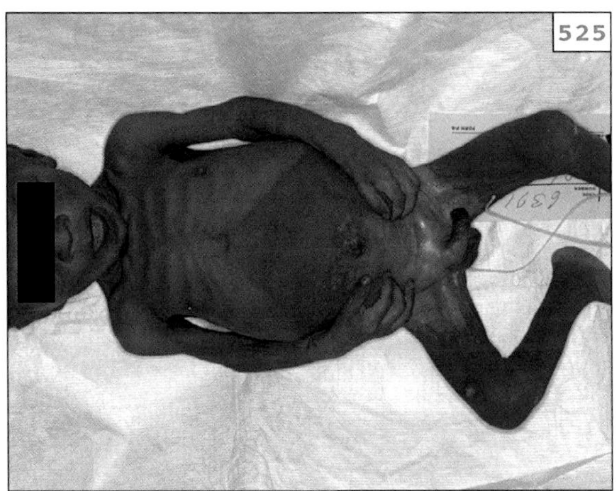

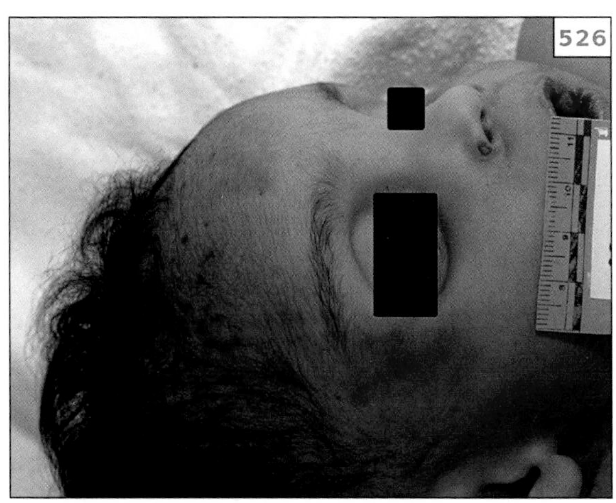

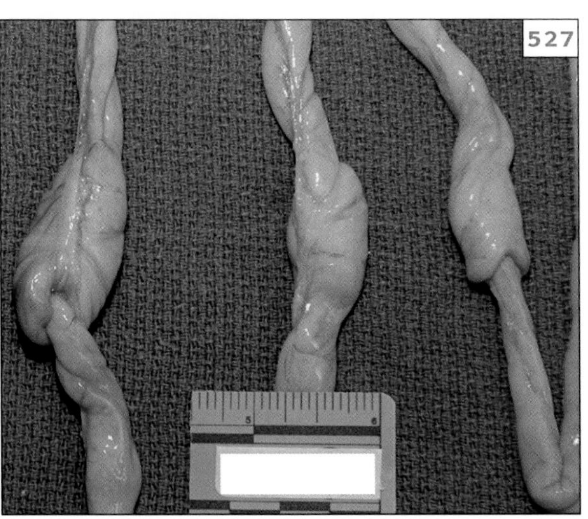

525 Infant suffering from extreme dehydration and malnutrition. The loss of subcutaneous tissue is obvious as is the chronic diaper/nappy rash so characteristic of neglect.

526 Infant showing extreme dehydration. The enophthalmos is evident.

527 Small bowel showing true intussusception (on left) and agonal intussusception (middle and right). It is much easier to reduce the agonal intussusceptions so care has to be used when documenting them or they will be lost.

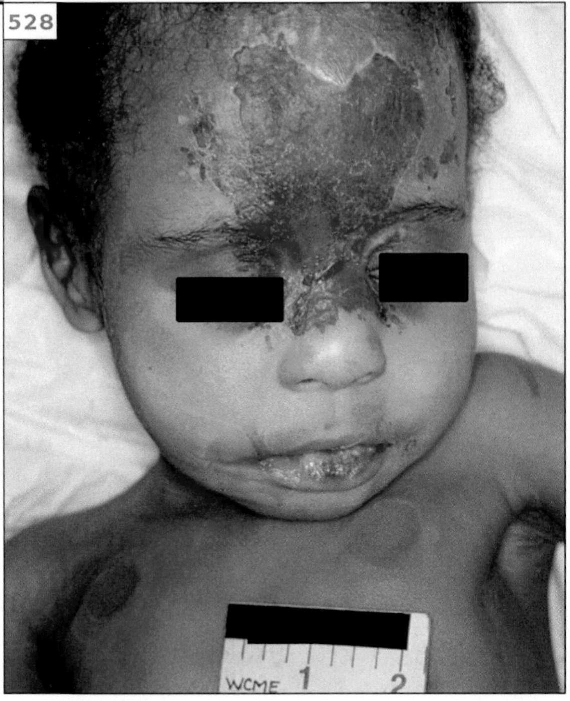

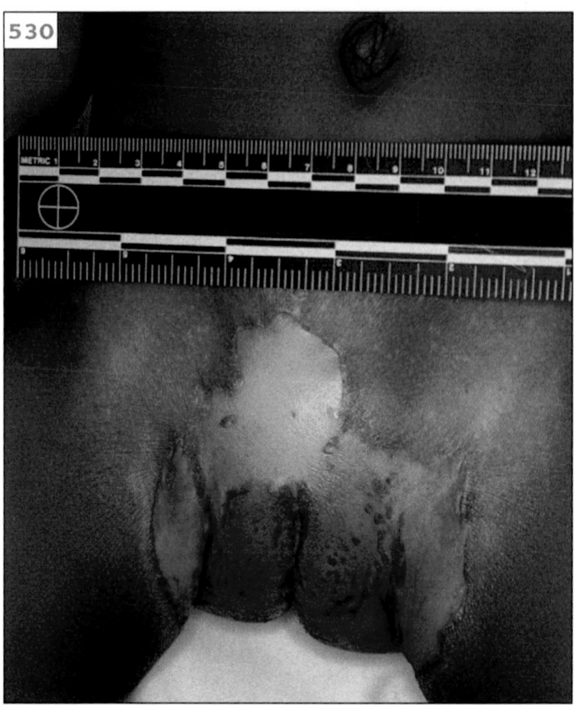

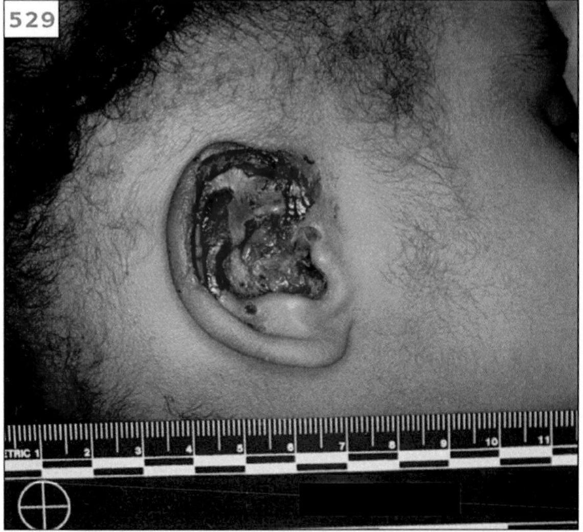

528 Forehead erosions in a child with self-mutilation syndrome. The symmetry in the forehead erosion is evident.

529 Ear erosions in a child with self-mutilation syndrome. The other ear had a similar erosive pattern.

530 Perineal erosions in child with self-mutilation syndrome. As in 528 and 529, the symmetry and locations of the erosions helped confirm this was self-inflicted.

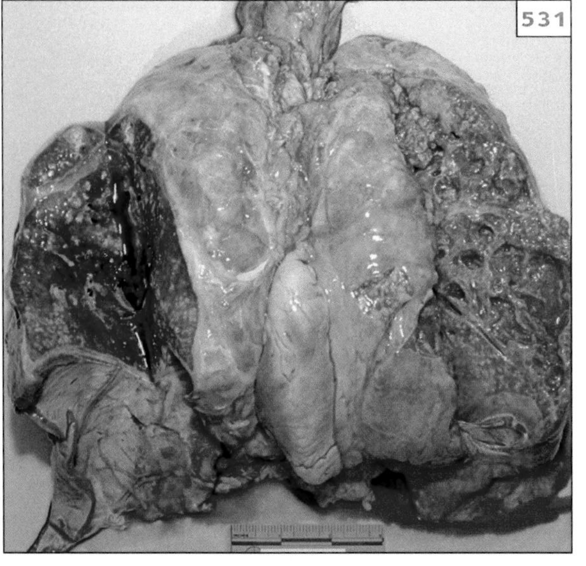

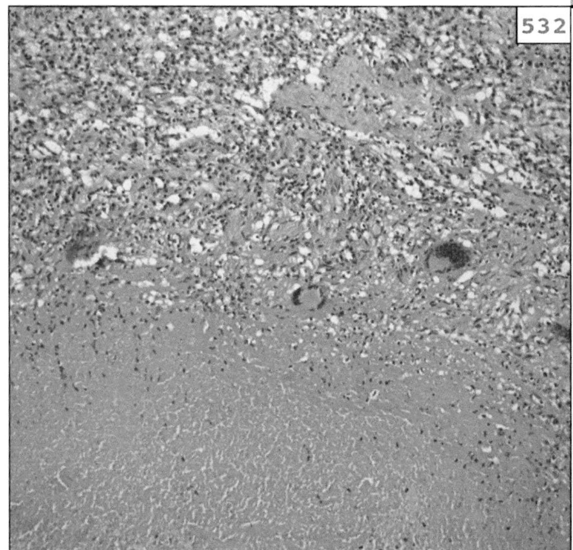

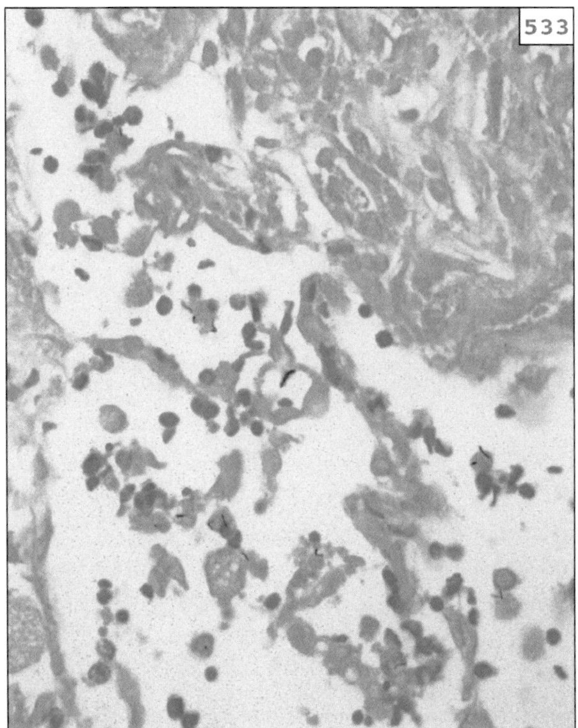

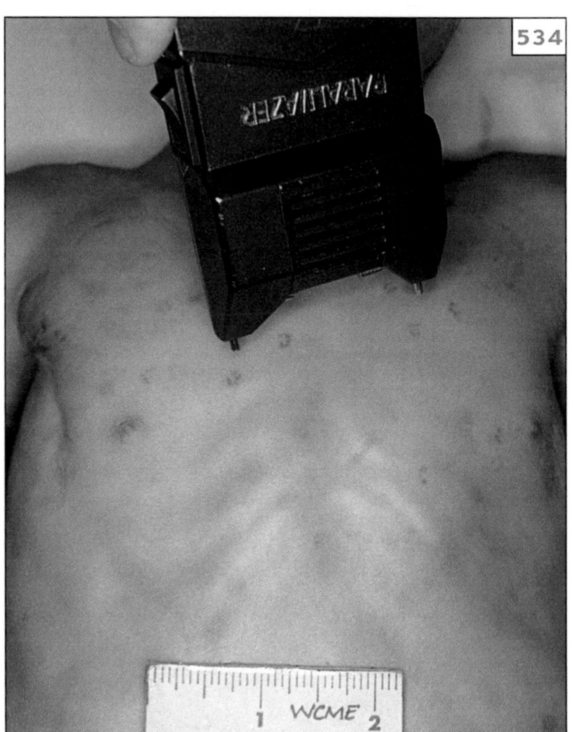

531 Consolidated lungs with tuberculous pneumonia and cavitation. The involvement was diffuse.

533 Tuberculous granuloma with Langhans-type giant cells. The latter are at the periphery of the granuloma.

532 *Mycobacterium tuberculosis* demonstrated with acid-fast stain.

534 Torture marks due to an electrical device. The superimposed device matches the electrodes with the lesions.

Fatal burns

Burns do not usually result in a child's death. When they do, they are usually from a house fire or similar catastrophic event that is an accident rather than abuse. There is commonly some survival time after the fire starts resulting in inhalation of carbon monoxide and loss of consciousness. Carboxyhemoglobin tinges mucous membranes a bright pink-red hue as seen in **535**. **536** shows soot in the airway. Findings like these, along with the presence of carboxyhemoglobin, are indicators that the child was alive after the fire started. If a burned body has no signs of identifiable carboxyhemoglobin, this is evidence that the death occurred before the body was exposed to a fire. It can also happen after a flash fire where death happens too quickly for carboxyhemoglobin to accumulate.

The most common kind of burn encountered in fatal child abuse is scalding with hot water[1,2]. This is covered in Chapter 3, Abusive burns. However, a scalding pattern is ordinarily identifiable as seen in **537**. This developmentally disabled child was placed in a bath partially filled with hot water. This left a distinct burn line indicating the level of submersion along the legs, back, and arms. **538** and **539** show a toddler who was held under a tap with hot, running water accounting for the unusual oblique truncal scald pattern. Not all infants with a scalded appearance are burned. **540** shows an *in utero* death with maceration that was confused with a scalding burn in the emergency room. Apart from the context in which this child was found, there was overlapping of the cranial bones as part of the process of maceration.

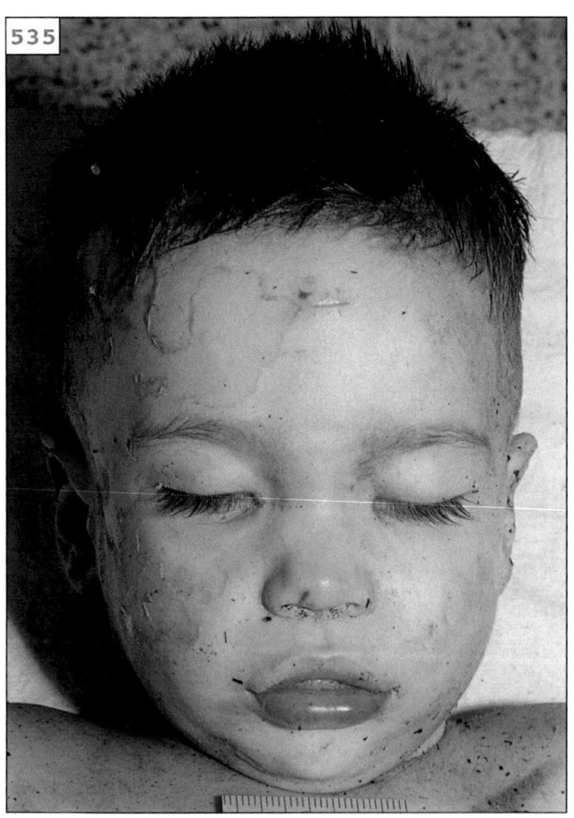

535 Pink–red hue due to carbon monoxide intoxication. It is most apparent in mucous membranes and areas of epithelial transition, such as the lips.

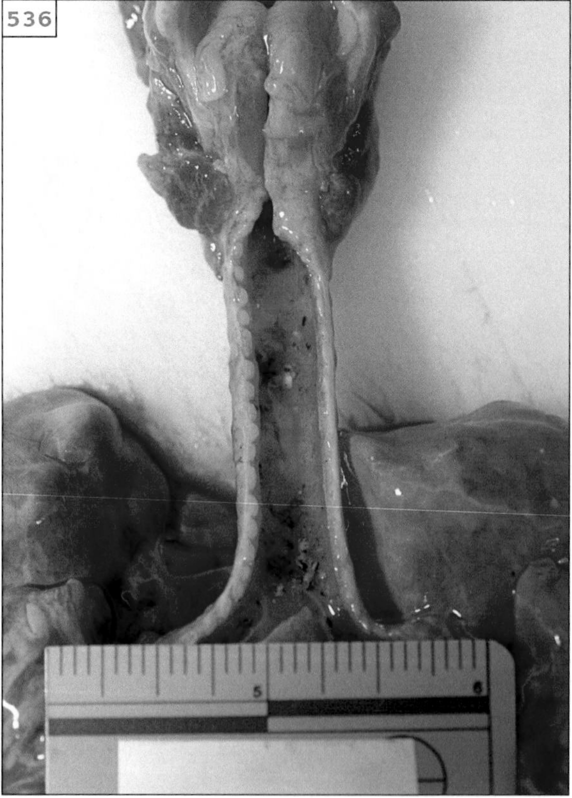

536 Soot in the airway due to inhalation of the products of combustion. The tissue retains the bright-red hue seen in mucous membranes.

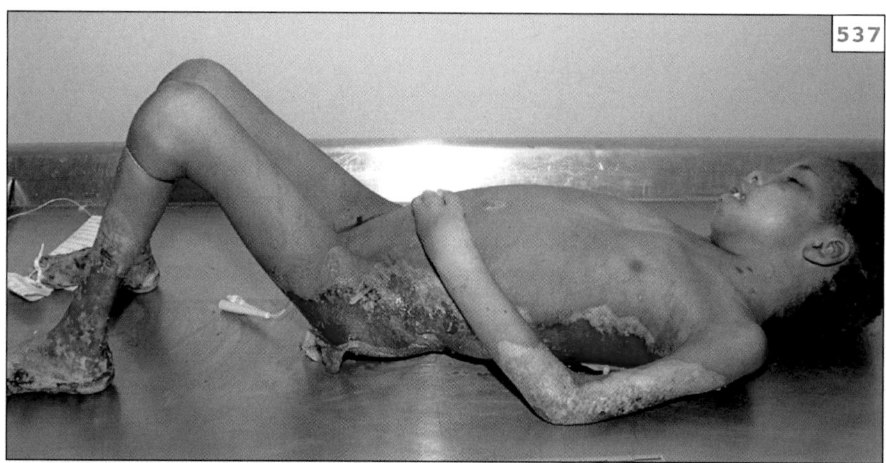

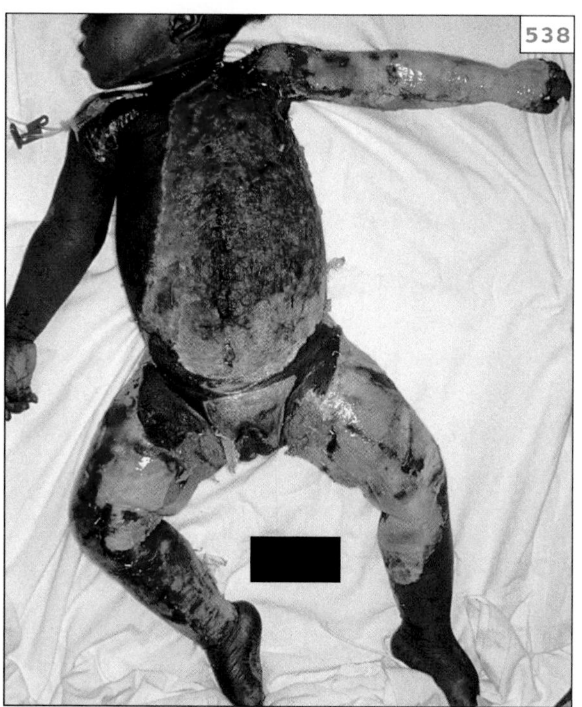

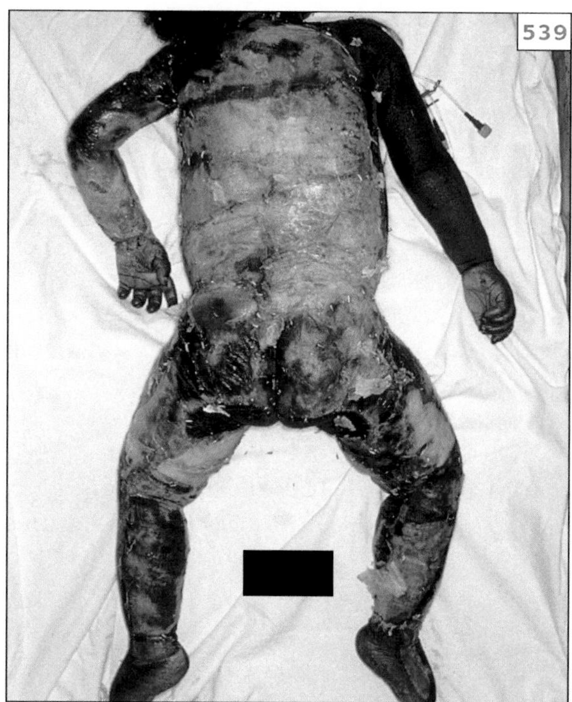

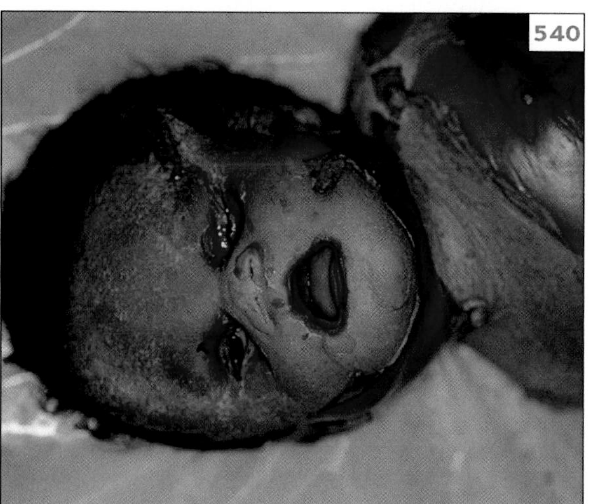

537 Scalding pattern after child was placed in a bath with hot water. The margin of injury in the flexed lower extremities matches the scald line on the trunk.

538 Scalding due to running water. This is an atypical pattern that was caused by placing the child under a running hot water tap.

539 Scalding due to running water. The full depth burns are apparent.

540 Maceration in a stillborn fetus. This is not to be confused with scalding injuries. The overriding cranial bones aid in the diagnosis.

Blunt force injuries

Most fatal child abuse is caused by blunt trauma more frequently to the head and less so to the abdomen, although they are often found together. When fatal abusive head trauma results from impact to the head, there is usually evidence of that impact in the form of ecchymoses and lacerations that are easily observed. **541** shows the scalp of a toddler who suffered multiple impacts to the head.

Sometimes there is no sign of impact on the head, and this can lead to controversy over whether the infant was shaken or suffered a blunt impact over a broad surface area, such as a soft surface like bedding, that allowed the energy to be dissipated such that no discrete ecchymosis could be identified[20–22]. Regardless, these children are still victims of abusive head trauma, with the intracranial consequences of absorbing a great deal of energy. One of the major consequences of head trauma is cerebral edema, which can be so intense it causes diastatic separation of the sutures as seen in **542**. On opening the skull, subdural hemorrhage was found as seen in **543**, although it may be more patchy as seen in **544**.

Frequently, peri-optic nerve sheath hemorrhage is grossly visible, as seen in **545**. Sometimes, peri-optic nerve sheath hemorrhage is not evident grossly, but can be identified microscopically, as seen in **546**, which clearly depicts the hemorrhagic boundary between the nerve and the sheath. This highlights the need to remove the eyes during autopsy and take sections for microscopy in every case of potentially abusive head trauma, since optic nerve sheath hemorrhage is usually present. Retinal hemorrhages can be seen microscopically (**547**), with hemorrhagic infiltration of the retina anteriorly near the ciliary body, a site where hemorrhages due to abusive head trauma typically appear. There are often discrepancies between what a pathologist and clinicians see during examination, and it is possible to identify retinal hemorrhages microscopically that were not seen clinically[23–25]. **548** is typical of the cerebral edema encountered in abusive head trauma. There is flattening of gyri, effacement of sulci, and bilateral grooving of the hippocampus.

Children with severe abusive head trauma sometimes survive for many years, albeit with profound neurological deficits. **549** shows the impressive atrophy and degeneration that can occur in the brain after the severe hypoxia–ischemia that accompanies head trauma. This was a 6-year-old child who had sustained head injury at the age of 1 year.

Blunt trauma to the chest and abdomen can present a diagnostic challenge to the clinician because it is possible to inflict severe injury to a child without evidence of external bruising[1,2]. This means that there can be severe visceral injury that may not be evident clinically at a time when potentially treatable. **550** shows the chest and upper abdomen of a 3-year-old female who arrived in the hospital unconscious. Careful inspection of the chest shows a few barely visible ecchymoses. **551** illustrates the extensive pulmonary contusions that this child suffered in spite of the fact that the lungs are protected by the ribs. **552** shows the liver that was split in half when trauma was inflicted.

553 shows the extensive injuries sustained by a 6-year-old boy who had survived long enough to undergo a laparotomy. The visible bruising does not indicate the severity of mesenteric and intestinal injuries (**554**). This child was also sexually assaulted (**555**), with rectal tears superimposed on the profound ecchymoses. **556** shows the extensive, confluent subcutaneous hemorrhage often present in extensively traumatized children, and is a good example of how, even in the extremities, subcutaneous hemorrhage may be a more accurate descriptor of the inflicted trauma than are externally visible bruises.

The infliction of severe abdominal trauma usually requires that the child's body be supported against a firm surface so that the energy transferred by the blow is absorbed by the abdominal organs rather than be dissipated by motion of the child's body. **557** shows a liver with semicircular imprints due to the ribs, while **558** shows a fractured pancreas, split in half against the spine over which it lies. In both of these instances, the abused children were held against a firm surface while they were punched. Sometimes multiple blunt trauma has a distinct, repeating pattern that allows one to identify the instrument with which the child was beaten. **559** shows the back of an 8-year-old boy who was chronically beaten, since many of the lesions had scarred. **560** shows a close-up of the electrical cord with which the injuries were inflicted.

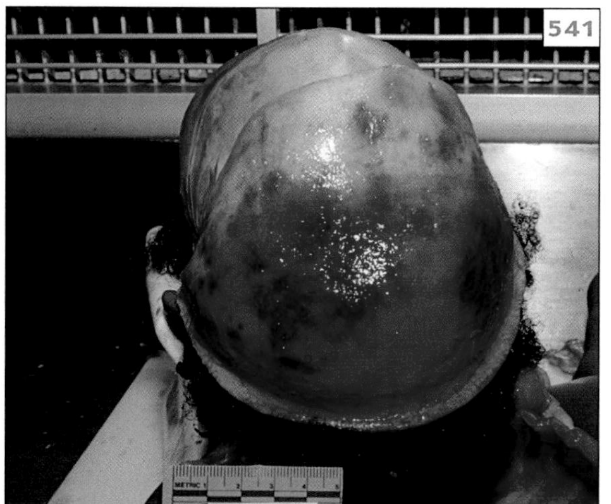

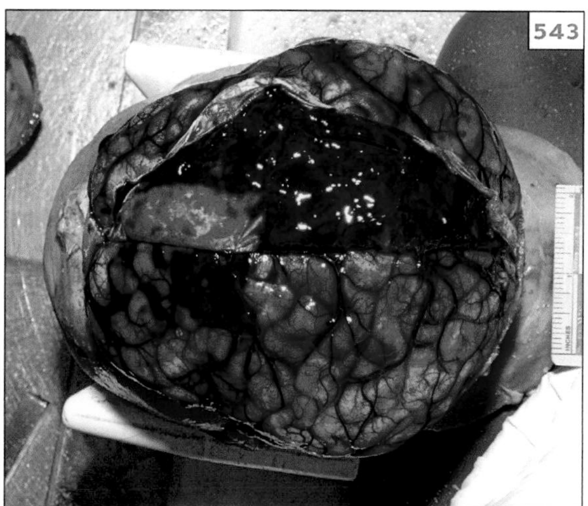

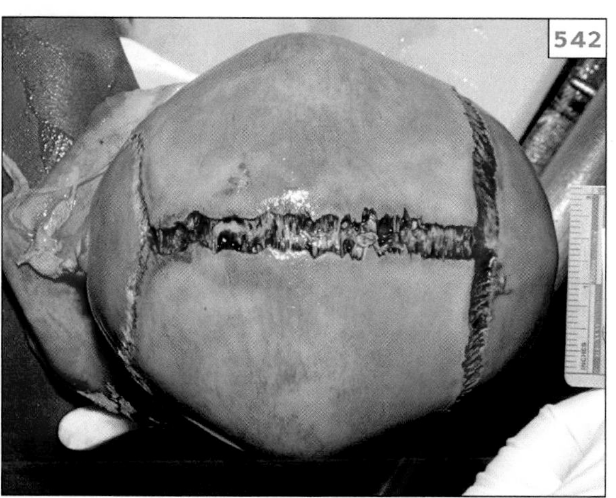

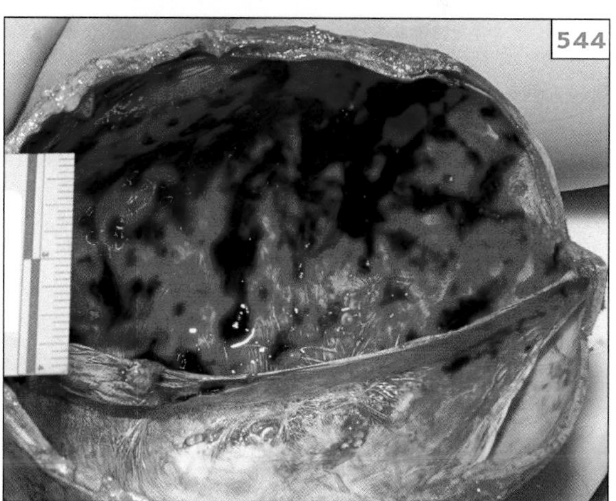

541 Reflected scalp showing multiple impact sites. The extensive, confluent hemorrhagic infiltration and their distribution is a clue to multiple impacts.

542 Diastatic separation of cranial sutures due to intense cerebral edema. It is more apparent in the sagittal and coronal sutures and in spite of closure of the fontanelles.

543 Reflected dura and brain with subdural clot. Beneath the dural clot, subarachnoid hemorrhage is also present.

544 Patchy subarachnoid hemorrhage attached to the inner surface of the dura. There is extensively distributed hemorrhage.

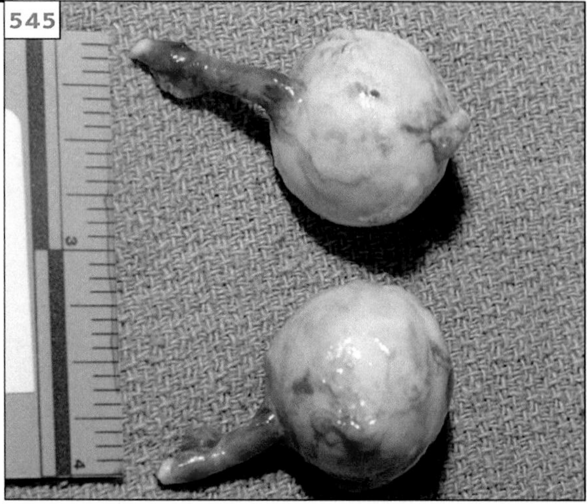

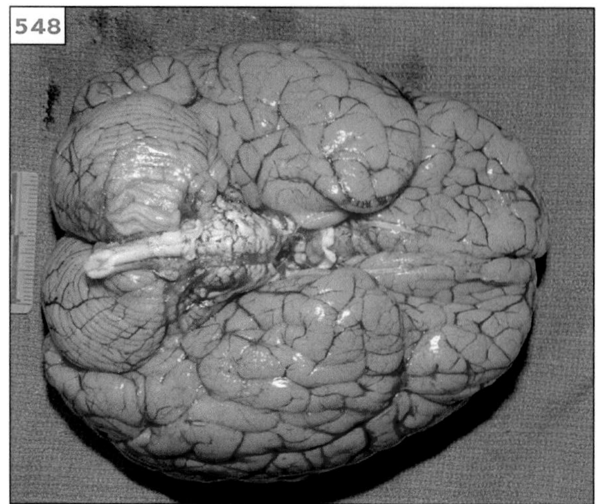

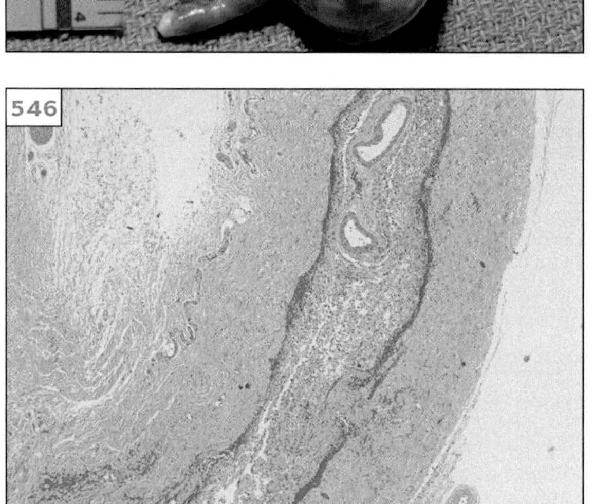

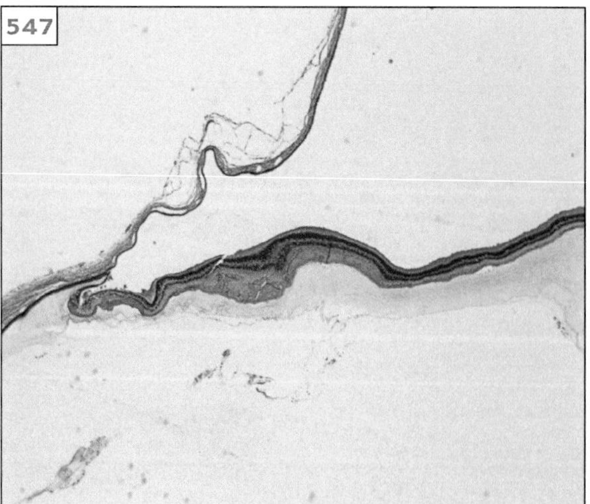

545 Peri-optic nerve sheath hemorrhage. Another manifestation of the violence suffered by this child.

546 Microscopic peri-optic nerve sheath hemorrhage. A bilateral line of hemorrhage separates the sheath from the optic nerve.

547 Hemorrhage in the retina. Although best seen in the center of the picture, other areas of hemorrhagic infiltration are evident on close inspection of the retina.

548 Intense cerebral edema. The gyri are flattened and there is bilateral grooving of the hippocampus.

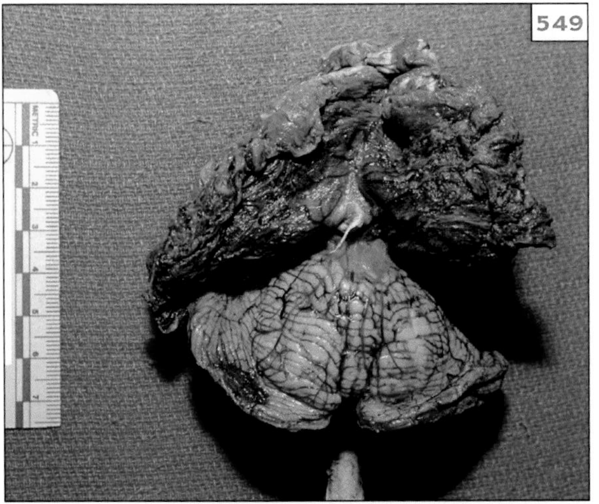

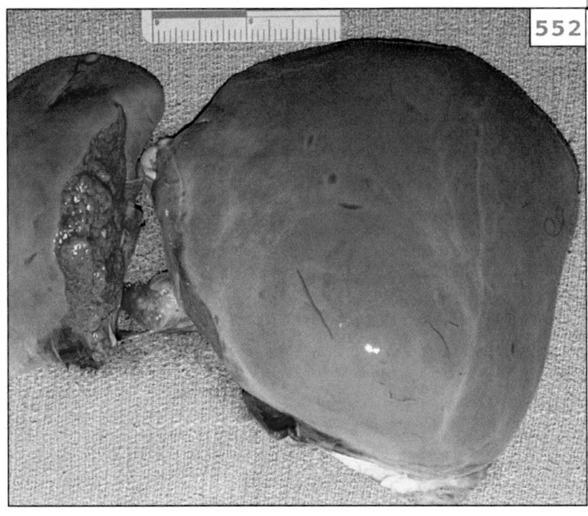

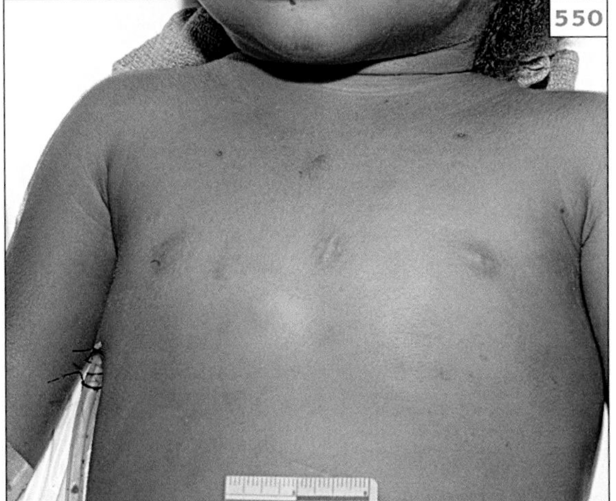

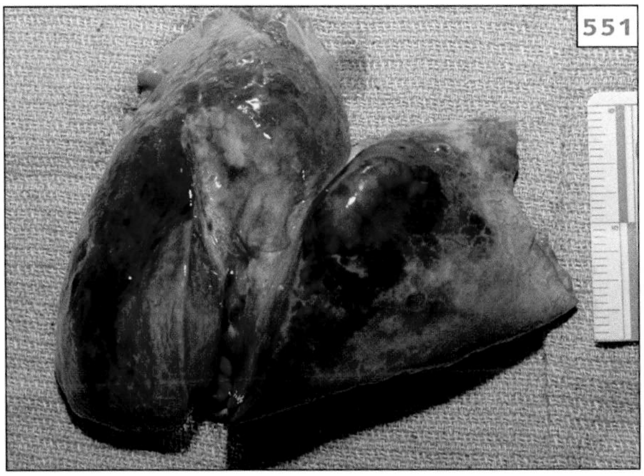

549 Intense gliosis and atrophy of the brain after severe hypoxia–ischemia. Only the cerebellum appears unaffected.

550 Barely visible bruising on the chest and abdomen. This can conceal extensive visceral injury.

551 Pulmonary contusions found in the child described in 550. The confluence of the hemorrhagic areas provide insight into the violence suffered by this child.

552 Bisected liver from the child described in 550. The left lobe is attached to the right only by a thin strip of Glisson's capsule.

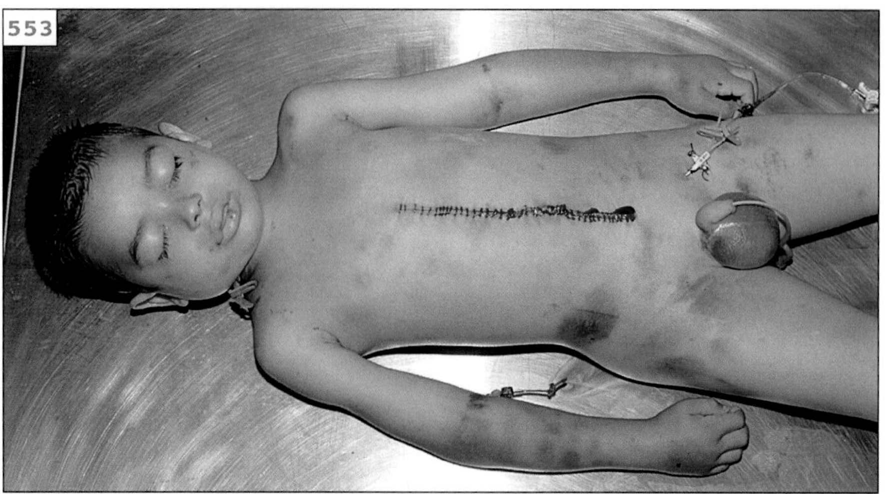

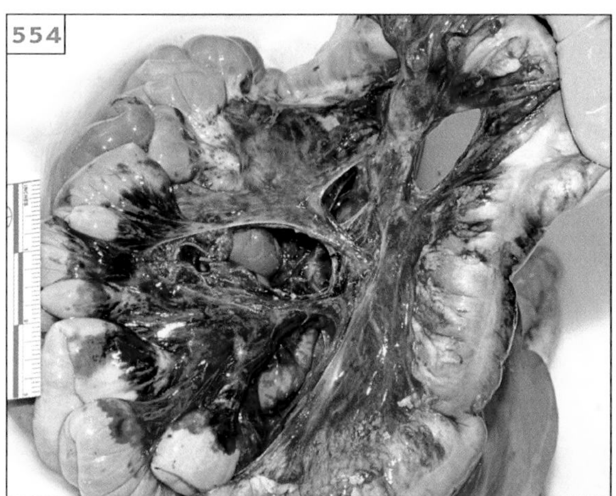

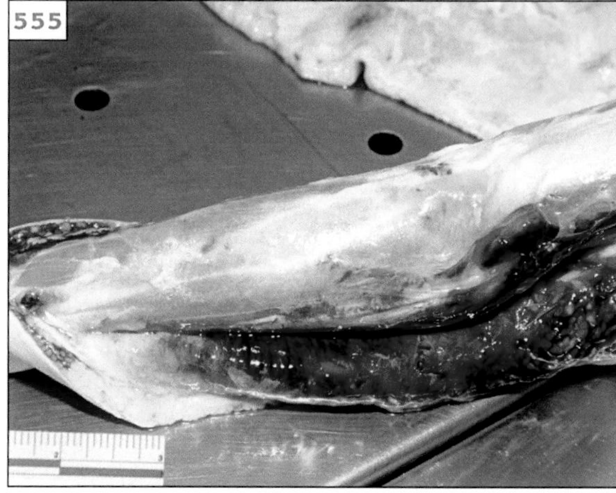

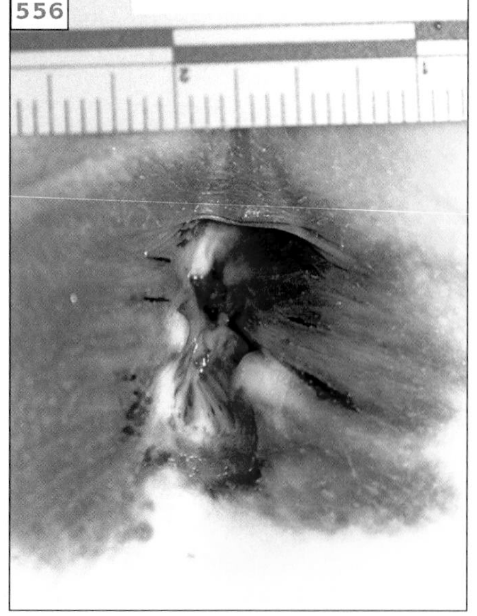

553 External aspect of a 6-year-old boy beaten multiple times and sexually assaulted. There is widespread distribution of injuries.

554 Mesenteric and enteric injuries from the child described in 553. There are multiple mesenteric tears and bowel ecchymoses.

555 Confluent subcutaneous hemorrhage in the right forearm of the child described in 553. The extent of the hemorrhage indicates multiple blows to the forearm.

556 Rectal bruising and tears from the child described in 553. The rectal hemorrhagic infiltration is apparent.

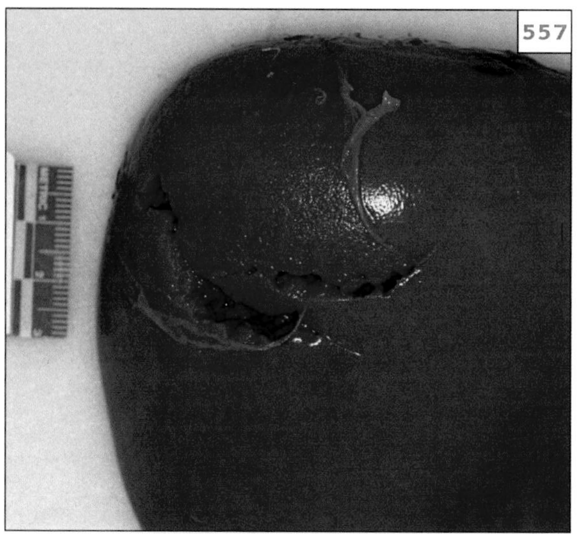

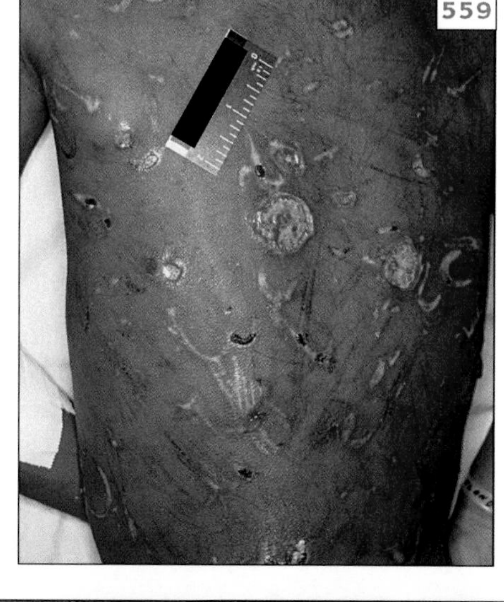

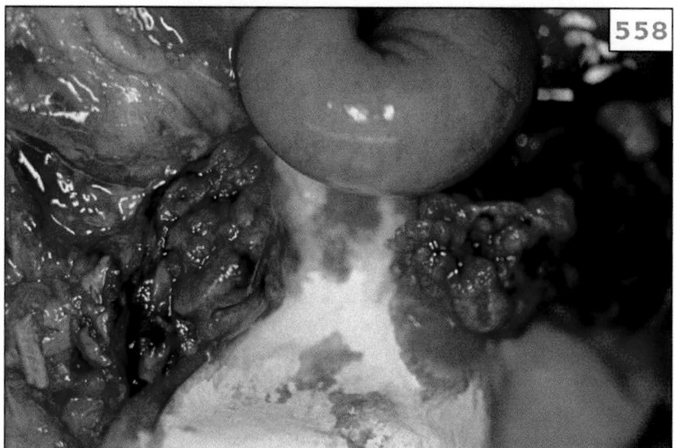

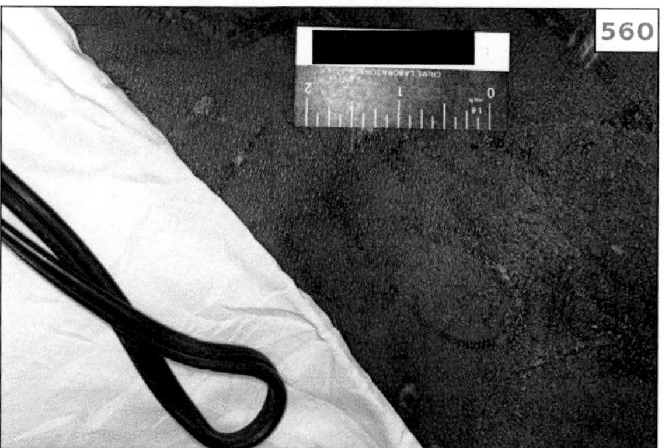

557 Liver with semicircular tears caused by the ribs pressing on its surface. The semicircular outline of the anterior ribs is highlighted.

558 Fractured pancreas in a child held against a wall and punched. This kind of visceral injury occurs when the body is supported against a firm surface.

559 The back of a child beaten multiple times with an electrical cord. The different stages of healing of the lesions indicate multiple beatings at different times.

560 Close-up of injury matching it to the electrical cord that caused it. It is always helpful to try to match the outline of the causative object with that of the injury.

Sharp force injuries

These kinds of injuries are not often seen in abused children. **561** shows a 6-year-old girl who was tortured with a knife, as seen by the various superficial incised wounds, and then stabbed multiple times. These wounds have well-defined, sharply outlined edges. It is not possible to identify the weapon that caused a stab or incised wound unless there is an adjacent patterned injury, such as the parallel lines caused by a serrated knife dragged along the skin. Sharp force injuries due to animal bites, most often dogs, are not rare.[26] **562** shows a 2-year-old child who was bitten many times by a pit bull terrier. The injuries to the neck are deceptively superficial. **563** shows the spine split in two at the level of T2 with exposure of the spinal cord. This child also had a punctured larynx. This is a remarkable example of the force than can be exerted by a dog bite.

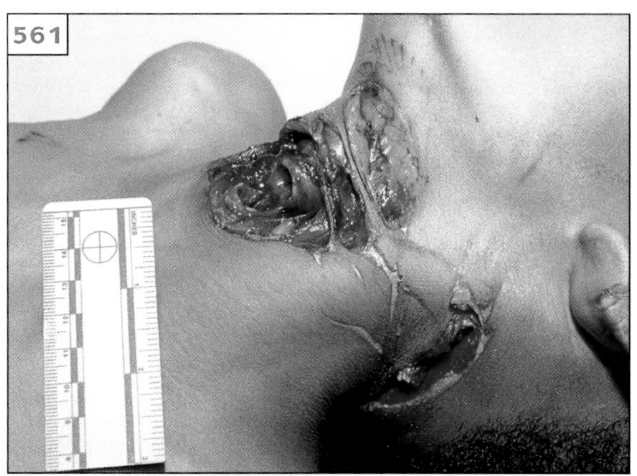

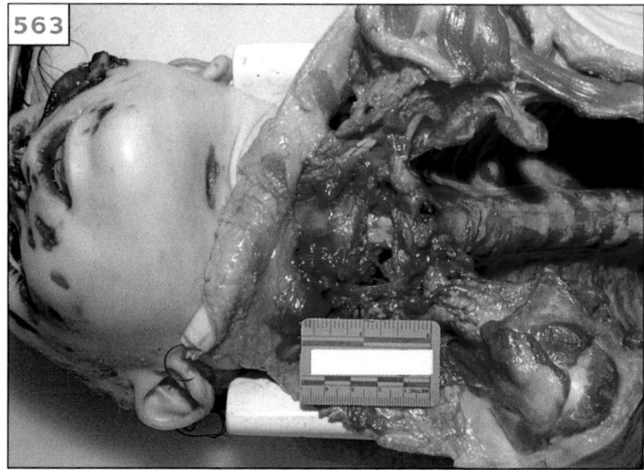

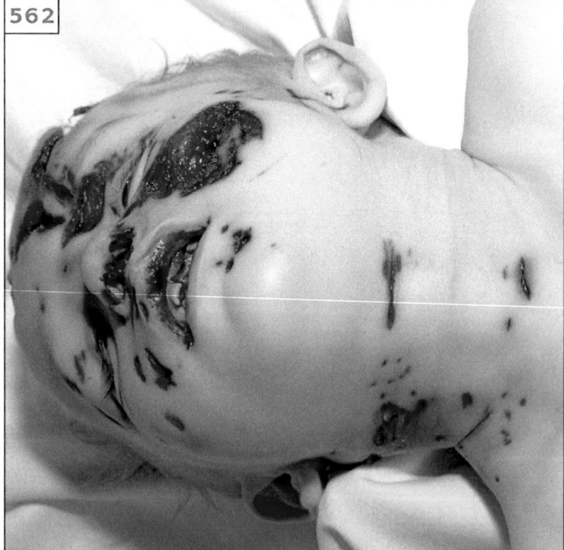

561 A 6-year-old girl stabbed multiple times, with transection of the trachea. Different, intersecting slashes are useful to assess the number of incisions and stab wounds.

562 A 2-year-old mauled by a pit bull dog. The puncture wounds in the neck do not reflect the extensive internal injuries.

563 Fractured spine with exposed cord due to a bite from a pit bull dog. This is a reflection of the energy of a dog bite.

Gunshot wounds

Gunshot wounds are usually the result of carelessness by an adult who leaves a weapon, often loaded, within the reach of a child. This problem is not new[27,28]. Many of these injuries are caused by weapons that the adult thought were hidden under a bed or in a closet. Unfortunately, children find guns easily and proceed to play with them. **564** shows a child with a gunshot wound to the left eye with dense stippling indicating the gun was fired at close range. Because guns are often discharged while playing with the weapon in close proximity, many of these wounds have signs of close range fire. A generic gun will leave stippling when fired within 2 feet (0.6 m) or less from the skin. **565** shows a gunshot wound where the gun was further away, as seen in the more widely dispersed stippling. **566** shows a stellate entrance wound with a rim of soot, which indicates this was a close contact gunshot wound. Since the muzzle of the gun was in contact with the skin, the gases from the burning powder traveled underneath the skin and caused the tears due to the sudden expansion of tissue. **567** shows a small caliber contact wound under the chin that exited through the left eye. This was a 12-year-old child who committed suicide with an easily available firearm.

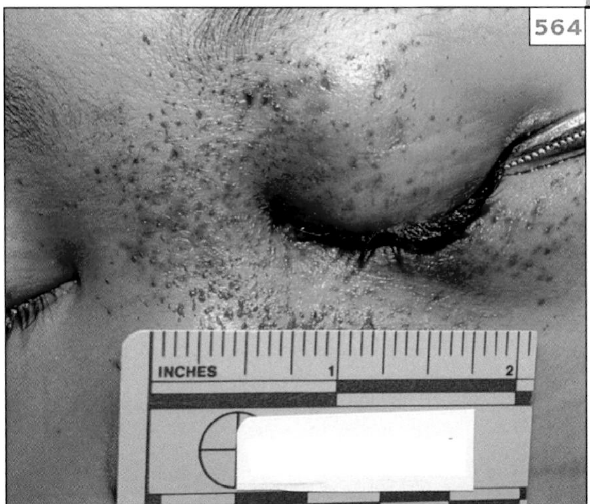

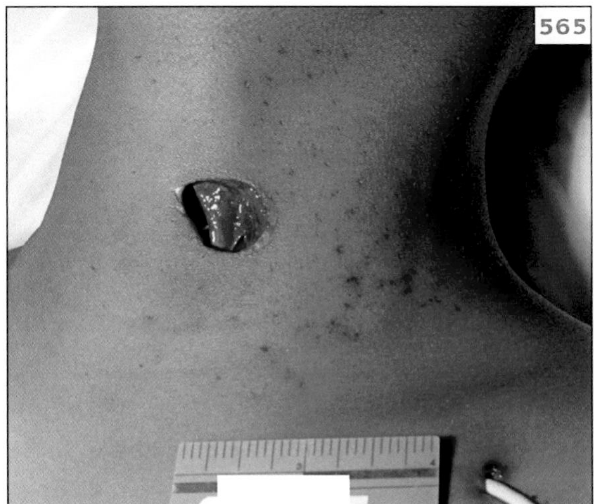

564 Gunshot wound of the left eye with dense stippling. The density of the stippling indicates that the gun was fired close to the skin.

565 Gunshot wound of the neck with less dense stippling. This reflects a gun that was fired further away from the skin than that in 564, but still close enough to cause the stippling. Larger guns with more gunpowder can leave stippling from a greater distance.

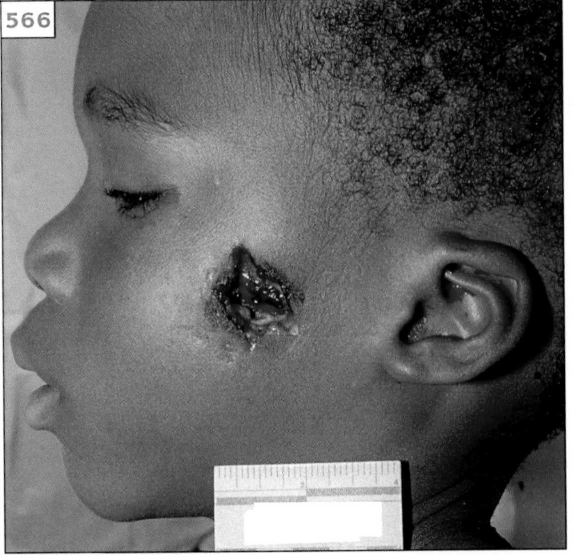

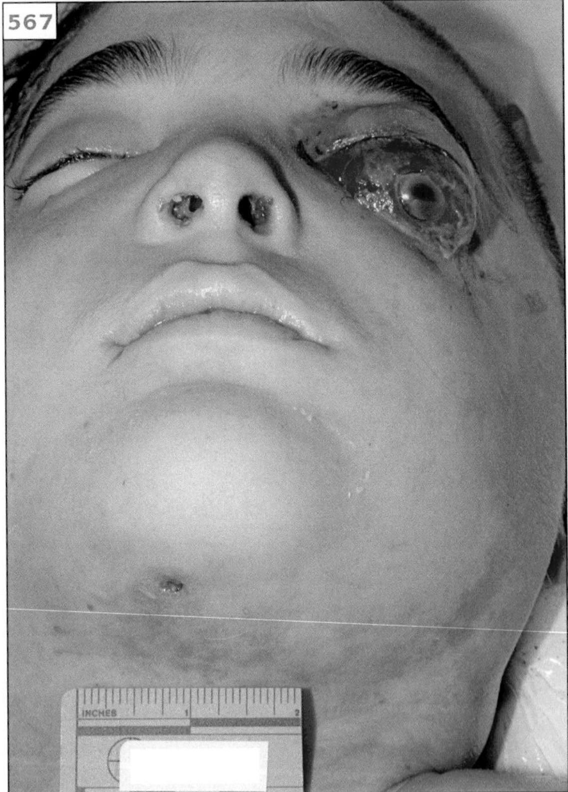

566 Contact gunshot wound of the left cheek. Notice the stellate appearance of the entrance wound and the blackened wound edges.

567 Contact gunshot wound of the chin in a suicide. The extent of intracranial injury is proportionately much greater than the size of the entrance wound.

Teaching points

- Most pediatric deaths from 'accident' or abuse are preventable.
- Physicians evaluating infants with sudden death need to be aware of the risk factors suggesting fatal maltreatment and that the diagnosis of sudden infant death syndrome requires a thorough autopsy, scene investigation, and review of the medical history. Many of these deaths are actually caused by asphyxia related to unsafe sleep practices.
- Medical and physical neglect contribute to an important proportion of 'natural' deaths.
- Burns, blunt, sharp and gun-related trauma have patterns of injury which can be identifiable as inflicted and can lead to the proper determination of the manner of death.

Chapter 12
FAILURE TO THRIVE

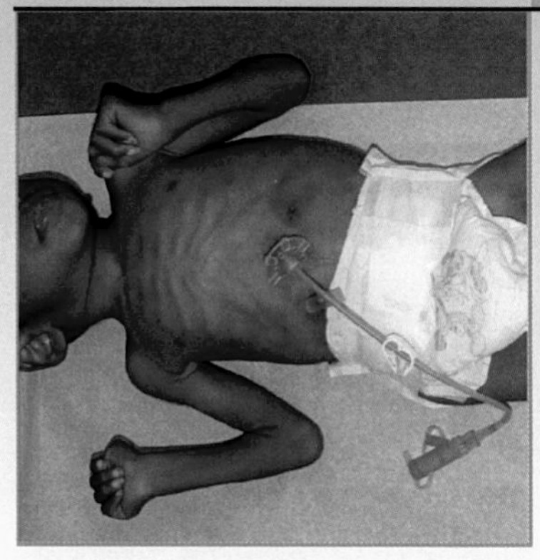

Lynn C. Smitherman
MD, FAAP

Failure to thrive (FTT) is a disorder commonly seen by primary care physicians. Although it is reported that FTT accounts for 1–5% of hospital admissions in the United States and in the UK,[1–3] and is seen in 8–10% of low income children, the prevalence in the general population is unknown[2,4]. It has also been noted that in inner city emergency departments, 15–30% of young children receiving acute care show growth deficits[3]. It is important to note that in itself, FTT is not a diagnosis, but a symptom of an underlying disorder. Children usually present either with parental concern about the child's growth, or it is noted by the provider during a routine examination. FTT in early infancy has been related to future growth and cognitive delays; therefore, early recognition is key to accurate diagnosis and treatment. The etiology of failure to thrive in many cases is multifactorial, with medical, behavioral, and social factors contributing to poor growth, but whatever the cause, failure to thrive reflects undernutrition of a child (**568**). The evaluation for FTT can become arduous and expensive, and in many cases, a clear-cut etiology is not found.

Introduction

In some circumstances, failure to thrive may be a presentation of child neglect. Neglect is defined as not meeting a child's basic needs, including adequate food and nurturing, which can result in actual or potential harm[5]. In the context of neglect, FTT may be due to inadequate nutrition, inadequate nurturing, or inadequate bonding between a child and his or her caregiver. When FTT is caused by neglect, certain risk factors are present, which are listed in *Table 19*. Risk factors for neglect as a cause of FTT may be secondary to parenting, infant, or family problems. Any of these risk factors may lead to inconsistent feeding patterns, decreased nutrition, decreased growth, and increased family stress[6]. It is important that these risk factors be positively identified and not simply assumed in the absence of a medical cause of FTT[5,7]. It is also important to note that these risk factors may be present in a child with medical problems which can also account for poor weight gain. Therefore, all potential causes must be investigated thoroughly.

If diagnosed and treated early, the prognosis of FTT may be favorable[8]. This chapter will examine the etiology, diagnosis, and management of failure to thrive, with special attention to its presentation in child neglect.

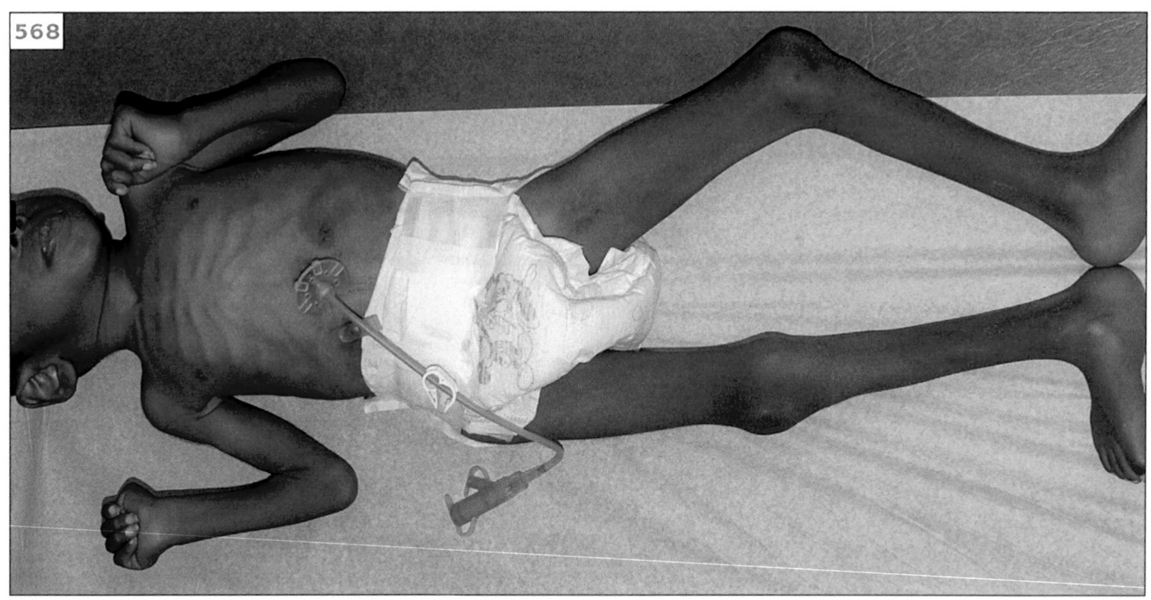

568 A 5-year-old boy who had normal growth until 2 months of age, when he developed intractable seizures. The etiology of the seizures remains unknown; however, growth remains poor despite gastrostomy tube feedings. This child exhibits typical features of long-standing failure to thrive: long, thin extremities, no subcutaneous fat, and a protuberant abdomen.

Table 19 **Risk factors present when failure to thrive is caused by neglect**

PARENTING PROBLEMS	INFANT PROBLEMS	FAMILY PROBLEMS
Parents with inadequate adaptive social behavior	Infant is preterm or born at a low birth weight	Lack of extended family
Parent is an adolescent	Infant was hospitalized during the postnatal period	Social isolation of the family
Parent has a history of abuse as a child	Difficult temperament	Substance abuse
Maternal depression		Family violence, single parenthood, employment instability, poverty

Definition

Failure to thrive is due to inadequate caloric intake (or utilization) resulting in inadequate weight gain. On the National Center for Health Statistics (NCHS) (United States) growth curves, this is manifested by being below the third percentile for height and weight, weight for length being less than 80% of ideal body weight, or by crossing two major percentile lines below the previously established rate of growth[2,3,6,9,10]. This condition is generally seen in infants and young children, and many authors limit this definition to include children younger than age 2 years[3,11]. Failure to thrive is usually accompanied by normal height velocity. However, when failure to thrive becomes chronic, there is an associated deceleration in height. In severe cases, there is a decrease in head circumference growth velocity due to poor brain growth. In itself, failure to thrive is not a diagnosis, but rather a sign of an underlying condition contributing to a child's poor growth[3,12].

Previously, the terms 'organic failure to thrive' and 'nonorganic failure to thrive' had been used to distinguish between medical causes and environmental causes of growth failure, respectively. This distinction has been abandoned as being simplistic. It is rare that this condition is caused by any one etiology, but rather it is reflective of the effects of organic disease combined with concurrent psychosocial problems[4,6,13]. In fact, the majority of cases of FTT are not due to strictly medical conditions, but rather due to social/behavioral issues or a combination of both (**569**)[3,4,8].

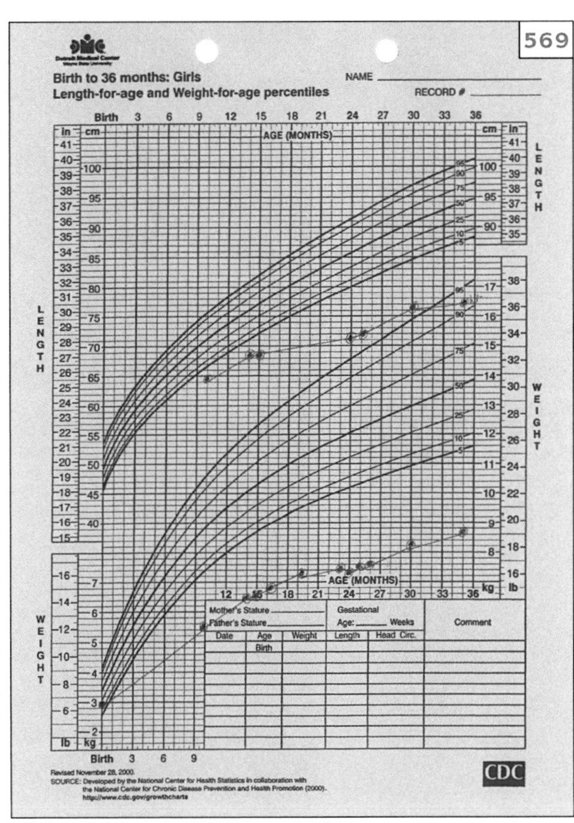

569 The growth chart of a patient born prematurely to a drug-dependent mother. She also had developmental delay, mild bronchopulmonary dysplasia, and gastroesophageal reflux disease. The patient was placed in the care of a relative. Her rate of growth remains poor.

In the case of child neglect, failure to thrive is the failure to maintain an established pattern of growth and development by providing adequate nutrition and emotional support to the patient[5,6].

Etiology

Failure to thrive is due to malnutrition and the failure to support normal growth and development in an infant or young child. This condition usually results from the interaction between the environment and the child's health, development, and behavior[8]. There are three major pathways that lead to FTT: (1) inadequate caloric intake, (2) decreased caloric absorption, or (3) increased caloric expenditure (*Table 20*). In some cases, a child may have an underlying medical condition that is exacerbated by the social environment leading to poor growth.

Children who fail to thrive because of inadequate caloric intake may have difficulties with obtaining food, the appropriate selection and preparation of food, or the actual mechanics of eating. In the context of neglect and abuse, children may not produce, or their parents may not perceive, hunger cues. This may account for children of adolescent parents being at an increased risk of neglect and growth failure[14]. In extreme cases, food may be intentionally withheld. Children who have growth failure secondary to inadequate caloric absorption may lose calories through vomiting, diarrhea, or impaired absorption from the gastrointestinal tract. Children who do not gain weight due to increased caloric needs may have an increased metabolic rate or inefficient use of calories, which is seen in several chronic medical conditions listed in *Table 20* and illustrated in **570**.

Along with the causes of FTT, there are several social and behavioral factors that may contribute to a child's poor growth (*Tables 19* and *21*). It is well established that poverty, maternal depression, and neglect are all linked with FTT[4,15–17]. Children living at or below the US federal poverty line are at a higher risk for failure to thrive due to inadequate access to food. Poverty has been associated with not only social problems (parental mental health disorders, inadequate food supplies), but also with chronic medical conditions. Lead poisoning and anemia, for example, as well as chronic medical conditions may take longer to be diagnosed due to

Table 20 **Major pathways leading to failure to thrive**

INADEQUATE CALORIC INTAKE	INADEQUATE CALORIC ABSORPTION	INCREASED CALORIC EXPENDITURE
Inadequate food supplies	Malabasorption	Cardiac disease
Child abuse/neglect	Gastrointestinal diseases	Renal disease
Improper formula mixing	Chronic diarrhea	Pulmonary disease
Breastfeeding problems	Food protein allergies	Malignancy
Excessive juice intake	Vitamin/nutrient deficiencies	Cerebral palsy
Neurologic disease		Metabolic diseases
Oromotor dysfunction		Chronic infections
Sensory food aversions		Chromosomal anomalies
Behavior disorders		

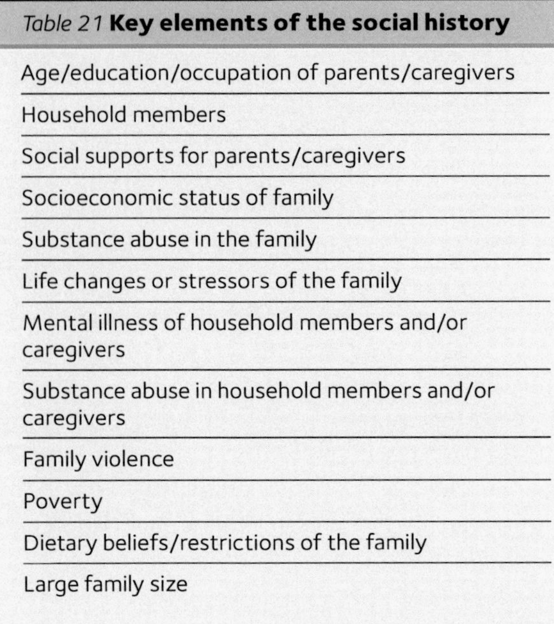

Table 21 **Key elements of the social history**
Age/education/occupation of parents/caregivers
Household members
Social supports for parents/caregivers
Socioeconomic status of family
Substance abuse in the family
Life changes or stressors of the family
Mental illness of household members and/or caregivers
Substance abuse in household members and/or caregivers
Family violence
Poverty
Dietary beliefs/restrictions of the family
Large family size

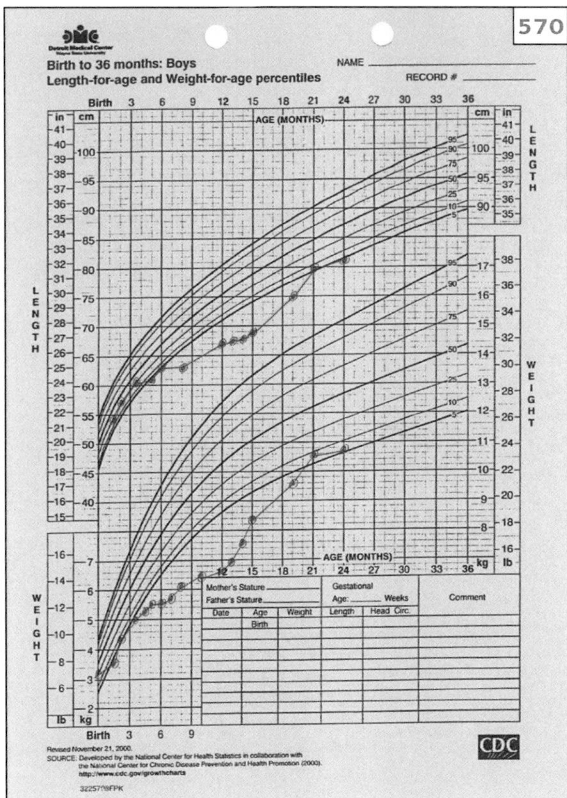

570 Growth chart of an infant boy who presented with decreased appetite and weight loss. The parents stated that the patient was irritable and preferred drinking water to formula. Laboratory testing confirmed type IV renal tubular acidosis. Polycitra (an alkalinizing solution) was started at 7 months of age. An increase in growth quickly followed.

poor access to care. Delays in obtaining treatment or surgical correction arise because of this. Parents who have unusual beliefs regarding what children should or should not eat may cause inadequate oral intake. For example, parents who believe in highly restrictive diets may cause their children to lack the nutrients necessary for growth. Certain folk medicines or traditional remedies may in fact have toxins that may cause growth failure. Children with behavioral or temperamental issues may exhibit feeding difficulties. Parents obsessed with neatness will prevent their children from normal feeding and food exploration, which may be messy, thus discouraging a child to feed. Parents who are depressed or have other mental illnesses may not be capable of properly preparing food and feeding the child at regular intervals. Parent–child dyads with poor attachment may result in failure to thrive. Physicians should assess a child's social environment along with investigating the medical etiology to determine the cause of a child's growth failure.

It is important to take into account that there are normal patterns of low weight for age or low rate of weight gain. These occur due to genetic potential, constitutional growth delay, prematurity, and postnatal 'catch down' growth of large infants whose rate of height gain increases while rate of weight gain decreases. For children with short stature, it is important to rule out genetic and constitutional causes of poor linear growth. Infants with constitutional delay or who are premature may eventually catch up with their peers and attain a normal height and weight for age. Genetically small children usually have low weight and length/height for age, but are proportionate and grow parallel to the standard growth curve (**571**).

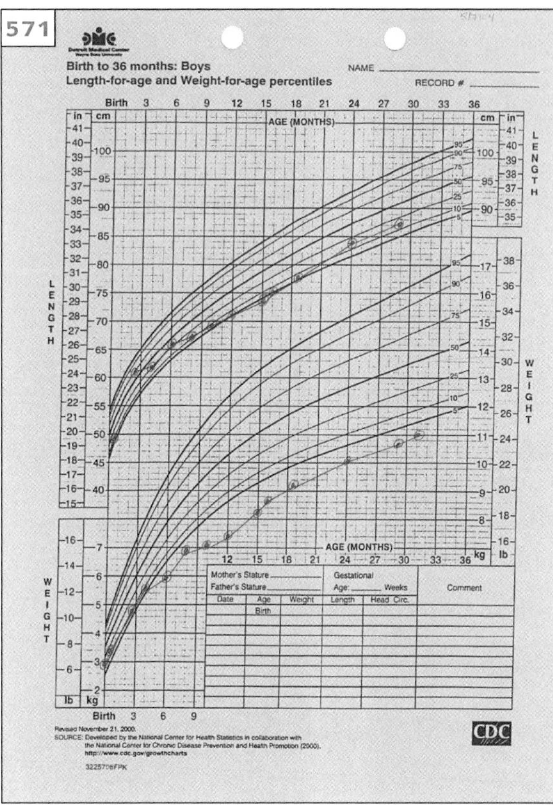

571 This figure shows the growth chart of an infant boy who was born at term without any complications. He remained healthy, but had a slow weight gain. He had a thorough evaluation for failure to thrive, which showed no abnormalities. Family history revealed that the patient's father had a similar growth pattern during infancy and early childhood. The patient was subsequently diagnosed with constitutional growth delay. Note how the growth percentiles parallel the 5th percentile line.

Clinical history

As with any illness, a thorough history and physical examination will assist in guiding physicians towards the correct etiology of failure to thrive. The prenatal history should focus on exposures and toxins that may interfere with normal fetal growth and development. Birth history complications may help distinguish between FTT and small for gestational age. A history of previous miscarriages and birth weights and lengths of previous children should also be documented.

Anthropomorphic measurements at birth should be carefully plotted so that reliable trends can be followed. It is important to know if the patient has always been small, or if there has been a steady decline from a certain time. It should be noted that the percentile for weight in healthy babies may vary until 13 months. Apgar scores, length of time in the hospital after birth, history of intubation, and gavage feeding may lead to clues regarding feeding and attachment problems. Knowledge of the newborn blood screen results may lead to an underlying metabolic or genetic disorder.

The nutritional history may also reveal clues as to an underlying medical or social/behavioral cause of FTT. Dietary recalls extending to 2–3 days are useful, especially if the utensils used at home are brought in to see the actual amounts of food being offered and fed. Types and changes of formulas, formula preparation, length of time breastfed, and the timing of the introduction of solids are also important to assess to know if the number of calories offered is adequate. Parents' understanding of how his/her child tolerates each feed, accepts new foods, and elimination patterns are important historical information. Finally, it is important to identify who feeds the baby and if there is a change in the child's behavior with different caregivers.

The feeding behavior of the patient with the caregiver is an important component that may shed light on the etiology of growth failure. Timing of growth failure in relation to the introduction of solid foods or restriction of self-feeding may be a clue to oromotor dysfunction or an eating disorder secondary to parental overinvolvement. It is also important to know if there is a history of vomiting or regurgitation that may indicate gastroesophageal reflux disease or rumination. A history of choking during feedings may indicate an anatomic defect, such as a vascular ring or tracheoesophageal fistula. A history of a weak suck may be seen in oromotor dysfunction, neurologic disease, or severe malnutrition. Infants who are disinterested in feeding may have an attachment disorder. A history of pica may lead to an underlying vitamin deficiency, anemia, or lead poisoning. Children at this young age who are labeled as 'picky' may actually have behavioral or temperamental problems. It has been previously shown that infants with difficult feeding behaviors (increased refusal of foods and decreased appetite) are more at risk for FTT[18–21]. In fact, parents whose children are difficult feeders may adversely affect weight gain by becoming overly involved in feeding[18].

A history of hospitalizations or surgery may give clues to a chronic underlying illness and decreased caloric intake. In addition, a history of accidents and injuries may suggest child abuse and neglect. Acute illness may also cause a decreased caloric intake leading to a temporary decrease in growth rate. However, in this instance, growth should improve without intervention and these children need to be monitored closely.

Family history, including growth parameters and patterns of parents, grandparents, and siblings may provide insight about the patient's genetic growth potential and chromosomal, metabolic, or inherited disorders. The history of FTT in other family members is also important.

Since the etiology of FTT is usually multifactorial, physicians should assess a child's social environment along with investigating possible medical causes to determine the etiology of a child's growth failure. The elements of the social history which should be documented are listed in *Table 21*. Members of the household and all caregivers of the patient should be ascertained. As mentioned above, poverty can contribute to FTT in a variety of ways and in particular inadequate access to food and medical care may place children at risk of poor growth. Unfortunately, because of poor access, many of these children do not get recognized as having growth failure until late, which may have a negative impact on prognosis. Parental beliefs regarding child rearing and food should also be explored, as this too may influence what and how children eat. Inquiring about stressors in the family, either due to or separate from the child's poor growth may give insight into either the causes or the exacerbating factors of FTT. It is important to know if any of the household members abuse alcohol or drugs, or have mental illness, which may be contributors to abuse or neglect in the home (**572**). Previous social work intervention or referral to protective services is also important to document when considering possible neglect or abuse.

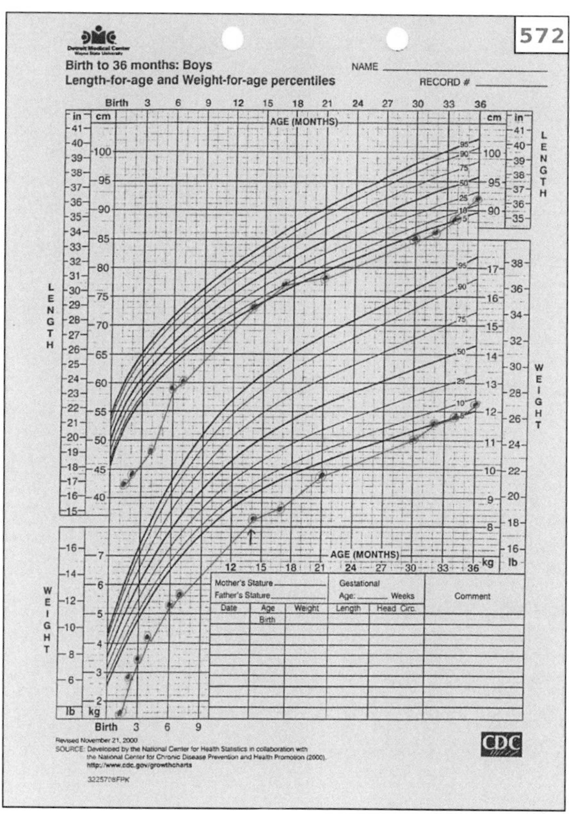

572 Growth chart of an infant whose mother was a substance abuser during and after her pregnancy. While he was living with his mother, his growth remained poor. At 14 months of age, the child's mother was incarcerated and he was placed in the custody of his maternal grandmother. His growth steadily improved thereafter.

The review of systems may also give clues to organic disease. A child's sleep history is important. Children who wake up frequently may have gastroesophageal reflux disease (GERD) or adenoid hypertrophy. Nocturnal cough may be due to uncontrolled asthma or chronic lung disease. Children with anorexia may have systemic disease, cardiac or respiratory compromise, or depression. Iatrogenic causes include medications and therapeutic diets. Children with hyperphagia may have GERD, diabetes mellitus, or diencephalic syndrome. Changes in mental status may be due to neurologic or metabolic disorders. Dysphagia may be due to oromotor dysfunction, vascular rings, esophageal webs, or neurologic conditions such as Arnold–Chiari malformation. Children with abnormal stools may have malabsorption, constipation, or inflammatory bowel disease. Children with recurrent fever may have chronic infection or a rheumatologic disorder. Children with dysuria or increased urinary frequency may have chronic renal infections, chronic renal disease, or diabetes mellitus. A decrease in activity level may be due to chronic pulmonary or cardiac disease.

Physical examination

A complete, comprehensive physical examination is essential in determining the etiology of failure to thrive. The goals of the physical examination are to identify dysmorphic features suggesting a genetic disorder, detection of an underlying disease that would impair growth, assessment for signs of possible abuse, and assessment for the severity and possible effects of malnutrition[8]. The first step is to measure the child's height, weight, and head circumference accurately and plot these values for age on an appropriate growth curve. Infants should be weighed in a dry diaper/nappy only, toddlers in underwear, and older children in light clothing or an examination gown. Recumbent length, not height, should be recorded until 2 years of age, and the head circumference until 3 years of age. Current growth parameters should be compared with previous growth measurements to assess growth trends. Children who are acutely malnourished tend to have low weight for height, and are referred to as 'wasted'. This is usually accompanied by normal height velocity. When a child is chronically malnourished, there is also a concomitant deceleration in height, which is termed 'stunting'[9]. Children with severe long-standing FTT may also show deceleration in head circumference. Premature infants should be corrected until 24 months for weight, 40 months for height, and 18 months for head circumference[9].

When assessing growth parameters, it should be noted that there are patterns of low weight for age that are not pathologic. The normal patterns of low weight for age are due to genetic potential, in which the parents are small in stature, constitutional growth delay, prematurity and postnatal 'catch down' growth. Genetic and constitutional causes of poor height growth should be ruled out in children with short stature before implicating chronic malnutrition[9]. These patterns are normal variants in which infants declare their growth curve by 6–12 months of age, and follow their individual curve as it parallels the standard growth curve. Infants with constitutional delay or who are premature may eventually catch up with their peers and attain a normal height and weight for age.

Children with pathologic growth patterns may either have normal weight for height (thus the growth parameters are proportional, but the child is small for age) or low weight for height. Genetically small children usually have low weight and height for age, but are proportional and grow parallel to the standard growth curve. Children with this pattern of growth may also have endocrine disorders, genetic disorders, long-standing failure to thrive or intrauterine growth retardation. These children should be evaluated for dysmorphology and parental heights estimated. Children who have low weight for height usually have inadequate energy intake, excessive energy losses, or malabsorption. The growth pattern of these children is such that weight falls off the growth curve first, followed by height, then head circumference. When only weight is affected, this is usually due to recent caloric deprivation. Children with this growth pattern may have any number of medical, social, or behavioral reasons for poor growth.

Physical examination findings that may indicate an etiology are outlined in *Table 22*. Along with the comprehensive physical examination, attention should also be paid to the maternal–child interaction, the overall hygiene of the child, and the child's development. Observation of certain behaviors may indicate that failure to thrive is secondary to neglect, such as gaze avoidance, decreased vocalization, or refusing to attach or respond to the caregiver[10]. Studies of observed interactions between mothers and infants with failure to thrive compared with infants with normal growth showed that the infants with failure to thrive had increased negative behaviors, including decreased vocalization, gaze aversion, unsociability, and increased fussiness. Mothers of these infants also characterized these behaviors as negative, which may impact the mother–child interaction during feeding and other times[21]. It is also important to note that some feeding behaviors leading to FTT may actually be due physical causes (**573**). Iron deficiency in infancy may cause anorexia, irritability, and lack of interest in surroundings. Likewise, zinc deficiency and lead toxicity may also be related to lack of appetite and decreased intake of food (**574**). Behaviors associated with neurologic disease, include arching, increased tone, and unusual body movements. Oromotor dysfunction (choking, gagging, weak suck) may be secondary to neuromuscular disease, whereas spitting and refusing the nipple may indicate a behavioral or social problem (**575**).

Table 22 **Findings of physical examination in failure to thrive**
Edema
Wasting
Hepatomegaly
Rash/skin changes
Hair changes (alopecia, texture)
Mental status changes
Dental caries
Palate deformities
Glossitis
Neck masses
Murmurs/arrthymias
Nail abnormalities
Spine/back problems
Abnormal deep tendon reflexes
Tone, gait, muscle mass
Dysmorphisms
Neurocutaneous findings
Abuse scars
Dehydration
Delayed tooth eruption

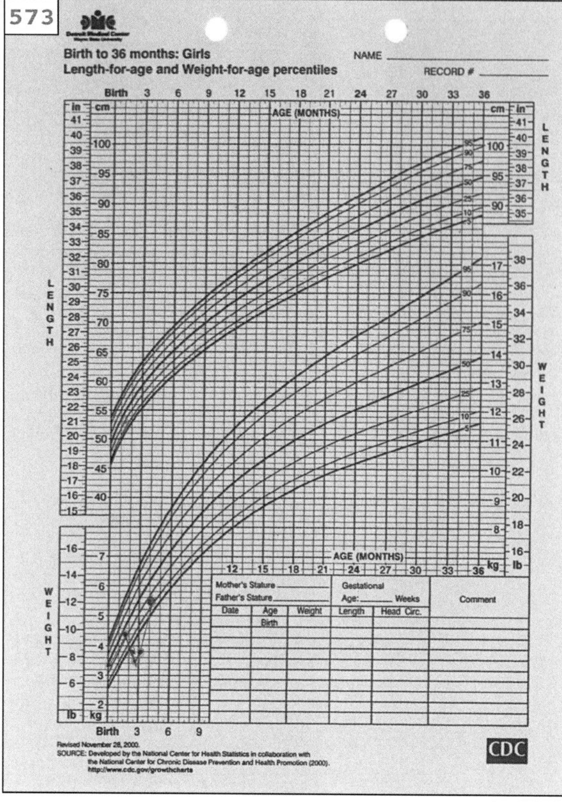

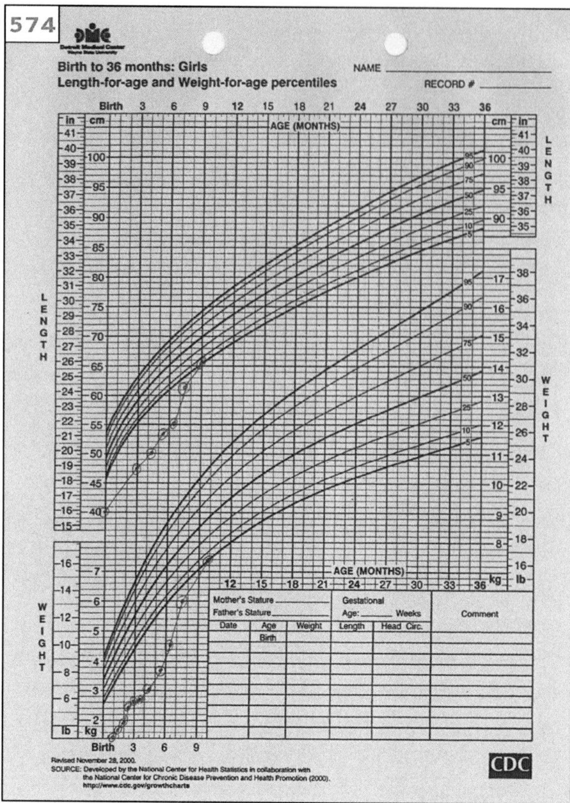

573 Growth chart of an infant who was initially healthy, and developed vomiting at 6 weeks of age, after being weaned from the breast. The baby was admitted because of severe weight loss, weakness, and an inefficient suck. Laboratory tests confirmed cow's milk protein allergy. The patient was initially treated with nasogastric tube feedings with a protein hydrolysate formula and intensive occupational therapy. The child gradually improved by nippling all feeds and gaining weight.

574 The growth chart of a patient born at 28 weeks gestational age. She was exclusively breastfed and demonstrated good catch-up growth until 2.5 months of age. The patient also had a persistent diaper/nappy dermatitis and peri-oral rash. Serum zinc levels were found to be low. Supplemental zinc was added at 4 months of age and the patient's growth improved.

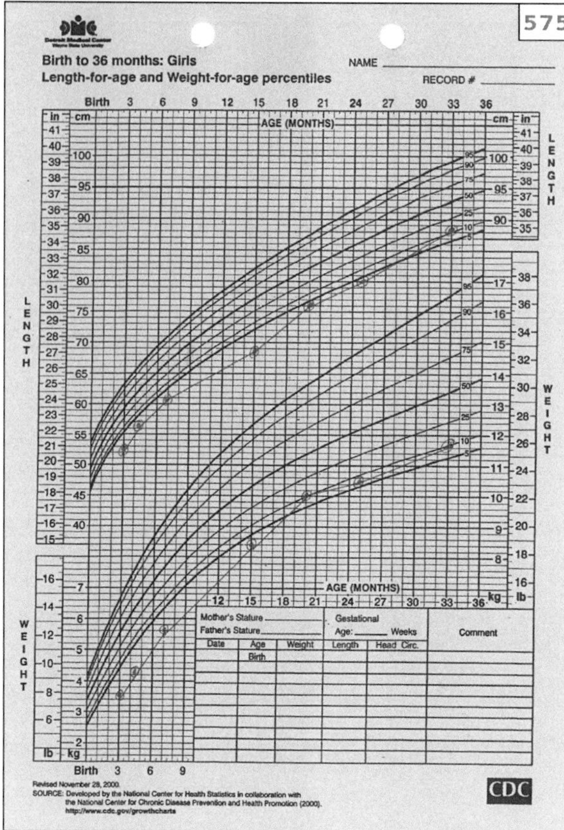

575 The growth chart of a patient born at 35 weeks gestational age to a drug-dependent mother. The child also has gastroesophageal reflux disease, and was started on medication at 1 month of age. The medication improved the reflux symptoms; however the patient refused oral feedings. Occupational therapy was initiated, but the patient was not able to take in sufficient calories orally to maintain adequate growth. A fundoplication and insertion of a gastrostomy feeding tube were performed at 8 months of age and subsequently the patient's rate of growth improved.

Differential diagnosis

As mentioned above, the differential diagnosis of failure to thrive is vast, and the comprehensive history and physical examination may point the physician in the direction of the etiology. There are some broad categories that can help narrow down the differential. For children who are also short, familial short stature, chromosomal abnormalities, skeletal dysplasias, endocrine disorders, constitutional growth delay, and long-standing failure to thrive should be considered. These children usually grow parallel to the fifth percentile curve. In those children whose weight is low for height, chronic diseases, systemic disorders, and social/behavioral disorders should be ruled out. Children with microcephaly should be evaluated for TORCH (toxoplasmosis, rubella, cytomegalovirus, herpes simplex virus) infections, teratogenic/genetic disorders, brain injury, or long-standing failure to thrive. For those children with a history of intra-uterine growth retardation, metabolic syndromes, intra-uterine infections, and poor maternal nutrition should be considered as etiologies (*Table 23*).

Table 23 **Differential diagnosis of failure to thrive (FFT) based on growth patterns**

Low weight for height	Normal weight for height	Microcephaly
Chronic disease	Familial short stature	Intra-uterine infections
Systemic disorder	Intra-uterine growth retardation	Teratogens
Social/behavioral problem	Chromosomal anomalies	Brain injury
	Genetic disorders	Long-standing FTT
	Skeletal dysplasias	
	Endocrine diseases	
	Constitutional growth delay	
	Long-standing FTT	

Laboratory investigations

Laboratory investigations should be directed by the history and physical examination. Few routine tests are recommended if there is no direction suggested by the comprehensive history and physical examination. Should these suggest a chronic medical condition, general screening laboratory tests, including a complete blood count with differential, free erythrocyte protoporphyrin, urinalysis, blood urea nitrogen, serum creatinine, and electrolytes should be ordered. If there are signs of protein wasting on examination, liver function tests, including transaminases and alkaline phosphatase should be undertaken. Additional investigations, including HIV titers, tuberculin skin testing, sweat chloride test (for cystic fibrosis), serum zinc levels, metabolic/endocrine testing, stool studies, thyroid function tests, serum immunoglobulin levels, insulin-like growth factor-1 (IGF-1), insulin-like growth factor binding protein (IGF-BP3), tissue transglutaminase antibody (TTG-IgA), IgA-endomysial antibody, immunoglobulin G antigliadin antibodies (AGA-IgG) (these last three to detect celiac disease), and imaging studies, such as skeletal survey, head computed tomography/magnetic resonance imaging or bone age, should be considered where appropriate[4,9–13].

Management

The goal of treatment of failure to thrive is two-fold: to treat the underlying pathology and to attain catch-up growth. Management should begin at the time this condition first becomes apparent, by increasing caloric density of formula and foods. The diet should provide 1.5 times to twice the recommended daily allowance of calories. Multivitamins should be included and some authors recommend the addition of supplemental zinc as part of the management[11].

All caregivers should be included in the treatment program, which includes education regarding the condition, optimal feeding strategies, and ensuring adequate resources for obtaining formula and supplies. Any social conditions that may influence caloric intake should also be addressed. Referral to a dietician is useful to help with the management plan. If the child shows any developmental delays, a community intervention program should be involved in the care as well. If oromotor dysfunction is a problem, occupational therapists should be consulted to evaluate and improve these skills.

All patients with FTT should be followed closely, initially weekly, then monthly for monitoring of growth and coordinating the care with community agencies or subspecialists. There are some circumstances in which hospitalization is warranted. Patients with severe malnutrition or dehydration should be hospitalized for close monitoring and possible intravenous therapy. Those children who are being abused and require immediate removal from the family should be hospitalized (**576**). Children with serious intercurrent illness may require hospitalization for close observation until weight has stabilized. Children whose parents are overwhelmed, extremely anxious, or impaired should be admitted. Those who have failed to respond to outpatient management in 2–3 months will require inpatient treatment.

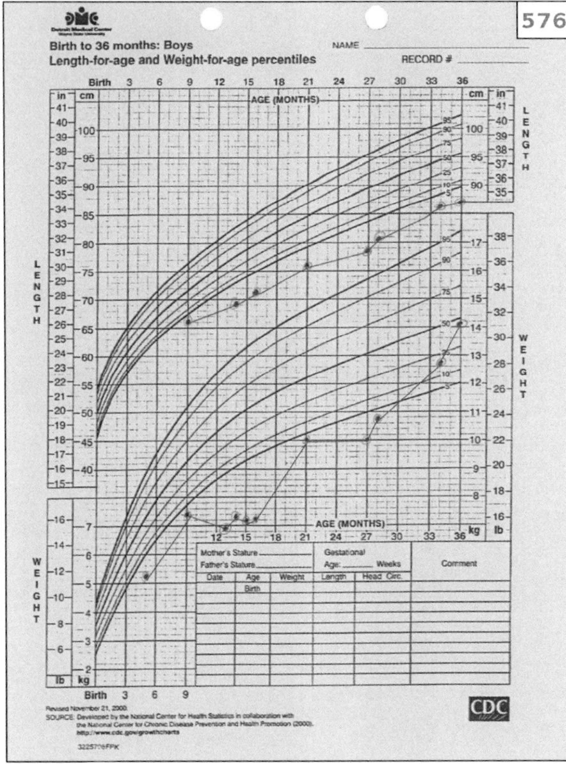

576 This figure shows the growth chart of a young boy who presented with severe gastroesophageal reflux disease (GERD) and recurrent septicemia. The patient's growth steadily declined despite medical and surgical interventions. Because of his poor response to treatment, the patient was scheduled to undergo a small-bowel transplant at 12 months of age. The day before surgery, the mother was witnessed contaminating the patient's central line with feces. The diagnosis of Munchausen syndrome by proxy was made. The patient's mother was incarcerated and the child was placed in custody of his father. No further medical problems were reported and the child's weight improved steadily.

Prognosis

Long-term outcome can be promising if intervention and treatment are initiated early. For patients with failure to thrive secondary to organic disease, detection, and treatment of the underlying disorder will improve the outcome significantly. Studies have been undertaken in infants and young children with social/emotional failure to thrive to look at long-term outcome. Many of the studies report that by the time these children enter school at age 4 years, they are smaller than same-aged peers and score slightly lower in cognitive scores. By the time these children reached age 5–6 years, they were still smaller than their peers, but there were no differences in IQ (intelligence quotient) scores[22]. However, these children scored lower than normal-sized peers in mathematics, reading, and memory skills and had increased internalizing behaviors in the classroom[23,24]. Of note, these studies showed that the maternal IQ was the strongest predictor of a child's IQ, especially when recovering from FTT. Children with FTT who were also poor and/or a victim of neglect also had lower cognitive scores compared with their peers, thus indicating that accumulation of risk factors may be detrimental to cognitive function[25]. In general, children who received multidisciplinary interventions, especially programs that include home visits, seem to have a better prognosis in the long run[26–29].

Teaching points

- Failure to thrive can be caused by medical or social/behavioral problems in children.
- In many instances, the cause is multifactorial and the etiology is usually not very clear.
- Once a patient presents with poor growth, a comprehensive history and physical examination must be undertaken and the patient should be started on a high-calorie diet and vitamin supplements.
- Good outcomes are usually associated with early detection and intervention.
- Children with failure to thrive usually remain smaller than their peers; however, differences in cognitive functioning may improve with age.

Chapter 13

MUNCHAUSEN SYNDROME BY PROXY

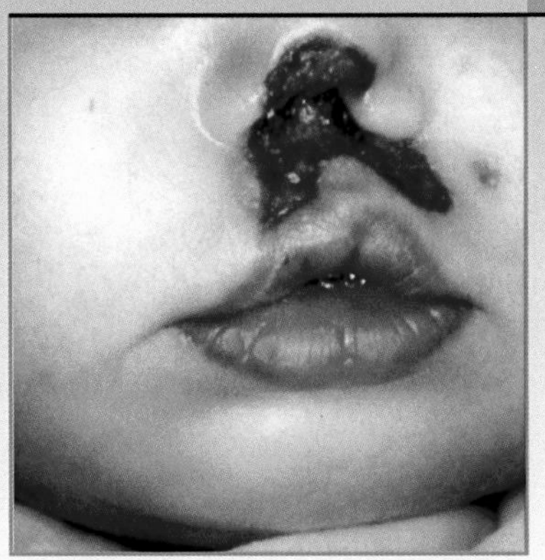

Howard Fischer MD

Munchausen syndrome by proxy (MBP) is a form of child abuse. In this premeditated form of abuse, a parent fraudulently convinces physicians that the child has medical problems, for which the physician orders unnecessary investigations and treatment, which may include surgery. MBP was first described in 1977 by Roy Meadow, a pediatric nephrologist[1]. He had been treating a child for recurrent hematuria, but was unable to find the cause. After much investigations and thought, Dr Meadow realized that the urine specimens that had been handled by the mother contained blood, whereas those collected in the mother's absence did not. The only possible explanation was that the mother was deliberately tampering with the child's urine samples. Dr Meadow called this Munchausen syndrome by proxy, borrowing the term 'Munchausen syndrome' from an earlier publication by Asher[2] in which the syndrome was named after Baron Von Munchausen, a fictitious notorious liar, and referred to adult patients fabricating their medical history and symptoms. When a parent lies about child's medical problems, the 'by proxy' is added to the definition.

Introduction

Case report

Two 6-month-old twin boys were transferred from a local emergency department to a children's hospital for evaluation of nasal destruction. Other than stating that both children had been dropped on their faces in separate incidents on the same day, 8 weeks before this presentation, the boys' mother had no explanation for the injuries. Before this admission, she had brought the children for medical evaluation three times in 7 weeks.

The twins were the product of an uncomplicated term pregnancy and a normal labor and delivery. On physical examination, they were thin, in no distress, and had normal vital signs. Twin A, the more severely injured of the two, had a loss of the nasal tip, columella, and distal septum, with collapse of the nares. There was crusted excoriation flanking the philtrum bilaterally (**577**). His brother's nasal injuries were less extensive. The remaining physical examinations were normal. Investigations included complete hemograms, blood cultures, serologic tests for syphilis, wound cultures, facial bone and skeletal survey radiographs. All were normal.

After investigation by child protective services, the children were placed in foster care. There was no further progression of the injuries.

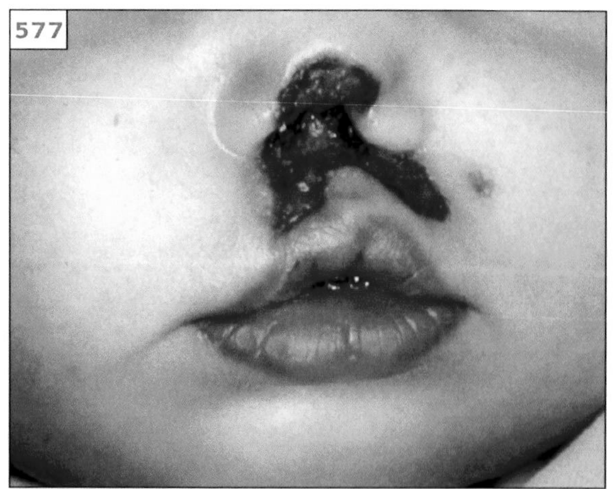

577 Nasal destruction. Reproduced with permission from Fischer H, Allasio D (1996). Nasal destruction due to child abuse. Clinical Pediatrics **35**:165–166[26].

Definition

Meadow and others[3,4] have suggested the following criteria for the diagnosis of MBP:

- Illness in a child that is simulated (faked) and/or produced by a parent or someone who is *in loco parentis*
- Presentation of the child for medical assessment and care, usually persistently, often resulting in multiple medical procedures
- Denial of knowledge by the perpetrator of the etiology of the child's illness
- Cessation of symptoms and signs when the child is separated from the perpetrator

Some authors[5,6] find it useful to separate the child abuse component of MBP (pediatric condition falsification) from the presumed parental motive (factitious disorder by proxy). This assignment of diagnoses to both parent and child may be helpful in reinforcing to the child protection and legal systems that to protect the child, both components of the diagnosis must be addressed.

Incidence and prevalence

Over 700 cases of MBP have been reported from 52 countries[7], but its prevalence is not known. McClure *et al.*[8] published a survey completed by consultant pediatricians, in the United Kingdom and Republic of Ireland. They estimated an annual incidence of about 2.8/100,000 children under 1 year of age and about 0.5/100,000 children under 16 years of age. If extrapolated to the United States population, we should expect about 625 new cases per year. As physicians become more aware of the condition's existence and presentations, more cases will probably be diagnosed[5,8,9]. It is worth remembering that MBP is based on deception; physicians will suspect and diagnose MBP only when the deception fails[10].

Victims and perpetrators

A literature review of 117 cases in 1987 by Rosenberg[11] provides much of the demographic data on MBP[12]. Males and females are equally victimized. More than one child in a family may be involved. Infants and toddlers (i.e. preverbal children) are frequent victims, but the age group of affected children ranges from newborn to 20 years. There is usually a delay of 14 months or more between the onset of symptoms and the correct diagnosis. In 95% of cases the perpetrators are biological mothers. The remaining 5% include grandmothers, foster mothers, and occasionally biological fathers[8].

Clinical presentation

In MBP an illness may be exaggerated, fabricated (i.e. lied about), simulated (e.g. samples may be altered to give the appearance of disease, such as adding blood to the stool or urine) or produced (i.e. the child is actually made ill, by poisoning, injection of contaminated material into an intravenous line, or other means). Sometimes the production of illness results in the death of the child. Common clinical symptoms and their prevalence, as reported by Rosenberg[11], are given in *Table 24*.

The prevalence adds up to more than 100% because many children had more than one presenting problem. Several of these symptoms may not be associated with clinical signs. Diagnosis is often based on parental history. The actual variety of symptoms, signs, and laboratory findings reported in MBP is enormous, and is limited only by the perpetrator's imagination. These are given in *Table 25*, which also includes a few personal cases not reported in the literature[11–13].

Table 24 **Common presentations and prevalence in Munchausen syndrome by proxy[11]**

	%
Bleeding	44
Seizures	42
Central nervous system depression	19
Diarrhea	11
Vomiting	10
Fever	10
Rash	9

Table 25 **Symptoms, signs, and laboratory findings in Munchausen syndrome by proxy[11–13]**

Abdominal pain	Failure to thrive	Otitis media, externa
Anorexia	Feculent vomiting	Personality change
Apnea	Feeding problems	Poisoning
Arthralgia	Fever	Polydipsia
Arthritis	Food allergy	Polymicrobial bacteremia
Asthma	Glucosuria	Polyphagia
Ataxia	Hallucination	Polyuria
Bacteriuria	Headache	Pyelonephritis
Biochemical chaos	Hearing loss	Pyuria
Bleeding diathesis	Hematemesis	Rash
Bleeding: ears, mouth, rectum, vagina, upper respiratory tract	Hematochezia	Renal failure
Bradycardia	Hematuria	Renal calculi

(*continues*)

Table 25 **Symptoms, signs, and laboratory findings in Munchausen syndrome by proxy[11–13] (*continued*)**

Catheter sepsis	Hemophilia	Respiratory distress
Chest pain	Hemoptysis	Seizures
Cerebral palsy	HIV infection	Septic arthritis
Cutaneous abscess	Hyperactivity	Shock
Cyanosis	Hypernatremia	Sickle cell anemia[a]
Cystic fibrosis	Hypertension	Stupor
Contaminated urine	Hypokalemia	Unconsciousness
Coma	Hyponatremia	Unimicrobial bacteremia
Dehydration	Hypothermia	Urinary gravel
Delirium	Hypotonia	Vaginitis
Dermatitis artefacta	Hypochromic, microcytic anemia	Ventricular tachycardia
Diabetes	Immunodeficiency	Vomiting
Diaphoresis	Insomnia	Weakness
Dysuria	Irritability	Weight loss
Easy bruising	Lethargy	
Eczema	Leukemia[a]	
Edema	Leukopenia	
Epistaxis	Myalgia	
Esophageal burns	Nystagmus	

[a]Unreported data (H. Fischer).

The harm done

Victims of MBP suffer physical, emotional, and psychological harm[14]. According to the study by Rosenberg, all children have short-term morbidity, defined as pain or illness without permanent disfigurement or impairment[11]. Long-term morbidity, that is, permanent disfigurement or impairment of function, was seen in 8%. Much of it was iatrogenic, surgically produced; some was the result of parent-induced hypoxia. Deliberate noncompliance with treatment for a true medical condition may lead to exacerbation of the condition or to more invasive diagnostic or therapeutic approaches[15]. Mortality of victims and their siblings ranges from 9 to 30%. Hyperactivity and school problems may also result from MBP. The most long-lasting psychological effect is the violation of a child's trust in the parent–child relationship[7].

Perpetrator motivation

It is not clear why mothers injure or kill their children. They seem to need to be the center of attention and to be praised for their patience and fortitude in coping with such ill children. Some perpetrators have no empathy for their children and use them as means to an end, namely for focusing attention on themselves[7] or for manipulating physicians[9]. In some cases, falsified childhood illness is used by the mother to keep a disinterested father involved in the family[16]. MBP, unlike physical abuse, is not reactive to frustration or anger, but is premeditated and repetitive. It results from calculated and deliberate behaviors of a perpetrator[17]. In any case, the motive of the caregiver is not important in making the diagnosis of this form of child abuse[6].

Suspecting MBP

The greatest hurdle in diagnosis is the failure to consider MBP in the differential diagnosis of an illness. Physicians may not realize that the presence of a real illness does not preclude the coexistence of MBP[5]. They may acknowledge that MBP exists, but do not consider it in their own patients. Some physicians think it is not possible that mothers would deliberately harm their children[18]. As pediatricians, we are trained to view the mother as our ally and chief source of reliable history about the child's illness.

There are several warning signs, which should make the pediatrician suspect the possibility of MBP. These warning signs, when taken individually are nonspecific, but could indicate MBP when taken collectively. They may be thought of as illness-related signs (*Table 26*), perpetrator warning signs (*Table 27*), and parent–child relationship warning signs (*Table 28*)[7].

Table 26 **Illness-related warning signs for Munchausen syndrome by proxy[7]**
Unexplained, recurrent, or prolonged illness leading to several hospitalizations and multiple medical procedures
Discrepancy between reported history and child's appearance, examination, and laboratory results
Symptoms are difficult to verify
Poor response to usual treatments

Table 27 **Perpetrator warning signs for Munchausen syndrome by proxy[7]**
Mother usually very attentive, loving, and cooperative
Intense desire to maintain close relationship with medical staff
Overly involved with others (parents, patients) on ward
Inappropriate affect involving child's medical condition
Immediate acceptance of recommendation for invasive or painful procedures
Failure to express relief at negative test findings
Increased uneasiness as child recovers
Resistance to having child discharged from hospital
Has a medical history similar to that of her child
History of factitious disorder
Familiar with medical terminology or has medical background
Reports numerous dramatic life events
No obvious psychopathology

Table 28 **Parent–child relationship warning signs for Munchausen syndrome by proxy**
Mother always at child's bedside
Mother insists on doing routine medical or nursing care in hospital
Child may exhibit passive tolerance for painful procedures
Child's symptoms diminish or cease when away from mother
Child responds to usual medical treatment when away from mother
Older child may collude with mother

Differential diagnosis

Most parents persistently present their child for medical care because the child is ill. The child may also suffer from[14]:

- Psychogenic illness (emotional origin)
- An anxious parent (no fabrication)
- A parent using the child for financial gain (malingering: fabrication present)
- Vulnerable child syndrome. The child's health has been threatened in the past. The parent continues to be deeply concerned about the child's health (no fabrication: misperception present).
- Parental symptom overemphasis. The parent does not accept credible reassurance regarding minor symptoms. 'Doctor shopping' occurs (no fabrication; misperception and some exaggeration).
- Parental extreme illness exaggeration (fabrication; a form of MBP).

Confirming the diagnosis

The presence of several warning signs should make the pediatrician consider the diagnosis of MBP. In a minority of cases there will be objective evidence, for example, poison identified in the child's blood or urine, laboratory evidence that the blood in the child's stool, urine or vomit is of parental origin, observing the parent tampering with a specimen or inducing illness[16]. Unfortunately, it is usually not that easy. In the majority of cases, the next step is a comprehensive review of the child's medical records. Records must be obtained from every physician and medical facility that has diagnosed and/or treated the child. Mothers are generally willing to sign release-of-information forms and often an enormous amount of material is obtained. It needs to be reviewed with several questions in mind, which should include the following:

- Were the diagnoses made on objective evidence or only on maternal history and persistence?
- Has anyone else witnessed the symptoms described by the mother?
- Are there inconsistencies or overt lies revealed in the histories the mother has given over time (e.g. a full-term infant being described as the product of a 30-week gestation)?

If the suspecting physician has access to a hospital Child Protection Team (CPT), it is useful (and much more convenient) for the suspecting pediatrician to enlist the help of the CPT physician (who has never seen the patient) in reviewing the records[7].

Should the record indicate MBP, the Child Protective Service agency in the community (county) in which the physician saw the child must be notified of this case of suspected child abuse. The Child Protective Service system will want some form of 'proof' that MBP is present. To provide this proof, and to protect the child from further harm, it is important to establish that the mother's presence is necessary for the child's symptoms to occur. The child needs to be separated from the mother (and the immediate family)[5,8]. The hallmark of MBP is that the symptoms cease when the child is separated from the perpetrator[3,19]. Such a confirmatory separation may be accomplished by a planned hospitalization in which the mother has no unsupervised access to the child. The other form of confirmatory separation, to which protective service is less likely to agree, is placement of the child in foster care, but not with family members[20].

Covert video surveillance (CVS) of suspected abusive parents harming their children in the hospital has proven confirmatory in several series. It has, equally importantly, also exonerated several parents under suspicion[21,22]. Some experts advise that 'all tertiary care children's hospitals should develop protocols and facilities to perform CVS to detect MBP'[22]. Consultation with a child psychiatrist or pediatric psychologist is needed to evaluate the mother–child relationship, the developmental functioning of the child, and the psychiatric status of the mother[5,7].

Treatment and re-unification

In general, treatment outcome of MBP perpetrators has not been successful[23]. However, some recent success has been reported using a treatment model that guides the mother towards taking responsibility for her actions and developing empathy for her child-victim[24]. Treatment may take 3 years and is most successful if the mother starts treatment with some acknowledgment of the abuse and where mother–child contact is restricted during the early part of treatment[21]. Re-unification should not occur until the perpetrator has confessed, other family members acknowledge that abuse has occurred, and they agree to protect the child in the future. The court must require the mother, child, and family to participate in a treatment program acceptable to the CPT and must establish a monitoring system to make sure that it happens[9,23,25].

Teaching points

- MBP is a form of child abuse. It is not as rare as one might think.
- The physician must realize that MBP occurs. It should be included in differential diagnoses of unexplained recurrent illness.
- MBP may coexist with real illnesses.
- In most cases, an extensive medical record review is needed and is often helpful.
- Confirmation of the diagnosis and case management is a multidisciplinary effort.

ABBREVIATIONS

ABFO	American Board of Forensic Odontology
ALT	Alanine transaminase
ALSPAC	Avon Longitudinal Study of Parents and Children
AP	Anterior–posterior
AST	Aspartate transaminase
BSA	Body surface area
CSF	Cerebrospinal fluid
CPT	Child Protection Team
CML	Classic metaphyseal lesion
CT	Computer tomography
CVS	Covert video surveillance
CPK	Creatine phosphokinase
FTT	Failure to thrive
FSE	Fast spin echo
FLAIR	Fluid attenuating inversion recovery
FAST	Focused abdominal sonography for trauma
GERD	Gastroesophageal reflux disease
HEENT	Head, eyes, ears, nose, throat
HSP	Henoch–Schönlein purpura
HSV	Herpes simplex virus
HPV	Human papillomavirus
ITP	Immune thrombocytopenic purpura
IQ	Intelligence quotient
LSA	Lichen sclerosis et atrophicus
MRI	Magnetic resonance imaging
MRSA	Methicillin-resistant *Staphylococcus aureus*
MBP	Munchausen syndrome by proxy
NCANDS	National Child Abuse and Neglect Data System
NCHS	National Center for Health Statistics

NAT	Nonaccidental trauma
NOFTT	Nonorganic failure to thrive
NSAID	Nonsteroidal anti-inflammatory drug
NAAT	Nucleic acid amplification tests
OI	Osteogenesis imperfecta
OTC	Over-the-counter
PA	Posterior–anterior
PTT	Partial thromboplastin time
PT	Prothrombin time
PM	Psychological maltreatment
STI	Sexually transmitted infections
SDH	Subdural hematoma
SIDS	Sudden infant death syndrome
SUIDI	Sudden Unexpected Infant Death Investigation
TPN	Total parenteral nutrition
TORCH	Toxoplasmosis, rubella, cytomegalovirus, herpes simplex virus
US	Ultrasound
UGI	Upper gastrointestinal
UA	Urinalysis

REFERENCES

Chapter 1

1. Kempe CH, Silverman FN, Steele BF, *et al.* (1962). The battered child syndrome. *Journal of the American Medical Association* **181**:17–24.
2. Anne E. Casey Foundation (2001). *Kids Count Data Book: State Profiles of Child Well-being, 2000.* Author, Baltimore, MD.
3. Sirotnak AP, Grigsby T, Krugman RD (2004). Physical abuse of children. *Pediatrics in Review* **25**:264–277.
4. Finkelhor D, Jones L (2006). Why have child maltreatment and child victimization declined? *Journal of Social Issues* **62**:685–716.
5. Pratt HD, Greydanus DE (2003). Violence: Concepts of its impact on children and youth. *Pediatric Clinics of North America* **50**:963–1003.
6. US Department of Health and Human Services, Administration for Children and Families, Administration on Children, Youth and Families, Children's Bureau (2008). *Child Maltreatment 2006: Reports from the States to the National Child Abuse and Neglect Data System*. US Government Printing Office, Washington, DC.
7. Spady DW, Saunder DL, Schopflocher DP, Svenson LW (2004). Patterns of injury in children: A population-based approach. *Pediatrics* **113**:522–529.
8. Gessner BD, Moore M, Hamilton B, Muth PT (2004). The incidence of physical abuse in Alaska. *Child Abuse and Neglect* **28**:9–23.
9. Cahill LT, Kaminer RK, Johnson PG (1999). Developmental, cognitive and behavioral sequelae of child abuse. *Child and Adolescent Psychiatric Clinics of North America* **8**:827–843.
10. Kaplan SJ, Labruna V, Pelcovitz D, *et al.* (1999). Physically abused adolescents: Behavior problems, functional impairment, and comparison of informants' reports. *Pediatrics* **104**:43–49.
11. Kairys SW, Johnson CF, and the American Academy of Pediatrics (2002). The psychological maltreatment of children – technical report. *Pediatrics* **109**:68–70.
12. Dube SR, Anda RF, Felitti VJ, *et al.* (2001). Childhood abuse, household dysfunction and the risk of attempted suicide throughout the lifespan: Findings from the Adverse Childhood Experiences study. *Journal of the American Medical Association* **286**:3089–3096.
13. Kendall-Tackett K (2002). The health effects of childhood abuse: Four pathways by which abuse can influence health. *Child Abuse and Neglect* **26**:715–729.
14. Davis L, Siegel LJ (2000). Posttraumatic stress disorder in children and adolescents: A review and analysis. *Clinical Child and Family Psychology Review* **3**:135–154.

15. Sibert JR, Payne EH, Kemp AM, *et al.* (2002). The incidence of severe physical child abuse in Wales. *Child Abuse and Neglect* **26**:267–276.
16. May-Chahal C, Cawson P. (2005). Measuring child maltreatment in the United Kingdom: A study of the prevalence of child abuse and neglect. *Child Abuse and Neglect* **29**:969–984.
17. Sidebotham P, Heron J, Golding J, The ALSPAC Study Team (2002). Child maltreatment in the 'children of the nineties': deprivation, class, and social networks in a UK sample. *Child Abuse and Neglect* **26**:1243–1259.
18. Sidebotham P, Heron J, The ALSPAC Study Team of Bristol (2006). Child maltreatment in the 'children in the nineties': A cohort study of risk factors. *Child Abuse and Neglect* **30**:497–522.
19. Palusci VJ (2003). The role of the health care professional in response to victimization. In: *The Victimization of Children: Emerging Issues*. JL Mullings, JW Marquart, DJ Hartley (eds). The Haworth Maltreatment & Trauma Press, Binghamton, NY, pp. 133–171.
20. Block RW, Palusci VJ (2006). Child abuse pediatrics: A new pediatric subspecialty. *Journal of Pediatrics* **148**: 711–712.
21. Flaherty EM, Sege R, Price LL, *et al.* (2006). Pediatrician characteristics associated with child abuse identification and reporting: Results from a national survey of pediatricians. *Child Maltreatment* **11**:361–369.
22. Briere J, Berliner L, Bulkley JA, *et al.* (eds). (1996). *The APSAC Handbook on Child Maltreatment*. Sage, Thousand Oaks, CA.
23. Ricci LR (2001). Photodocumentation of the abused child. In: *Child Abuse Medical Diagnosis and Management*, 2nd edn. RM Reese, S Ludwig (eds). Lipincott, Williams & Wilkins, Philadelphia, PA, pp. 385–404.
24. Kleinman PK (1998). *Diagnostic Imaging of Child Abuse*, 2nd edn. Mosby, St Louis, MO.
25. Jenny C. and the American Academy of Pediatrics (2006). Evaluating infants and young children with multiple fractures. *Pediatrics* **118**:1299–1303.
26. Berger RP, Hymel K, Gao W (2006). The use of biomarkers after inflicted traumatic brain injury: Insight into etiology, pathophysiology, and biochemistry. *Clinical Pediatric Emergency Medicine* **7**:186–193.
27. Kellogg N, and the American Academy of Pediatrics (2005). The evaluation of sexual abuse in children. *Pediatrics* **116**:506–512.
28. Caffey J (1946). Multiple fractures of the long bones of infants suffering from chronic subdural hematoma. *American Journal of Roentgenology* **56**:163–173.
29. Caffey J (1972). On the theory and practice of shaking infants. Its potential residual effects of permanent brain damage and mental retardation. *American Journal of Diseases in Children* **124**:161–169.
30. Caffey J (1974). The whiplash shaken baby syndrome: A manual shaking by the extremities with whiplash-induced intracranial and intraocular bleeding, linked with residual permanent brain damage and mental retardation. *Pediatrics* **54**:396–403.
31. Woolley PV, Evans WA (1955). Significance of skeletal lesions in infants resembling those of traumatic origin. *Journal of the American Medical Association* **158**:539–547.
32. Helfer ME, Kemp RS, Krugman RD (eds) (1997). *The Battered Child*, 5th edn. University of Chicago Press, Chicago, IL.
33. Silverman FM (1953). The roentgen manifestations of unrecognized skeletal trauma in infants. *American Journal of Radiology* **69**:413–426.
34. Silverman FM (1972). Unrecognized trauma in infants, the battered child syndrome, and the syndrome of Ambroise Tardieu. *Radiology* **104**:347–353.
35. American Academy of Pediatrics (1966). Maltreatment of children: The physically abused child. *Pediatrics* **37**:377–381.
36. American Academy of Pediatrics (1998). Gonorrhea in prepubertal children. *Pediatrics* **101**:134–135.
37. American Academy of Pediatrics (1998). The role of the pediatrician in recognizing and intervening on behalf of abused women. *Pediatrics* **101**:1091–1092.
38. Cupoli JM, Sewell PM (1988). One thousand fifty-nine children with a chief complaint of sexual abuse. *Child Abuse and Neglect* **12**:151–162.

39. Dubowitz H (2002). Preventing child neglect and physical abuse: A role for pediatricians. *Pediatrics in Review* **23**:191–195.
40. Duhaime AC, Alario AJ, Lewander MD (1992). Head injury in very young children: Mechanisms, injury types, and ophthalmologic findings in 100 hospitalized patients younger than 2 years of age. *Pediatrics* **90**:179–185.
41. Finkelhor D (1979). Sexually victimized children. The Free Press, New York, NY.
42. Ommaya AK, Fass F, Yarnell P (1968). Whiplash injury and brain damage: An experimental study. *Journal of the American Medical Association* **204**:285–289.
43. Rimsza ME, Niggermann EH (1982). Medical evaluation of sexually abused children: A review of 311 cases. *Pediatrics* **69**:8–14.
44. Ewing-Cobbs L, Kramer L, Prasad M, *et al.* (1998) Neuroimaging, physical and developmental findings after inflicted and non-inflicted brain injury in young children. *Pediatrics* **102**:300–307.
45. Woodling BA, Heger A (1986). The use of the colposcope in the diagnosis of sexual abuse in the pediatric age group. *Child Abuse and Neglect* **10**:111–114.
46. Herr S, Fallat ME (2006). Abusive abdominal and thoracic trauma. *Clinical Pediatric Emergency Medicine* **7**:149–152.
47. Siegel PT, Fischer H (2001). Munchausen syndrome by proxy: Barriers to detection, confirmation and intervention. *Children's Services: Social Policy, Research and Practice* **4**:31–50.
48. World Health Organization (1999). *Report of the Consultation on Child Abuse Prevention*. World Health Organization, Geneva.
49. Hennes H, Kini N, Palusci VJ (2001). The epidemiology, clinical characteristics and public health implications of shaken baby syndrome. *Journal of Aggression, Maltreatment and Trauma* **5**:19–40.
50. American Academy of Pediatrics (2001). Shaken baby syndrome: Rotational cranial injuries – technical report. *Pediatrics* **108**:206–210.
51. Newton AW, Vandeven AM (2006). Unexplained infant and child death: A review of sudden infant death syndrome, sudden unexplained infant death, and child maltreatment fatalities including shaken baby syndrome. *Current Opinion in Pediatrics* **18**:196–200.
52. American Medical Association Council on Scientific Affairs (1985). AMA diagnostic and treatment guidelines concerning child abuse and neglect. *Journal of the American Medical Association* **254**:796–800.
53. American Academy of Pediatrics, Section on Radiology (1991). Diagnostic imaging of child abuse. *Pediatrics* **87**:262–264.
54. Kini N, Lazoritz S (1998). Evaluation for possible physical or sexual abuse. *Pediatric Clinics of North America* **45**:205–219.
55. Wells RG, Vetter C, Laud P (2002). Intracranial hemorrhage in children younger than 3 years: Prediction of intent. *Archives of Pediatric and Adolescent Medicine* **156**:252–257.
56. American Academy of Pediatrics (2002). When skin injuries constitute child abuse. *Pediatrics* **110**:644–645.
57. Allasio D, Fischer H (2005). Immersion scald burns and the ability of young children to climb into a bath tub. *Pediatrics* **115**:1419–1421.
58. Adams JA, Harper K, Knudson S, Revilla J (1994). Examination findings in legally confirmed child sexual abuse: It's normal to be normal. *Pediatrics* **94**:310–317.
59. Adams JA, Kaplan RA, Starling SP, *et al.* (2007). Guidelines for medical care of children who may have been sexually abused. *Journal of Pediatric and Adolescent Gynecology* **20**:163–172.
60. American Professional Society on the Abuse of Children (1995). *Descriptive Terminology in Child Sexual Abuse Medical Evaluations*. Author, Chicago, IL.
61. Centers for Disease Control and Prevention (2006). Sexually transmitted diseases treatment guidelines, 2006. *Morbidity and Mortality Weekly Report* **55**(RR-11):1–94.
62. Giedinghagen DH, Hoff GL, Biery RM (1992). Gonorrhea in children: Epidemiologic unit analysis. *Pediatric Infectious Disease Journal* **11**:973–974.
63. Hammerschlag MR (1998). The transmissibility of sexually transmitted diseases in sexually abused children. *Child Abuse and Neglect* **22**:623–635.
64. Ingram DL, Everett VD, Flick LAR, *et al.* (1997). Vaginal gonococcal cultures in sexual abuse

evaluations: Evaluation of selective criteria for preteenaged girls. *Pediatrics* **99**:e8.

65. Ingram DL, Everett VD, Lyna PR, *et al.* (1992). Epidemiology of adult sexually transmitted disease agents in children being evaluated for sexual abuse. *Pediatric Infectious Disease Journal* **11**:945–950.

66. Robinson AJ, Watkeys JE, Ridgway GL (1998). Sexually transmitted organisms in sexually abused children. *Archive of Disease in Childhood* **79**:356–358.

67. Shapiro RA, Schubert CJ, Siegel RM (1999). *Neisseria gonorrhea* infections in girls younger than 12 years of age evaluated for vaginitis. *Pediatrics* **104**:e72.

68. Sicoli RA, Losek JD, Hudlett JM, Smith D (1995). Indications for *Neisseria gonorrhoeae* cultures in children with suspected sexual abuse. *Archives of Pediatric and Adolescent Medicine* **149**:86–89.

69. Siegel RM, Schubert CJ, Myers PA, Shapiro RA (1995). The prevalence of sexually transmitted diseases in children and adolescents evaluated for sexual abuse in Cincinnati: Rationale for limited STD testing in prepubertal girls. *Pediatrics* **96**:1090–1094.

70. Palusci VJ, Reeves M (2003). Testing for genital gonorrhea infection in prepubertal females. *Pediatric Infectious Disease Journal* **22**:618–623.

71. Muram D, Jones CE (1993). The use of videocolposcopy in the gynecologic examination of infants, children and young adolescents. *Adolescent and Pediatric Gynecology* **6**:154–156.

72. Bechtel K, Podrazik M (1999). Evaluation of the adolescent rape victim. *Pediatric Clinics of North America* **46**:809–823.

73. Palusci VJ, Cox EO, Shatz EM, Schultze J (2006). Urgent medical assessment after child sexual abuse. *Child Abuse and Neglect* **30**:367–380.

74. Greydanus DE, Shaw RD, Kennedy EL (1987). Examination of sexually abused adolescents. *Seminars in Adolescent Medicine* **3**:59–66.

75. Adams JA (2004). Medical evaluation of suspected child sexual abuse. *Journal of Pediatric and Adolescent Gynecology* **17**:191–197.

76. Palusci VJ, Cyrus TA (2001). Reaction to videocolposcopy in the assessment of child sexual abuse. *Child Abuse and Neglect* **25**:1535–1546.

77. Gushurst CA (2003). Child abuse: Behavioral aspects and other associated problems. *Pediatric Clinics of North America* **50**:919–938.

78. Drach KM, Wientzen J, Ricci LR (2001). The diagnostic utility of sexual behavior problems in diagnosing sexual abuse in a forensic child abuse evaluation. *Child Abuse and Neglect* **29**: 489–503.

79. Cahill L, Sherman P (2006). Child abuse and domestic violence. *Pediatrics in Review* **27**:339–345.

80. Sugar NF, Graham EA (2006). Common gynecologic problems in prepubertal girls. *Pediatrics in Review* **27**:213–223.

81. Ammerman RT, Hersen M, Van Hasselt, *et al.* (1989). Abuse and neglect in psychiatrically hospitalized, multihandicapped children. *Child Abuse and Neglect* **13**:335–343.

82. Helfer RE (1990). The neglect of our children. *Pediatric Clinics of North America* **37**:923–942.

83. Dubowitz H, Papas MA, Black MM, Starr RH (2002). Child neglect: Outcomes in high-risk urban preschoolers. *Pediatrics* **109**:1100–1107.

84. Liu J, Raine A, Venables PH, *et al.* (2003). Malnutrition at age 3 years and lower cognitive ability at age 11 years. *Archives of Pediatrics and Adolescent Medicine* **157**:593–600.

85. Sedlak AJ, Broadhurst DD (1996). *The Third National Incidence Study of Child Abuse and Neglect (NIS-3)*. US Department of Health and Human Services, Washington, DC.

86. Dubowitz H (2000). Child neglect: Guidance for pediatricians. *Pediatrics in Review* **21**:111–116.

87. Michigan Child Death Review State Advisory Team (2001). Child deaths in Michigan: Second annual report. Michigan Public Health Institute, Okemos, MI.

88. Coohey C (2003). Defining and classifying supervisory neglect. *Child Maltreatment* **8**:145–156.

89. Hymel KP and the American Academy of Pediatrics (2006). When is lack of supervision neglect? *Pediatrics* **118**:1296–1298.

90. Block RW, Krebs NF, and the American Academy of Pediatrics (2005). Failure to thrive as a manifestation of child neglect. *Pediatrics* **116**:1234–1237.

91. Bays J, Chadwick D (1993). Medical diagnosis of the sexually abused child. *Child Abuse and Neglect* **17**:91–110.

92. Johnson CF (1999). Medical evaluation of child abuse. *Children's Health Care* **28**:91–108.
93. Palusci VJ, Cox EO, Cyrus TA, *et al.* (1999). Medical assessment and legal outcome in child sexual abuse. *Archives of Pediatric and Adolescent Medicine* **153**:388–392.
94. Zitelli BJ, Davis HW (eds) (1987). *Atlas of Pediatric Physical Diagnosis*. CV Mosby, St Louis, MO.
95. Palusci VJ, Palusci JV (2006). Screening for sexual abuse. *Journal de Pediatrics (Rio J)* **82**:409–410.
96. US Department of Health and Human Services, Centers for Disease Control and Prevention, National Center for Health Statistics (1998). *ICD-10: International Statistical Classification of Diseases and Related Health Problems*, 10th rev. US Government Printing Office, Washington, DC.
97. Council of the American Academy of Child and Adolescent Psychiatry (1997). Statement: Practice parameters for the forensic evaluation of children and adolescents who may have been physically or sexually abused. *Journal of the American Academy of Child and Adolescent Psychiatry* **36**:423–442.
98. Newman Dorland WA (ed) (1974). *Dorland's Illustrated Medical Dictionary*, 25th edn. WB Saunders, Philadelphia, PA, pp. 435.
99. Fontana VJ (1989). Child abuse: The physician's responsibility. *New York State Journal of Medicine* **89**:152–155.
100. Paradise JE, Bass J, Forman SD, *et al.* (1995). Minimum criteria for reporting child abuse from health care settings. *Pediatric Emergency Care* **11**:335–339.
101. Migley G, Wiese D, Salmon-Cox S (1996). *World Perspectives on Child Abuse: The Second International Resource Book*. International Society for Prevention of Child Abuse and Neglect, Chicago, IL.
102. Morris JL, Johnson CF, Clasen M (1985). To report or not to report: Physicians' attitudes toward discipline and child abuse. *American Journal of Diseases of Children* **139**:194–197.
103. Johnson CF (1993). Physicians and medical neglect: Variables that affect reporting. *Child Abuse and Neglect* **17**:605–615.
104. Myers JEB (2002). Keep the lifeboat afloat. *Child Abuse and Neglect* **26**:561–567.

Further reading

American Academy of Pediatrics (2001). *Visual Diagnosis of Child Abuse* (CD-ROM). Author, Elk Grove Village, IL.
Briere J, Berliner L, Bukley JA, *et al.* (eds) (1996). *The APSAC Handbook on Child Maltreatment*. Sage, Thousand Oaks, CA.
Bross DC, Krugman RD, Lenherr MR, *et al.* (1988). *The New Child Protection Team Handbook*. Garland Publishing, New York, NY.
Frasier LD, Rauth-Farley K, Alexander R, Parrish RN (2006). *Abusive Head Trauma in Infants and Children*. GW Medical Publishing, St Louis, MO.
Helfer ME, Kemp RS, Krugman RD (eds) (1997). *The Battered Child*, 5th edn. University of Chicago Press, Chicago, IL.
Heger A, Emans SJ, Muram D (2000). *Evaluation of the Sexually Abuse Child*, 2nd edn. Oxford University Press, Oxford.
Kleinman PK (1998). *Diagnostic Imaging of Child Abuse*, 2nd edn. Mosby, St Louis, MO.
Lazoritz S, Palusci VJ (eds) (2001). *Shaken Baby Syndrome: A Multidisciplinary Approach*. Haworth Press, Philadelphia, PA.
Mullings JL, Marquart JW, Hartley DJ (eds) (2003). *The Victimization of Children: Emerging Issues*. The Haworth Maltreatment and Trauma Press, Binghamton, NY.
Reece RM, Ludwig S (2001). *Child Abuse: Medical Diagnosis and Treatment*. Lippincott Williams & Wilkins, Philadelphia, PA.
Reece RM, Nicholson CE (eds) (2003). *Inflicted Childhood Neurotrauma*. American Academy of Pediatrics, Elk Grove Village, IL.
US Department of Health and Human Services, Administration for Children and Families, Administration on Children, Youth and Families, Children's Bureau (2008). *Child Maltreatment 2006: Reports from the States to the National Child Abuse and Neglect Data System*. US Government Printing Office, Washington, DC.

Chapter 2

1. Kellogg ND and the American Academy of Pediatrics (2007). Evaluation of suspected child physical abuse. *Pediatrics* **119**:1232–1241.

2. AAP Committee on Child Abuse and Neglect (2002). When inflicted skin injuries constitute child abuse. *Pediatrics* **110**:644–645.
3. Sugar NF, Taylor JA, Feldman KW (1999). Bruises in infants and toddlers: Those who don't cruise rarely bruise. Puget Sound Pediatric Research Network. *Archives of Pediatrics and Adolescent Medicine* **153**:399–403
4. Schmitt B (1987). The child with non-accidental trauma. In: *The Battered Child*, 4th edn. RE Helfer, RS Kempe (eds). University of Chicago Press, Chicago, pp. 178–183.
5. Kos L, Shwayder T (2006). Cutaneous manifestations of child abuse. *Pediatric Dermatology* **23**:311–320.
6. Feldman KW (1992). Patterned abusive bruises of the buttocks and the pinnae. *Pediatrics* **90**:633–636.
7. McGuire S, Hunter B (2007). Diagnosing abuse: A systematic review of torn frenum and intraoral injuries. *Archives of Disease in Childhood* **92**: 1113–1117.
8. Wilson EF (1977). Estimation of the age of cutaneous contusions in child abuse. *Pediatrics* **60**: 750–752.
9. Langlois NEI, Gresham GA (1991). The ageing of bruises: A review and study of the color changes with time. *Forensic Science International* **50**: 227–238.
10. Stephenson T, Bialis Y (1996). Estimation of the age of bruising. *Archives of Disease in Childhood* **74**:53–55.
11. Maguire S, Mann MK, Sibert J, Kemp A (2005). Are there patterns of bruising in childhood which are diagnostic or suggestive of abuse? A systematic review. *Archives of Disease in Childhood* **90**:182–186.
12. Maguire S, Mann MK, Siebert J, Kemp A (2005). Can you age bruises accurately in children? A systematic review. *Archives of Disease in Childhood* **90**:187–189.
13. Carpenter RF (1999). The prevalence and distribution of bruising in babies. *Archives of Disease in Childhood* **80**:363–366.
14. Khair K, Liesner R (2006). Bruising and bleeding in infants and children – a practical approach. *British Journal of Haematology* **133**: 221–231.
15. Thomas AE (2004). The bleeding child: Is it NAI? *Archives of Disease in Childhood* **89**: 1163–1167.
16. Ricci LR (1991). Photographing the physically abused child. *American Journal of Diseases of Children* **145**:275–281.
17. Bohnert M, Baumgartner R, Pollak S. Spectrophotometric evaluation of the colour of intra- and subcutaneous bruises. *International Journal of Legal Medicine* **113**:343–348.
18. Vogeley E, Pierce MC, Bertocci PE (2002). Experience with Wood lamp illumination and digital photography in the documentation of bruises on human skin. *Archives of Pediatrics and Adolescent Medicine* **156**:265–268.

Further reading

Giardino AP, Christian CW, Giardino ER (1997). *A Practical Guide to the Evaluation of Child Physical Abuse and Neglect*. Sage, Thousand Oaks, CA.
Ludwig S, Kornberg AE (1992). *Child Abuse: A Medical Reference*, 2nd edn. Churchill Livingstone, New York.
Paller AS, Mancini AJ. (2006) *Hurwitz Clinical Pediatric Dermatology*. Elsevier Saunders, Philadelphia, PA.
Reece RM, Ludwig S (2001). *Child Abuse: Medical Diagnosis and Treatment*. Lippincott Williams & Wilkins, Philadelphia, PA.
Wissow LS (1990). *Child Advocacy for the Clinician*. Williams & Wilkins, Baltimore, MD.

Chapter 3

1. Hobbs CJ (1989). Burns and scalds. *British Medical Journal* **298**:1302–1306.
2. Monteleone JA, Brodeur AE (1998). *Child Maltreatment: A Clinical Guide and Reference*. GW Medical Publishing Inc, St Louis, MO.
3. Showers J, Garrison KM. (1988). Burn abuse: A four-year study. *Journal of Trauma* **28**:1581–1583.
4. Thompson S (2005). Burns: Accidental or inflicted? *Pediatric Annals* **34**:372–381.
5. Hobbs C, Wynne JM (2001). *Physical Signs of Child Abuse: A Colour Atlas*. WB Saunders, London.
6. Smith ML (2000). Pediatric burns: Management of thermal, electrical and chemical burns and

burn-like dermatologic conditions. *Pediatric Annals* **29**:367–378.

7. Stone N, Rinaldo L, Humphrey CR, Brown RH (1970). Child abuse by burning. *Surgical Clinics of North America* **50**:1419–1424.

8. Thombs B (2008). Patient and injury characteristics, mortality risk, and length of stay related to child abuse by burning, evidence from a national sample of 15,802 pediatric admissions. *Annals of Surgery* **247**:519–523.

9. Andronicus M, Oates RK, Peat J, *et al.* (1998). Non-accidental burns in children. *Burns* **24**:552–558.

10. Ayoub C, Pfeifer D (1979). Burns as a manifestations of child abuse and neglect. *American Journal of Diseases of Children* **133**:910–914.

11. Greenbaum A, Donne J, Wilson D, Dunn KW (2004). Intentional burn injury: An evidence based, clinical and forensic review. *Burns* **30**: 628–642.

12. Peck MD, Priolo-Kapel D (2002). Child abuse by burning: A review of the literature and an alogorithm for medical investigations. *Journal of Trauma* **53**:1013–1022.

13. Kumar P (1984). Child abuse by thermal injury – A retrospective survey. *Burns* **10**:344–348.

14. Helfer ME, Kempe RS, Krugman RD (eds) (1997). *The Battered Child.* University of Chicago Press, Chicago.

15. Allasio D, Fischer H, Mann-Gray S, *et al.* (2005). Immersion scald burns and the ability of young children to climb into a bathtub. *Pediatrics* **15**:1419–1421.

16. Chester DL, Jose RM, Aldlyami E, *et al.* (2006). Non-accidental burns in children – Are we neglecting neglect? *Burns* **32**:222–228.

17. Greenbaum AR, Horton JB, Williams CJ, *et al.* (2006). Burn injuries inflicted on children or the elderly: A framework for clinical and forensic assessment. *Plastic and Reconstructive Surgery* **118**:46–58.

Chapter 4

1. Kos L, Shwayder T (2006). Cutaneous manifestations of child abuse. *Pediatric Dermatology* **23**:311–320.

2. Stewart GM, Rosenberg NM (1996). Conditions mistaken for child abuse: Part II. *Pediatric Emergency Care* **12**:217–221.

3. Mudd SS, Findlay JS (2004). The cutaneous manifestations and common mimickers of physical child abuse. *Journal of Pediatric Health Care* **18**:123–129.

4. Dungy CI (1982). Mongolian spots, day care centers, and child abuse. *Pediatrics* **69**:672.

5. Peru H, Soylemezoglu O, Bakkaloglu SA, *et al.* (2008). Henoch Schonlein purpura in childhood: Clinical analysis of 254 cases over a 3-year period. *Clinical Rheumatology* **27**:1087–1092.

6. Grieg AV, Harris DL (2003). A study of perceptions of facial hemangiomas in professionals involved in child abuse surveillance. *Pediatric Dermatology* **20**:1–4.

7. Kruse RW, Harcke HT, Minch CM (1997). Osteogenesis imperfecta (OI) may be mistaken for child abuse. *Pediatric Emergency Care* **13**:244–245.

8. Shaw DG, Hall CM, Carty H (1995). Osteogenesis imperfecta: The distinction from child abuse and the recognition of a variant form. *American Journal of Medical Genetics* **56**:116–118.

9. Bawle EV (1994). Osteogenesis imperfecta vs. child abuse. *American Journal of Medical Genetics* **49**:131–132.

10. Hansen KK (1998). Folk remedies and child abuse: A review with emphasis on caida de mollera and its relationship to shaken baby syndrome. *Child Abuse and Neglect* **22**:117–127.

11. Amshel CE, Caruso DM (2000). Vietnamese 'coining': A burn case report and literature review. *Journal of Burn Care and Rehabilitation* **21**:112–114.

12. Ferrari AM (2002). The impact of culture upon child rearing practices and definitions of maltreatment. *Child Abuse and Neglect* **26**:793–813.

13. Coffman K, Boyce WT, Hansen RC (1985). Phytophotodermatitis simulating child abuse. *American Journal of Diseases of Children* **139**:239–240.

14. Hill PF, Pickford M, Parkhouse N (1997). Phytophotodermatitis mimicking child abuse. *Journal of the Royal Society of Medicine* **90**:560–561.

15. Carlsen K, Weismann K (2007). Phytophotodermatitis in 19 children admitted to hospital and their differential diagnoses: Child abuse and herpes

simplex virus infection. *Journal of the American Academy of Dermatology* **57**(5 Suppl):S88–S91.

16. Furniss D, Adams T (2007). Herb of grace: An unusual cause of phytophotodermatitis mimicking burn injury. *Journal of Burn Care and Research* **28**:767–769.

17. Khachemoune A, Khechmoune K, Blanc D (2006). Assessing phytophotodermatitis: Boy with erythema and blisters on both hands. *Dermatology Nursing* **18**:153–154.

18. Pomeranz MK, Karen JK (2007). Images in clinical medicine. Phytophotodermatitis and limes. *New England Journal of Medicine* **357**:e1.

19. Schmidt J (2007). Phytophotodermatitis. *Dermatology Nursing* **19**:486.

20. Kamat DM (2006). Photoclinic: Foresee your next patient: 'Popsicle' panniculitis. *Consultant for Pediatricians* **5**:729.

21. Day S, Klein BL (1992). Popsicle panniculitis. *Pediatric Emergency Care* **8**:91–93.

22. Forks TP. Brown recluse spider bites. *Journal of the American Board of Family Practitioners* **13**:415–423.

23. Nuthakki S, Schlievert R (2007). Child abuse – or mimic? Child with 'burns' on the tongue. *Consultant for Pediatricians* **6**:345–346.

24. Reinhart MA, Ruhs H (1985). Moxibustion. Another traumatic folk remedy. *Clinical Pediatrics* **24**:58–59.

25. Nazer D, Evans JB, Sawni A, Palusci VJ (2007). Child abuse or mimic? Child with bullous lesion on left side of groin. *Consultant for Pediatricians* **6**:240–246.

26. Garty BZ (1993). Garlic burns. *Pediatrics* **91**:658–659.

27. Dietz DM, Varcelotti JR, Stahlfeld KR (2004). Garlic burns: A not-so-rare complication of a naturopathic remedy? *Burns* **30**:612–613.

28. Friedman T, Shalom A, Westreich M (2006). Self-inflicted garlic burns: Our experience and literature review. *International Journal of Dermatology* **45**:1161–1163.

29. San Lazaro C (1990). Lichen sclerosis. *Archives of Disease in Childhood* **65**:1184.

30. Kanekura T, Kawamura K, Kanzaki T (1994). Lichen sclerosis et atrophicus with prominent telangiectasia. *Journal of Dermatology* **21**:447–449.

31. Pappano D (2007). Group A ß-hemolytic streptococcal vulvovaginitis. *Consultant for Pediatricians* **6**:428

Chapter 5

1. Caffey J (1946). Multiple fractures in the long bones of infants suffering from chronic subdural hematoma. *American Journal of Roentgenology* **56**:163–173.

2. Silverman FN (1953). Roentgen manifestations of unrecognized skeletal trauma in infants. *American Journal of Roentgenology* **69**:413–427.

3. Woolley PV, Evans WA (1955). Significance of skeletal lesions in infants resembling those of traumatic origin. *Journal of the American Medical Association* **158**:539–543.

4. Kempe CH, Silverman FN, Steele BF, *et al.* (1962). The battered-child syndrome. *Journal of the American Medical Association* **181**:105–112.

5. Kleinman PK (ed.) (1998). *Diagnostic Imaging of Child Abuse*, 2nd edn. Mosby, St Louis, MO.

6. Dalton HJ, Slovis T, Helfer RE, *et al.* (1990). Undiagnosed abuse in children younger than 3 years with femoral fracture. *American Journal of Diseases of Children* **144**:875–878.

7. Lonergan GJ, Baker AM, Morey MK, Boos SC (2003). Child abuse: Radiologic–pathologic correlation. *RadioGraphics* **23**:811–845.

8. Rao P, Carty H (1999). Non-accidental injury: Review of the radiology. *Clinical Radiology* **54**:11–24.

9. Nimkin K, Kleinman P (2001). Imaging of child abuse. *Pediatric Clinics of North America* **44**:615–635.

10. Chapman S (1990). Radiological aspects of non-accidental injury. *Journal of the Royal Society of Medicine* **83**:67–71.

11. Akbarnia B, Torg JS, Kirkpatrick J, Sussman S (1974). Manifestations of the battered-child syndrome. *Journal of Bone and Joint Surgery* **56A**:1159–1166.

12. Herndon WA (1983). Child abuse in a military population. *Journal of Pediatric Orthopedics* **3**: 73–76.

13. Johnson K, Chapman S, Hall CM (2004). Skeletal injuries associated with sexual abuse. *Pediatric Radiology* **34**:620–623.

14. Sty JR, Starshak RJ (1983). The role of bone scintigraphy in the evaluation of the suspected abused child. *Radiology* **146**:369–375.
15. American College of Radiology (2006). *Practice Guidelines and Technical Standards*. American College of Radiology, Reston, VA, pp. 17.
16. Merten DF, Radkwoski MA, Leonidas JC (1983). The abused child: A radiological reappraisal. *Radiology* **146**:377–381.
17. Carty HML (1993). Fractures caused by child abuse. *Journal of Bone and Joint Surgery* **75B**: 849–857.
18. Kleinman PK, Marks SC, Blackbourne B (1986). The metaphyseal lesion in abused infants: A radiologic–histopathologic study. *American Journal of Roentgenology* **146**:895–905.
19. Kleinman PK, Marks SC, Richmond JM, Blackbourne B (1995). Inflicted skeletal injury: A postmortem radiologic–histopathologic study in 31 infants. *American Journal of Roentgenology* **165**:647–650.
20. Kleinman PK (2008). Problems in the diagnosis of metaphyseal fractures. *Pediatric Radiology* **38**(Suppl 3):S388–S394.
21. Worlock P, Stower M, Barbor P (1986). Patterns of fractures in accidental and non-accidental injury in children: A comparative study. *British Medical Journal* **293**:100–102.
22. Thomas P (1977). Rib fractures in infancy. *Annales de Radiologie* **20**:155–122.
23. Kleinman PK, Marks SC, Nimkin K, *et al.* (1996). Rib fractures in 31 abused infants: Postmortem radiologic–histopathologic study. *Radiology* **200**:807–810.
24. Feldman KW, Brewer DK (1984). Child abuse, cardiopulmonary resuscitation and rib fractures. *Pediatrics* **74**:1075–1078.
25. Loder RT, Bookout C (1991). Fracture patterns in battered children. *Journal of Orthopedic Trauma* **5**:428–433.
26. Thomas SA, Rosenfeld NS, Leventhal JM, Markowitz RI (1991). Long-bone fractures in young children: Distinguishing accidental injuries from child abuse. *Pediatrics* **88**:471–476.
27. Kleinman PK, Nimkin K, Spevak MR, *et al.* (1996). Follow-up skeletal surveys in suspected child abuse. *American Journal of Roentgenology* **167**:893–896.
28. Zimmerman S, Makoroff, Care M, *et al.* (2005). Utility of follow-up skeletal surveys in suspected child physical abuse evaluations. *Child Abuse and Neglect* **29**:1075–1083.
29. Anilkumar A, Fender LJ, Broderick NJ, *et al.* (2006). The role of the follow-up chest radiograph in suspected non-accidental injury. *Pediatric Radiology* **36**:216–218.
30. Ablin DS, Greenspan A, Reinhart M, Grix A (1990). Differentiation of child abuse from osteogenesis imperfecta. *American Journal of Roentgenology* **154**:1035–1046.
31. Ablin DS, Sane SM (1997). Non-accidental injury: Confusion with temporary brittle bone disease and mild osteogenesis imperfecta. *Pediatric Radiology* **27**:111–113.
32. Taitz LS (1988). Child abuse and osteogenesis imperfecta (letter). *British Medical Journal* **296**:292.
33. Paterson CR, Burns J, McAllion SJ (1993). Osteogenesis imperfecta: The distinction from child abuse and the recognition of a variant form. *American Journal of Medical Genetics* **45**:187–192.
34. Miller ME (2003). The lesson of temporary brittle bone disease: All bones are not created equal. *Bone* **33**:466–474.
35. Smith R (1995). Osteogenesis imperfecta, non-accidental injury and temporary brittle bone disease. *Archives of Disease in Childhood* **72**: 169–176.
36. Chapman S, Hall CM (1997). Non-accidental injury or brittle bones. *Pediatric Radiology* **27**:106–110.
37. Caffey J (1972). On the theory and practice of shaking infants. *American Journal of Diseases of Children* **124**:161–169.
38. Caffey J (1974). The whiplash shaken infant syndrome: Manual shaking by the extremities with whiplash-induced intracranial and intraocular bleedings, linked with residual permanent brain damage and mental retardation. *Pediatrics* **54**:396–403.
39. Duhaime AC, Christian CW, Rorke LB, Zimmerman RA (1998). Non-accidental head injury in infants – the 'shaken baby syndrome'. *New England Journal of Medicine* **338**:1822–1829.
40. Jaspan T (2008). Current controversies in the interpretation of non-accidental head injury. *Pediatric Radiology* **38**(Suppl 3):S378–S387.

41. Merten DF, Osborne DRS (1984). Craniocerebral trauma in the child abuse syndrome: Radiological observations. *Pediatric Radiology* **14**:272–277.
42. Meservy CJ, Towbin R, McLaurin RL, *et al.* (1987). Radiographic characteristics of skull fractures resulting from child abuse. *American Journal of Roentgenology* **149**:173–175.
43. Hobbs CJ (1984). Skull fracture and the diagnosis of child abuse. *Archives of Disease in Childhood* **59**:246–252.
44. Helfer RE, Slovis TL, Black M (1977). Injuries resulting when small children fall out of bed. *Pediatrics* **60**:533–535.
45. Chadwick DL, Bertocci G, Castillo E, *et al.* (2008). Annual risk of death resulting from short falls among young children: less than 1 in 1 million. *Pediatrics* **121**:1213–1224.
46. David T (2008). Non-accidental head injury – the evidence. *Pediatric Radiology* **38**(Suppl 3): S370–S377.
47. Zimmerman RA, Bilaniuk LA, Bruce D, *et al.* (1978). Interhemispheric acute subdural hematoma: A computed tomographic manifestation of child abuse by shaking. *Neuroradiology* **16**:39–40.
48. Barnes PD, Robson CD (2000). CT findings in hyperacute nonaccidental brain injury. *Pediatric Radiology* **30**:74–81.
49. Dias MS, Backstrom J, Falk M, Li V (1998). Serial radiography in the infant shaken impact syndrome. *Pediatric Neurosurgery* **29**:77–85.
50. Tung GA, Kumar M, Richardson RC, *et al.* (2006). Comparison of accidental and nonaccidental traumatic head injury in children on noncontrast computed tomography. *Pediatrics* **118**:626–633.
51. Bradley WG Jr (1993). MR appearance of hemorrhage in the brain. *Radiology* **189**:15–26.
52. Han BK, Towbin RB, De Courten-Myers G, *et al.* (1990). Reversal sign on CT: Effect of anoxic/ischemic brain injury in children. *American Journal of Roentgenology* **154**:361–368.
53. Sato Y, Yuh WT, Smith WL, *et al.* (1989). Head injury in child abuse: Evaluation with MR imaging. *Radiology* **173**:653–657.
54. Kirks DR (1983). Radiological evaluation of visceral injuries in the battered-child syndrome. *Pediatric Annals* **12**:888–893.
55. Ledbetter DJ, Hatch EI Jr, Feldman KW, *et al.* (1988). Diagnostic and surgical implications of child abuse. *Archives of Surgery* **123**:1101–1105.
56. Sivit CJ, Taylor GA, Eichelberger MR (1989). Visceral injury in battered children: A changing perspective. *Radiology* **173**:659–661.
57. Ziegler DW, Long JA, Philippart AI, Klein MD (1988). Pancreatitis in childhood. Experience in 49 patients. *Annals of Surgery* **207**:257–261.
58. Cooney DR, Grosfeld JL (1975). Operative management of pancreatic pseudocysts in infants and children: A review of 75 cases. *Annals of Surgery* **182**:590–596.
59. Slovis TL, Berdon WE, Haller JO, *et al.* (1975). Pancreatitis and the battered child syndrome: Report of two cases with skeletal involvement. *American Journal of Roentgenology* **125**:456–461.
60. Cooper A, Floyd T, Barlow B, *et al.* (1996). Major blunt abdominal trauma due to child abuse. *Journal of Trauma* **28**:1463–1486.
61. McEniery J, Hanson R, Grigor W, Horowitz A (1991). Lung injury resulting from a non-accidental crush injury to the chest. *Pediatric Emergency Care* **7**:166–168.
62. Slovis TL, Haller JO, Joshi A (2004). *Pediatric imaging*, 3rd edn. Springer, Heidelberg.

Chapter 6

1. McGwin G Jr, Xie A, Owsley C (2005). Rate of eye injury in the United States. *Archives of Ophthalmology* **123**:970–976.
2. Brophy M, Sinclair SA, Hostetler SG, Xiang H (2006). Pediatric eye injury-related hospitalizations in the United States. *Pediatrics* **117**:e1263–e1271.
3. MacEwen CJ, Baines PS, Desai P (1999). Eye injuries in children: The current picture. *British Journal of Ophthalmology* **83**:933–936.
4. Niiranen M, Raivio I (1981). Eye injuries in children. *British Journal of Ophthalmology* **65**:436–438.
5. MacEwen CJ (1989). Eye injuries: A prospective survey of 5,761 cases. *British Journal of Ophthalmology* **73**:888–894.
6. Nelson LB, Wilson TW, Jeffers JB (1989). Eye injuries in childhood: Demography, etiology and prevention. *Pediatrics* **84**:438–441.

7. May DR, Kuhn FP, Morris CD, *et al.* (2000). The epidemiology of serious eye injuries from the United States Eye Injury Registry. *Graefes Archive for Clinical and Experimental Ophthalmology* **238**:153–157.

8. Motley WW 3rd, Kaufman AH, West CE (2003). Pediatric airbag-associated ocular trauma and endothelial cell loss. *Journal of the American Association of Pediatric Ophthalmology and Strabismus* **7**:380–383.

9. Baskin DE, Stein F, Coats DL, Paysse EA (2003). Recurrent conjunctivitis as a presentation of Munchausen syndrome by proxy. *Ophthalmology* **110**:1582–1584.

10. Jandeck C, Kellner U, Fornfeld N, Foerster MH (2000). Open globe injuries in children. *Graefes Archive for Clinical and Experimental Ophthalmology* **238**:420–426.

11. Blumenthal I (2002). Review: Shaken baby syndrome. *Postgraduate Medicine Journal* **78**: 732–735.

12. Green MA, Lieberman G, Milroy CM, Parsons MA (1996). Ocular and cerebral trauma in non-accidental injury in infancy: Underlying mechanisms and implications for paediatric practice. *British Journal of Ophthalmology* **80**:282–286.

13. Karkhaneh R, Naeeni M, Chams H, *et al.* (2003). Topical aminocaproic acid to prevent rebleeding in cases of traumatic hyphema. *European Journal of Ophthalmology* **13**:57–61.

14. Pieramici DJ, Goldberg MF, Melia M, *et al.* (2003). A phase III, multicenter, randomized placebo controlled clinical trial of topical aminocaproic acid in the management of traumatic hyphema. *Ophthalmology* **110**:2106–2112.

15. Dashti SR, Decker DD, Razzaq A, Cohen AR (1999). Current patterns of inflicted head injury in children. *Pediatric Neurosurgery* **31**:302–306.

16. Bechtel K, Stoessel K, Leventhal JM, *et al.* (2004). Characteristics that distinguish accidental from abusive injury in hospitalized young children with head trauma. *Pediatrics* **128**:340–344.

17. Mierisch RF, Frasier LD, Braddock SR, *et al.* (2004). Retinal hemorrhages in an 8-year-old child: An uncommon presentation of abusive injury. *Pediatric Emergency Care* **20**:118–120.

18. Morad Y, Kim YM, Armstrong DC, *et al.* (2002). Correlation between retinal abnormalities and intracranial abnormalities in the shaken baby syndrome. *American Journal of Ophthalmology* **134**:354–359.

19. Ewing-Cobbs L, Krame L, Prasad M, *et al.* (1998). Neuroimaging, physical and developmental findings after inflicted and noninflicted traumatic brain injury in young children. *Pediatrics* **102**:300–307.

20. Buys YM, Levin AV, Ensenaur RW, *et al.* (1992). Retinal findings after head trauma in infants and young children. *Ophthalmology* **99**:1718–1723.

21. Christian CW, Taylor AA, Hertle RW, Duhaime AC (1999). Retinal hemorrhages caused by accidental household trauma. *Journal of Pediatrics* **135**:125–127.

22. Herr S, Pierce MC, Berger RP, *et al.* (2004). Does valsalva retinopathy occur in infants? An initial investigation in infants with vomiting by pyloric stenosis. *Pediatrics* **113**:1658–1661.

23. Odom A, Christ E, Kerr N, *et al.* (1997). Prevalence of retinal hemorrhages in pediatric patients after in-hospital cardiopulmonary resuscitation: a prospective study. *Pediatrics* **99**:E3.

24. Mei-Zahav M, Useil Y, Raz J, *et al.* (2002). Convulsion and retinal haemorrhage: Should we look further? *Archives of Disease in Childhood* **86**: 334–335.

25. Kaur B, Taylor D (1992). Fundus hemorrhages in infancy. *Survey of Ophthalmology* **37**:1–17.

26. Emerson MV, Pieramicic DJ, Stoessel KM, *et al.* (2001). Incidence and rate of disappearance of retinal hemorrhage in newborns. *Ophthalmology* **108**:36–39.

27. Massicotte SJ, Folberg R, Torczynski E, *et al.* (1991). Vitreoretinal traction and perimacular retinal folds in the eyes of deliberately traumatized children. *Ophthalmology* **98**:1124–1127.

28. Lantz PE, Sinal SH, Stanton CA, Weaver RG (2004). Perimacular retinal folds from childhood head trauma. *British Medical Journal* **328**: 754–756.

29. Lueder GT, Turner JW, Paschall R (2006). Perimacular retinal folds simulating nonaccidental injury in an infant. *Archive of Ophthalmology* **124**:1782–1783.

30. Greenwald MJ, Weiss A, Oesterle CS, Friendly DS (1986). Traumatic retinoschisis in battered babies. *Ophthalmology* **93**:618–625.

31. Gaynon M, Koh K, Marmor M, Frankel LR (1988). Retinal folds in the shaken baby syndrome. *American Journal of Ophthalmology* **106**:423–425.
32. Mills M (1998). Fundoscopic lesions associated with mortality in shaken baby syndrome. *Journal of the American Association of Pediatric Ophthalmology and Strabismus* **2**:67–71.
33. Cackett P, Fleck B, Mulhivill A (2004). Bilateral fourth nerve palsy occurring after shaking injury in infancy. *Journal of the American Association of Pediatric Ophthalmology and Strabismus* **9**:53–56.
34. McCabe CF, Donohue SP (2000). Prognostic indicators for vision and mortality in shaken baby syndrome. *Archives of Ophthalmology* **118**:373–377.

Chapter 7

1. Manning SC, Casselbrant M, Lammers D (1990). Otolaryngologic manifestations of child abuse. *International Journal of Pediatric Otorhinolaryngology* **20**:7–16.
2. da Fonseca MA, Feigal RJ, ten Bensel RW (1992). Dental aspects of 1248 cases of child maltreatment on file at a major county hospital. *Pediatric Dentistry* **14**:152–157.
3. Crouse CD, Faust RA (2003). Child abuse and the otolaryngologist: Part I. *Otolaryngology and Head and Neck Surgery* **128**:305–310.
4. Sirotnak AP, Grigsby T, Krugman RD (2004). Physical abuse of children. *Pediatrics in Review* **25**:264–277.
5. Crouse CD, Faust RA (2003). Child abuse and the otolaryngologist: Part II. *Otolaryngology and Head and Neck Surgery* **128**:311–317.
6. Morris MW, Smith S, Cressman J, *et al.* (2000). Evaluation of infants with subdural hematoma who lack external evidence of abuse. *Pediatrics* **105**:549–553.
7. Kittle PE, Richardson DS, Parker JW (1986). Examining for child abuse and child neglect. *Pediatric Dentistry* **8**:80–82.
8. Kabbani H, Raghuveer TS (2004). Craniosynostosis. *American Family Physician* **69**:2863–2870.
9. Sugar NF, Taylor JA, Feldman KW (1999). Bruises in infants and toddlers: Those who don't cruise rarely bruise. Puget Sound Pediatric Research Network. *Archives of Pediatrics and Adolescent Medicine* **153**:399–403.
10. Carpenter RF (1999). The prevalence and distribution of bruising in babies. *Archives of Disease in Childhood* **80**:363–366.
11. Hanigan WC, Peterson RA, Njus G (1987). Tin ear syndrome: Rotational acceleration in pediatric head injuries. *Pediatrics* **80**:618–622.
12. Henderson JM, Salama AR, Blanchaert RH Jr (2000). Management of auricular hematoma using a thermoplastic splint. *Archives of Otolaryngology and Head and Neck Surgery* **126**: 888–890.
13. Feldman KW, Stout JW, Inglis AF Jr (2002). Asthma, allergy, and sinopulmonary disease in pediatric condition falsification. *Child Maltreatment* **7**:125–131.
14. Bennett AM, Bennett SM, Prinsley PR, *et al.* (2005). Spitting in the ear: A falsified disease using video evidence. *Journal of Laryngology and Otology* **119**:926–927.
15. Schlievert R (2006). Infant mandibular fractures: Are you considering child abuse? *Pediatric Emergency Care* **22**:181–183.
16. Siegel MB, Wetmore RF, Potsic WP, *et al.* (1991). Mandibular fractures in the pediatric patient. *Archives of Otolaryngology and Head and Neck Surgery* **117**:533–536.
17. Fischer H, Allasio D (1996). Nasal destruction due to child abuse. *Clinical Pediatrics* **35**:165–166.
18. Woolford TJ, Jones NS (2001). Repair of nasal septal perforations using local mucosal flaps and a composite cartilage graft. *Journal of Laryngology and Otology* **115**:22–25.
19. McGuire S, Hunter B, Hunter L, *et al.* (2007). Diagnosing abuse: A systematic review of torn frenum and intraoral injuries. *Archives of Disease in Childhood* **92**:1113–1117.
20. Jessee SA (1995). Orofacial manifestations of child abuse and neglect. *American Family Physician* **52**:1829–1834.
21. Brookhouser PE, Sullivan P, Scanlan JM, *et al.* (1986). Identifying the sexually abused deaf child: The otolaryngologist's role. *Laryngoscope* **96**:152–158.
22. Ramnarayan P, Qayyum A, Tolley N, *et al.* (2004). Subcutaneous emphysema of the neck in infancy: Under-recognized presentation of child

abuse. *Journal of Laryngology and Otology* **118**:468–470.

23. Ng CS, Hall CM, Shaw DG (1997). The range of visceral manifestations of non-accidental injury. *Archives of Disease in Childhood* **77**:167–174.

24. Ricci LR (1991). Photographing the physically abused child. Principles and practice. *American Journal of Diseases of Children* **145**:275–281.

Chapter 8

1. McDowell J, Kassebaum D, Stromboe S (1992). Recognizing and reporting victims of domestic violence. *Journal of the American Dental Association* **123**:44–50.

2. Judd R (1988). Child, spousal and elderly abuse: An overview. *Emergency Medical Services* **17**:43–45.

3. Wolfe D, Jaffe P, Wilson S, Zak L (1985). Children of battered women: The relation of child behavior to family violence and maternal stress. *Journal of Consulting and Clinical Psychology* **53**:657–665.

4. Council on Ethical and Judicial Affairs, American Medical Association (1992). Physicians and domestic violence: Ethical considerations. *Journal of the American Medical Association* **267**:3190–3193.

5. American College of Obstetricians and Gynecologists (1989). The battered woman. ACOG Technical Bulletin No. 124.

6. Appleton W (1980). The battered woman syndrome. *Annals of Emergency Medicine* **9**:84–91.

7. Council on Scientific Affairs (1987). Elder abuse and neglect. *Journal of the American Medical Association* **257**:966–971.

8. Guinan ME (1990). Domestic violence: Physicians a link to prevention. *Journal of the American Women's Association* **45**:231.

9. Chiodo G, Tilden V, Limandri BJ, Schmidt TA (1994). Addressing family violence among dental patients: Assessment and intervention. *Journal of the American Dental Association* **125**:69–75.

10. American Academy of Pediatrics Committee on Child Abuse and Neglect, American Academy of Pediatric Dentistry Council on Clinical Affairs (2005). *Guideline on Oral and Dental Aspects of Child Abuse and Neglect. Clinical guidelines*. Adopted 1999, revised 2005.

11. Ghent WR, DaSylva N, Farren ME (1985). Family violence: Guidelines for recognition and management. *Canadian Medical Association Journal* **132**:541–553.

12. Vicken RM (1982). Family violence: Aids to recognition. *Postgraduate Medicine* **71**:115–122.

13. McGuire S, Hunter B, Hunter L, *et al.* (2007). Diagnosing abuse: A systemic review of torn frenum and intra-oral injuries. *Archives of Disease in Childhood* **92**:1113–1117.

14. Naidoo S (2000). A profile of the oro-facial injuries in child physical abuse at a children's hospital. *Child Abuse and Neglect* **24**:521–534.

15. Bariciak E, Plint C, Gaboury I, Bennett S (2003). Dating of bruises in children: An assessment of physician accuracy. *Pediatrics* **112**:804–807.

16. Maguire S, Mann MK, Sibert J, Kemp A. (2005). Can you age bruises accurately in children? A systemic review. *Archives of Disease in Childhood* **90**:187–189.

17. Daily JC, Bowers CM (1997). Aging of bite marks: A literature review. *Journal of Forensic Sciences* **42**:792–795.

18. American Academy of Pediatrics, Committee on Child Abuse (1999). Guidelines for the evaluation of sexual abuse of children: A subject review. *Pediatrics* **103**:186–191.

19. Schlesinger SL, Borbotsina J, O'Neill L (1975). Petechial hemorrhages of the soft palate secondary to fellatio. *Oral Surgery, Oral Medicine, and Oral Pathology* **40**:376–378.

20. American Academy of Pediatric Dentistry (2003). Definition of dental neglect. *Pediatric Dentistry* **25**(Suppl):7.

21. American Society of Forensic Odontology (2006). Bite mark analysis and human abuse and neglect. In: *Manual of Forensic Odontology*, 4th edn. E Herschaft, M Alder, D Ord, *et al.* (eds). Impress Printing and Graphics, Albany, NY, pp. 172–179.

22. Hsieh N, Herzig K, Gansky SA, *et al.* (2006). Changing dentists' knowledge, attitudes, and behavior regarding domestic violence through an interactive multimedia tutorial. *Journal of the American Dental Association* **137**:596–603.

Chapter 9

1. Ledbetter DJ, Hatch EI, Feldman KW, Fligner CL (1988). Diagnostic and surgical implications of child abuse. *Archives of Surgery* **123**:1101–1105.
2. Cooper A, Floyd R, Barlow B, *et al.* (1988). Major blunt abdominal trauma due to child abuse. *Journal of Trauma* **28**:1483–1486.
3. Caniano DA, Beaver BL, Boles ET (1986). Child abuse. An update on surgical management in 256 cases. *Annals of Surgery* **203**:219–224.
4. Kirks DR (1983). Radiological evaluation of visceral injuries in the battered child syndrome. *Pediatric Annals* **12**:888–893.
5. Barnes PM, Norton CM, Dunstan FD, *et al.* (2005). Abdominal injury due to child abuse. *Lancet* **366**:234–235.
6. Canty TG, Canty TG, Brown C (1999). Injuries of the gastrointestinal tract from blunt trauma in children: A 12-year experience at a designated pediatric trauma center. *Journal of Trauma* **46**:234–240.
7. Philippart AI (1977). Blunt abdominal trauma in childhood. *Surgical Clinics of North America* **57**:151–163.
8. Huntimer CM, Muret-Wagstaff S, Leland NL (2000). Can falls on stairs result in small intestine perforations? *Pediatrics* **106**:301–305.
9. Kottmeier PD (1987). The battered child. *Pediatric Annals* **16**:343–351.
10. Pena SDJ, Medovy H (1973). Child abuse and traumatic pseudocyst of the pancreas. *Journal of Pediatrics* **83**:1026–1028.
11. Ziegler DW, Long JA, Philippart AI, Klein MD (1988). Pancreatitis in childhood: Experience with 49 patients. *Annals of Surgery* **207**:257–261.
12. Coant PN, Kornberg AE, Brody AS, Edwards-Holms K (1992). Markers for occult liver injury in cases of physical abuse in children. *Pediatrics* **89**:274–278.
13. Nijs E, Callahan MJ, Taylor GA (2005). Disorders of the pediatric pancreas: imaging features. *Pediatric Radiology* **35**:358–373.
14. Kleinman PK, Raptopoulos VD, Brill PW (198). Occult nonskeletal trauma in the battered-child syndrome. *Radiology* **141**:393–396.
15. Kleinman PK, Brill PW, Winchester P (1986). Resolving duodenal-jejunal hematoma in abused children. *Radiology* **160**:747–750.

Chapter 10

1. World Health Organization (1999). *Report of the Consultation on Child Abuse Prevention*. World Health Organization, Geneva, pp. 13–17.
2. Johnson CF (2006). Sexual abuse in children. *Pediatrics in Review* **27**:17–27.
3. Palusci VJ, Cox EO, Cyrus TA, *et al.* (1999). Medical assessment and legal outcome in child sexual abuse. *Archives of Pediatric and Adolescent Medicine* **153**:388–392.
4. Adams JA, Kaplan RA, Starling SP, *et al.* (2007). Guidelines for medical care of children who may have been sexually abused. *Journal of Pediatric and Adolescent Gynecology* **20**:163–172.
5. McCann J, Miyamoto S, Boyle C, Rogers K (2007). Healing of hymenal injuries in prepubertal and adolescent girls: A descriptive study. *Pediatrics* **119**:e1094–e1106.
6. Heger A, Ticson L, Velasquez O, Bernier R (2002). Children referred for possible sexual abuse: Medical findings in 2384 children. *Child Abuse and Neglect* **26**:645–659.
7. Palusci VJ, Cox EO, Shatz EM, Schultze JM (2006). Urgent medical assessment after child sexual abuse. *Child Abuse and Neglect* **30**: 367–380.
8. American Professional Society on the Abuse of Children (1995). *Practice Guidelines: Descriptive Terminology in Child Sexual Abuse Medical Evaluations*. Author, Chicago, IL.
9. Palusci VJ, Cyrus TA (2001). Reaction to video-colposcopy in the assessment of child sexual abuse. *Child Abuse and Neglect* **25**:1535–1546.
10. Kellogg N, the American Academy of Pediatrics (2005). The evaluation of sexual abuse of children. *Pediatrics* **116**:506–512.
11. Simmons KJ, Hicks DJ (2005). Child sexual abuse evaluation: Is there a need for routine screening for *N. gonorrhoeae* and *C. trachomatis*? *Journal of Pediatric and Adolescent Gynecology* **18**:343–345.
12. Sugar NF, Graham EA (2006). Common gynecologic problems in prepubertal girls. *Pediatrics in Review* **27**:213–223.
13. Wellington MA, Bonnez W (2005). Genital warts. *Pediatrics in Review* **26**:467–471.
14. Centers for Disease Control and Prevention (2006). Sexually transmitted diseases treatment

guidelines, 2006. *Morbidity and Mortality Weekly Report* **55**(RR-11):1–94.

15. Young KJ, Jones JG, Worthington T, *et al.* (2006). Forensic laboratory evidence in sexually abused children and adolescents. *Archives of Pediatrics and Adolescent Medicine* **160**:585–588.
16. Christian CW, Lavelle JM, De Jong AR, *et al.* (2000). Forensic evidence findings in prepubertal victims of sexual assault. *Pediatrics* **106**:100–104.
17. Santucci KA, Nelson DG, McQuillen KK, *et al.* (1999). Wood's lamp utility in the identification of semen. *Pediatrics* **104**:1342–1344.
18. Johnson K, Chapman S, Hall CM (2004). Skeletal injuries associated with sexual abuse. *Pediatric Radiology* **34**:620–623.
19. American Academy of Pediatrics (1998). *Visual diagnosis of child sexual abuse*. Author, Elk Grove Village, IL.

Chapter 11

1. DiMaio VJ, Dana SE (2007). *Handbook of Forensic Pathology*, 2nd edn. Taylor & Francis, Boca Raton, FL.
2. Dolinak D, Matshes EW, Lew EO (2005). *Forensic Pathology Principles and Practice*. Elsevier, Amsterdam.
3. Pasquale-Styles MA, Tackitt PL, Schmidt CJ (2007). Infant death scene investigation and the assessment of potential risk factors for asphyxia: A review of 209 sudden unexpected infant deaths. *Journal of Forensic Science* **52**:924–929.
4. American Academy of Pediatrics (2000). The changing concept of sudden infant death syndrome: Diagnostic coding shifts, controversies regarding the sleeping environment, and new variables to consider in reducing risk. *Pediatrics* **105**:650–656.
5. Krous HF, Beckwith JB, Byard RW, *et al.* (2004). Sudden infant death syndrome and unclassified sudden infant deaths: A definitional and diagnostic approach. *Pediatrics* **114**:234–238.
6. Centers for Disease Control and Prevention (2005). Racial/ethnic disparities in infant mortality – United States, 1995–2002. *Morbidity and Mortality Weekly Report (MMWR)* **54**:553–556.
7. Malloy MH (2004). SIDS – a syndrome in search of a cause. *New England Journal of Medicine* **351**:957–959.
8. Limerick SR, Bacon CJ (2004). Terminology used by pathologists in reporting on sudden infant deaths. *Journal of Clinical Pathology* **57**:309–311.
9. Tappin D, Ecob R, Brooke H (2005). Bedsharing, roomsharing, and sudden infant death syndrome in Scotland: A case–control study. *Journal of Pediatrics* **147**:32–37.
10. Knight LD, Hunsaker DM, Corey TS (2005). Cosleeping and sudden unexpected infant deaths in Kentucky: A 10-year retrospective case review. *American Journal of Forensic Medicine and Pathology* **26**:28–32.
11. Kemp JS, Unger B, Wilkins D, *et al.* (2000). Unsafe sleep practices and an analysis of bedsharing among infants dying suddenly and unexpectedly: Results of a four-year, population-based, death-scene investigation study of sudden infant death syndrome and related deaths. *Pediatrics* **106**:E41.
12. Paluszynska DA, Harris KA, Thach BT (2004). Influence of sleep position experience on ability of prone-sleeping infants to escape from asphyxiating microenvironments by changing head position. *Pediatrics* **114**:1634–1639.
13. Spitz WU, Spitz DJ (2006). *Spitz and Fisher's Medicolegal Investigation of Death*, 4th edn. Charles C. Thomas, Springfield, FL.
14. McCoy RC, Hunt CE, Lesko SM, *et al.* (2004). Frequency of bed sharing and its relationship to breastfeeding. *Journal of Developmental and Behavioral Pediatrics* **25**:141–149.
15. Nakamura SW (2001). Are cribs the safest place for infants to sleep? Yes: bed sharing is too hazardous. *Western Journal of Medicine* **174**:300.
16. Sachdeva DK, Stadnyk JM (2005). Are one or two dangerous? Opioid exposure in toddlers. *Journal of Emergency Medicine* **29**:77–84.
17. Li L, Fowler D, Liu L, *et al.* (2005). Investigation of sudden infant deaths in the State of Maryland (1990–2000). *Forensic Science International* **148**:85–92.
18. Gilbert-Barness E, Hegstrand L, Chandra S, *et al.* (1991). Hazards of mattresses, beds and bedding in deaths of infants. *American Journal of Forensic Medicine and Pathology* **12**:27–32.
19. Bass M, Kravath RE, Glass L (1986). Death-scene investigation in sudden infant death. *New England Journal of Medicine* **315**:100–105.
20. Case ME (2007). Abusive head injuries in infants and young children. *Legal Medicine* **9**:83–87.

21. Case ME, Graham MA, Handy TC, *et al.* (2001). Position paper on fatal abusive head injuries in infants and young children. *American Journal of Forensic Medicine and Pathology* **22**:112–122.
22. American Academy of Pediatrics: Committee on Child Abuse and Neglect. (2001). Shaken baby syndrome: Rotational cranial injuries – technical report. *Pediatrics*. **108**:206–210.
23. Lambert SR, Johnson TE, Hoyt CS (1986). Optic nerve sheath and retinal hemorrhages associated with the shaken baby syndrome. *Archives of Ophthalmology* **104**:1509–1512.
24. Wygnanski-Jaffe T, Levin AV, Shafiq A, *et al.* (2006). Postmortem orbital findings in shaken baby syndrome. *American Journal of Ophthalmology* **142**:233–240.
25. Salehi-Had H, Brandt JD, Rosas AJ, Rogers KK (2006). Findings in older children with abusive head injury: Does shaken-child syndrome exist? *Pediatrics* **117**:e1039–1044.
26. Loewe CL, Diaz FJ, Bechinski J (2007). Pitbull mauling deaths in Detroit. *American Journal of Forensic Medicine and Pathology* **28**:356–360.
27. Hartzog TH, Timerding BL, Alson RL (1996). Pediatric trauma: Enabling factors, social situations, and outcome. *Academic Emergency Medicine* **3**:213–220.
28. Ordog GJ, Wasserberger J, Schatz I, *et al.* (1988). Gunshot wounds in children under 10 years of age. A new epidemic. *American Journal of Diseases of Children* **142**:618–622.

Chapter 12

1. Sullivan PB (2004). Commentary: The epidemiology of failure to thrive in infants. *International Journal of Epidemiology* **33**:1.
2. Frank DA, Zeisel SH (1988). Failure to thrive. *Pediatric Clinics of North America* **35**:1187–1206.
3. Zenel JA (1997). Failure to thrive: A general pediatrician's perspective. *Pediatrics in Review* **18**:371–378.
4. Frank D (2005). Failure to thrive. In: *Developmental and Behavioral Pediatrics: A Handbook for Primary Care*. S Parker, B Zuckerman, M Augustyn (eds). Lippincott Williams & Wilkins, Philadelphia, PA pp. 183–187.
5. Dubowitz H, Giardino A, Gustavson E (2000). Child neglect: Guidance for pediatricians. *Pediatrics in Review* **21**:111–116.
6. Block RW, Krebs NF, American Academy of Pediatrics (2005). Failure to thrive as a manifestation of child neglect. *Pediatrics* **116**:1234–1237.
7. Blair PS, Drewett, RF, Emmett PM, *et al.*, ALSPAC Study Team (2004). Family, socioeconomic and prenatal factors associated with failure to thrive in the Avon Longitudinal Study of Parents and Children. *International Journal of Epidemiology* **33**:839–847.
8. Krugman SD, Dubowitz H (2003). Failure to thrive. *American Family Physician* **68**:879–886.
9. Committee on Nutrition American Academy of Pediatrics (2004). Failure to thrive (pediatric undernutrition). In: *Pediatric Nutrition Handbook*, 5th edn. RE Kleinman (ed). American Academy of Pediatrics, Oak Grove Village, IL, pp. 443–457
10. Schwarz DI (2000). Failure to thrive: An old nemesis in the new millennium. *Pediatrics in Review* **21**:257–264.
11. Gahagan S (2006). Failure to thrive: A consequence of undernutrition. *Pediatrics in Review* **27**:1–11.
12. Maggioni A, Lifshitz F (1995). Nutritional management of failure to thrive. *Pediatric Clinics of North America* **42**:791–809.
13. Schlecter M (2000). Weight loss/failure to thrive. *Pediatrics in Review* **21**:238–239.
14. Stier DM, Leventhal JM, Berg AT, *et al.* (1993). Are children born to young mothers at increased risk of maltreatment? *Pediatrics* **91**:642–648.
15. Dubowitz H, Papas M, Black MM, Starr RH Jr (2002). Child neglect: Outcomes in high-risk urban preschoolers. *Pediatrics* **109**:1100–1107.
16. O'Brien LM, Heycock EG, Hanna M, *et al.* (2004). Postnatal depression and faltering growth: A community study. *Pediatrics* **113**:1242–1247.
17. Skuse DH, Gill D, Reilly S, *et al.* (1995). Failure to thrive and the risk of child abuse: A prospective population survey. *Journal of Medical Screening* **2**:145–159.
18. Wright CM, Parkinson KN, Drewett RF (2006). How does maternal and child feeding behavior relate to weight gain and failure to thrive? Data from a prospective birth cohort. *Pediatrics* **117**:1262–1269.

19. Drewett RF, Kasese-Hara M, Wright C (2003). Feeding behaviour in children who fail to thrive. *Appetite* **40**:55–60.
20. Wright C, Birks E. (2000). Risk factors for failure to thrive: A population-based study. *Child Care Health and Development* **26**:5–16.
21. Powell GF, Low JF, Speers MA (1987). Behavior as a diagnostic aid in failure to thrive. *Developmental and Behavioral Pediatrics* **8**:18–24.
22. Mackner LM, Black MM, Starr RH Jr (2003). Cognitive development of children in poverty with failure to thrive: A prospective study through age 6. *Journal of Child Psychology and Psychiatry* **44**:743–751.
23. Dykman RA, Casey PH, Ackerman PT, McPherson WB (2001). Behavioral and cognitive status in school-aged children with a history of failure to thrive during early childhood. *Clinical Pediatrics* **40**:63–70.
24. Boddy J, Skuse D, Andrews B (2000). The developmental sequelae of nonorganic failure to thrive. *Journal of Child Psychology and Psychiatry* **41**:1003–1014.
25. Mackner LM, Starr RH Jr, Black MM (1997). The cumulative effect of neglect on failure to thrive and cognitive functioning. *Child Abuse and Neglect* **21**:691–700.
26. Drewett, RF, Corgett SS, Wright CM (2006). Physical and emotional development, appetite and body image in adolescents who failed to thrive as infants. *Journal of Child Psychology and Psychiatry* **46**:524–531.
27. Reif S, Beler B, Villa Y, Spirer Z (1995). Long-term follow-up and outcome of infants with non-organic failure to thrive. *Israel Journal of Medical Sciences* **31**:483–489.
28. Pearce A, Finlay F (1998). Children investigated for failure to thrive: Where are they now? *Professional Care of Mother and Child* **8**:5–6.
29. Black MM, Dubowitz H, Krishnakumar A, Starr RH Jr (2007). Early intervention and recovery among children with failure to thrive: Follow-up at age 8. *Pediatrics* **120**:59–69.

Chapter 13

1. Meadow R (1997). Munchausen syndrome by proxy: The hinterland of child abuse. *Lancet* **2**:343–345.
2. Asher R (1951). Munchausen's syndrome. *Lancet* **2**:343–345.
3. Meadow R (1953). The history of Munchausen syndrome by proxy. In: *Munchausen Syndrome by Proxy: Issues in Diagnosis and Treatment*. AV Levin, MS Sheridan (eds). Lexington Books, New York, pp. 3–11.
4. Parnell TF (1998). Defining Munchausen syndrome by proxy. In: *Munchausen by Proxy Syndrome: Misunderstood Child Abuse*. TF Parnell, DO Day (eds). Sage Publications, Thousand Oaks, CA, pp. 9–46.
5. Ayoub CC, Alexander R (1998). Definitional issues in Munchausen by proxy. *APSAC Advisor* **11**:7–10.
6. Stirling JM, American Academy of Pediatrics (2007). Beyond Munchausen syndrome by proxy: Identification and treatment of child abuse in a medical setting. *Pediatrics* **119**:1026–1030.
7. Siegel PT, Fischer H (2001). Munchausen by proxy syndrome: Barriers to detection, confirmation and intervention. *Children's Services: Social Policy, Research and Practice* **4**:31–50.
8. McClure RJ, Davis PM, Meadow SR, Sibert JR (1996). Epidemiology of Munchausen syndrome by proxy, non-accidental poisoning and non-accidental suffocation. *Archives of Diseases in Childhood* **75**:57–61.
9. Schreier HA, Libow JA (1993). *Hurting for Love*. Guilford Press, New York.
10. Feldman KM (1994). Denial in Munchausen syndrome by proxy. *International Journal of Medicine* **24**:121–128.
11. Rosenberg DA (1977). Web of deceit: A literature review of Munchausen syndrome by proxy. *Child Abuse and Neglect* **11**:547–563.
12. Siebel MA, Parnell TF. The physician's role in confirming the diagnosis. In: *Munchausen by Proxy Syndrome: Misunderstood Child Abuse*. TD Parnell, DP Day (eds). Sage Publications, Thousand Oaks, CA pp. 68–94.
13. Ayass M, Bussing R, Mehta P (1993). Munchausen syndrome presenting as hemophilia: A convenient and economical 'steal' of disease and treatment. *Pediatric Hematology and Oncology* **10**:241–244.
14. Rosenberg DA (1994). Munchausen syndrome by proxy. In: *Child Abuse: Medical Diagnosis*

and Management. Reece RM (ed). Lea Febiger, Philadelphia, PA, pp. 266–278.

15. Rosenberg DA (1995). From lying to homicide: The spectrum of Munchausen syndrome by proxy. In: *Munchausen Syndrome by Proxy: Issues in Diagnosis and Treatment*. Levin AV, Sheridan MS (eds). Lexington Books, New York, pp. 13–37.
16. Skau K, Mouridsen SE (1995). Munchausen syndrome by proxy: A review. *Acta Pediatrica* **84**:977–982.
17. Bryk M, Siegel PT (1997). My mother caused my illness: The story of a survivor of Munchausen by proxy syndrome. *Pediatrics* **100**:1–7.
18. Parnell TF (1998). An overview. In: *Munchausen by Proxy Syndrome: Misunderstood Child Abuse*. TF Parnell, DO Day (eds). Sage Publications, Thousand Oaks, CA, pp. 3–8.
19. Parnell TF (1998). Guidelines for identifying cases. In: *Munchausen by Proxy Syndrome: Misunderstood Child Abuse*. TF Parnell, DO Day (eds). Sage Publications, Thousand Oaks, CA, pp. 47–67.
20. Wilkinson R, Parnell TF (1998). The criminal prosecutor's perspective. In: *Munchausen by Proxy Syndrome: Misunderstood Child Abuse*. TP Parnell, DO Day (eds). Sage Publications, Thousand Oaks, CA, pp. 219–252.
21. Southall DP, Plunkett MCB, Banks MW, *et al.* (1997). Covert video recordings of life threatening child abuse: Lessons for child protection. *Pediatrics* **100**:735–760.
22. Hall DE, Eubanks L, Meyyazhagan S, *et al.* (2000). Evaluation of covert video surveillance in the diagnosis of Munchausen syndrome by proxy: Lessons from 41 cases. *Pediatrics* **105**:1305–1312.
23. Seidl T (1995). Is family preservation, reunification, and successful treatment, a possibility? A round table. In: *Munchausen Syndrome by Proxy: Issues in Diagnosis and Treatment*. Levin AV, Sheridan MS (eds). Lexington Books, New York pp. 411–412.
24. Day DO, Parnell TF (1998). Setting the treatment framework. In: *Munchausen by Proxy Syndrome: Misunderstood Child Abuse*. TF Parnell, DO Day (eds). Sage Publications, Thousand Oaks, CA, pp. 151–166.
25. Meadow R (1990). Suffocation, recurrent apnea and sudden infant death. *Journal of Pediatrics* **117**:351–357.
26. Fischer H, Allasio D (1996). Nasal destruction due to child abuse. *Clinical Pediatrics* **35**:165–166.

INDEX

Note: Page numbers in *italic* refer to tables

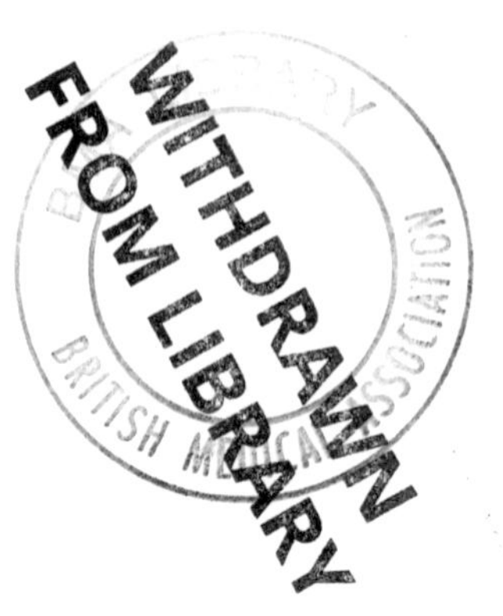